Life in a Time of Pestilence

From the Middle Ages onwards, deadly epidemics swept through portions of Spain repeatedly, but the Castilian plague at the end of the sixteenth century was especially terrible. In late 1596 a ship carrying the plague docked in Santander, and over the next five years the disease killed some 500,000 people in Castile, around 10 percent of the population.

Plague is traditionally understood to have triggered chaos and madness. By contrast, Ruth MacKay focuses on the sites of everyday life, exploring how beliefs, practices, laws, and relationships endured even under the onslaught of disease. She takes an original and holistic approach to understanding the impact of plague, and explores how the epidemic was understood and managed by everyday people. Offering a fresh perspective on the social, political, and economic history of Spain, this original and engaging book demonstrates how, even in the midst of chaos, life carried on.

RUTH MACKAY has worked as a university lecturer, newspaper editor, writer, translator, and interpreter, having been awarded fellowships from the American Council of Learned Societies, the National Endowment for the Humanities, and the Fulbright Commission, among others. She is the author of *The Limits of Royal Authority: Resistance and Obedience in Seventeenth-Century Castile* (1999), *"Lazy Improvident People": Myth and Reality in the Writing of Spanish History* (2006), and *The Baker Who Pretended to Be King of Portugal* (2012).

Life in a Time of Pestilence

The Great Castilian Plague of 1596–1601

Ruth MacKay

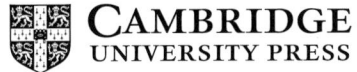
CAMBRIDGE
UNIVERSITY PRESS

CAMBRIDGE
UNIVERSITY PRESS

University Printing House, Cambridge CB2 8BS, United Kingdom

One Liberty Plaza, 20th Floor, New York, NY 10006, USA

477 Williamstown Road, Port Melbourne, VIC 3207, Australia

314–321, 3rd Floor, Plot 3, Splendor Forum, Jasola District Centre, New Delhi – 110025, India

79 Anson Road, #06–04/06, Singapore 079906

Cambridge University Press is part of the University of Cambridge.

It furthers the University's mission by disseminating knowledge in the pursuit of education, learning, and research at the highest international levels of excellence.

www.cambridge.org
Information on this title: www.cambridge.org/9781108498203
DOI: 10.1017/9781108632720

First published 2019

Printed in the United Kingdom by TJ International Ltd, Padstow Cornwall

A catalogue record for this publication is available from the British Library.

ISBN 978-1-108-49820-3 Hardback

We insist, it seems, on living.

Virginia Woolf [*The Waves*]

Contents

Maps

Figures

Acknowledgments

The American Council of Learned Societies once again showed their faith in me by generously funding this project, and I am very grateful. I relied upon the patience and ingenuity of archivists at the Archivo General de Simancas, Archivo Histórico Nacional, Archivo de Villa, and a long list of smaller but equally important municipal, provincial, and regional archives throughout Spain. I also would like to thank, as I have done after writing my previous books, the interlibrary loan service of the San Francisco Public Library, whose staff sometimes looked puzzled as they handed me my books, but always intrigued. Our public libraries are treasures.

Colleagues and friends who provided assistance of varying sorts include Javier Álvarez Dorronsoro, Jim Amelang, Laura Bass, Ted Bergman, José Ignacio Fortea, Maria Fusaro, Mike Hannigan, Tamar Herzog, Karin Maag, Katrina Olds, Geoffrey Parker, Carla and William Phillips, Barbara Pitkin, Lisa Surwillo, Tony Thompson, Lourdes Unceta Satrustegui, María Unceta Satrustegui, Kate Van Liere, Nükhet Varlik, Betsy Wright, and Juan Zubillaga. They made it easier, they made it possible.

Abbreviations

ACC	*Actas de las Cortes de Castilla*
AFB	Archivo Foral de Bizcaya (Bilbao)
AGN TR	Archivo General de Navarra, Tribunales Reales
AGS	Archivo General de Simancas
AHMA	Archivo Histórico Municipal de Ávila
AHN	Archivo Histórico Nacional
AMAH	Archivo Municipal de Alcalá de Henares
AMB	Archivo Municipal de Burgos
AMS	Archivo Municipal de Segovia
AMT	Archivo Municipal de Toledo
AMVA	Archivo Municipal de Valladolid
AMVal	Archivo Municipal de Valdemoro (Madrid)
ARCM	Archivo Regional de la Comunidad de Madrid
ARCV	Archivo de la Real Chancillería de Valladolid
ASV	Archivio di Stato (Venice)
AV	Archivo de Villa (Madrid)
BL	British Library
BN	Biblioteca Nacional de España (Madrid)
CC	Cámara de Castilla
CH	Cajas Históricas
CJH	Consejos y Juntas de Hacienda
CODOIN	*Colección de documentos inéditos de la historia de España*
CR	Consejo Real
CS	Consejos Suprimidos
E	Estado
Eg.	Egerton
EH	Expedientes de Hacienda
GyM	Guerra y Marina
HI	Sección Histórica
Inq.	Inquisición
IVDJ	Instituto de Valencia de Don Juan (Madrid)
LA	Libros de Actas

PR	Patronato Real
RAE	Real Academia Española
RAH	Real Academia de la Historia
RBP	Real Biblioteca del Palacio (Madrid)

Maps

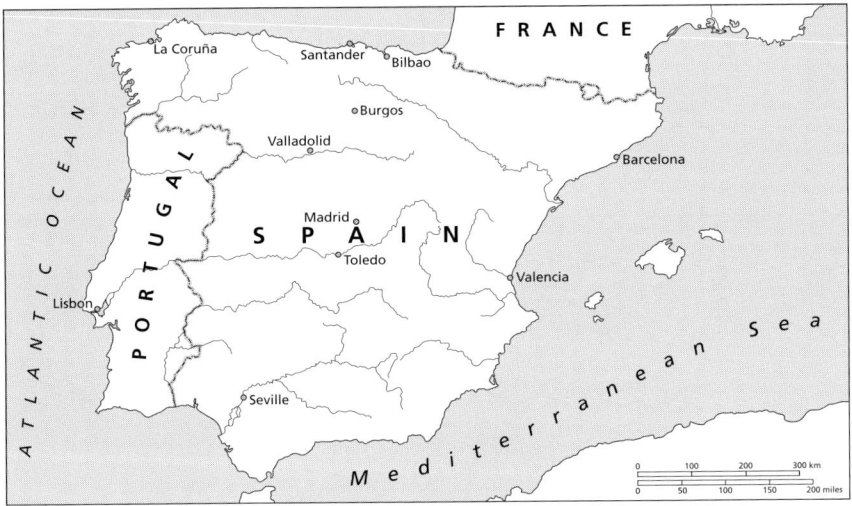

1. Map of selected towns mentioned

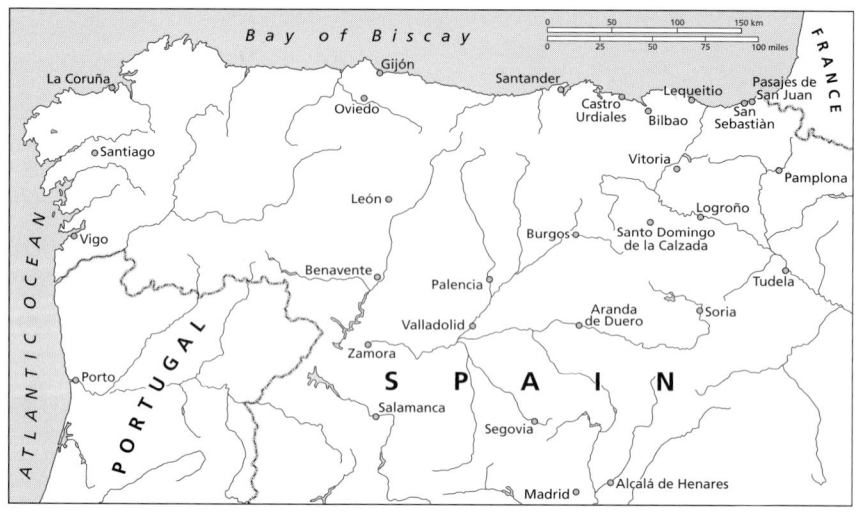

Bay of Biscay

FRANCE

La Coruña
Gijón
Santander
Lequeitio
Pasajes de San Juan
Oviedo
Castro Urdiales
Bilbao
San Sebastiàn
Santiago
Vitoria
Pamplona
León
Logroño
Vigo
Burgos
Santo Domingo de la Calzada
Benavente
Tudela
Palencia
Aranda de Duero
Soria
Valladolid
SPAIN
Zamora
Porto
ATLANTIC OCEAN
PORTUGAL
Salamanca
Segovia
Madrid
Alcalá de Henares

0   50   100   150 km
0   25   50   75   100 miles

2. Map of northern Iberian Peninsula

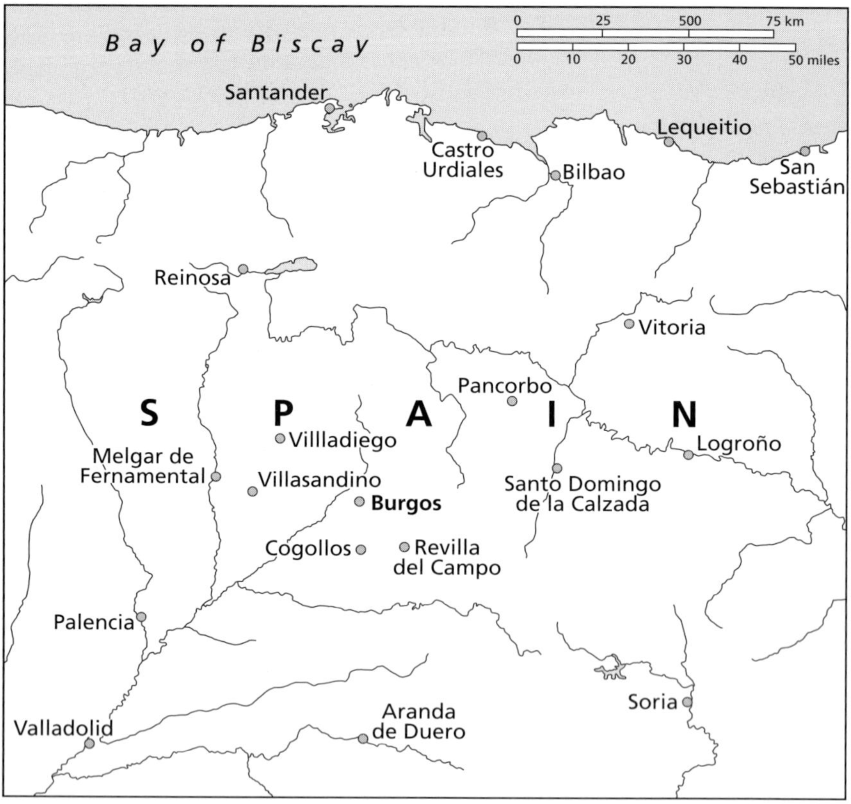

Bay of Biscay

0   25   500   75 km
0   10   20   30   40   50 miles

Santander
Castro Urdiales
Lequeitio
Bilbao
San Sebastián
Reinosa
Vitoria
Pancorbo
S   P   A   I   N
Villladiego
Logroño
Melgar de Fernamental
Villasandino
Santo Domingo de la Calzada
Burgos
Cogollos
Revilla del Campo
Palencia
Soria
Valladolid
Aranda de Duero

3. Map of Burgos and its towns

Introduction

From high above the Castilian meseta, a swallow gliding and wheeling in and out in search of food or shelter or friends might see a clump of buildings, then wide open space, then more clumps, then more space, the occasional river or wetlands, the inevitable church steeples at the heart of the clumps, with dwellings and a town hall huddled around them, and large or small squares where, if the bird swooped low, it might see people going about their business, lingering to talk, fingering the merchandise. Some towns were more beautiful than others, richer, more important, but they all had the same elements, noises, smells, purpose. There was probably some sort of wall, or there had been at some point. There were shrines scattered about the outlying countryside, among the fields, along the roads leading to neighboring towns and villages and then to the city. There were mills on the riverside, poorer neighborhoods on the outskirts. The local aristocrat might have a grand home in the town, or an estate outside. The kingdom was a body, according to the old commonplace, and each of these iterations, each of its parts, echoed the meaning and organization of the whole.

In the late sixteenth century, this assemblage of structures both physical and mental was visited by plague. It was not the first, it would not be the last, but it was probably the most awful such visitation. On the simplest level, this book is an attempt to figure out what it was like. I wanted to find the ordinary amidst the extraordinary and to see how both poles were embedded in fabrics of law, custom, memory, and the common good. I have tried to follow people as they spoke and surmised and bought and moved while their world crashed and burned. They continued getting up in the morning, milking the cows, dressing their children, gossiping, working, getting along tolerably, suing each other. To the extent that they could, they behaved normally, because that's generally what people want to do. I have followed my people around their towns and cities, but I lose sight of them more than I see them. Was there still any sort of school as the plague approached? How many layers of clothes did they wear when it was cold? What did they talk about with their neighbors? What were their prayers like in the absence of church gatherings, and did they even say them? What did they most look forward to? What was the farthest away from their town they had ever been? I don't know how to find those stories, and unless they're very lucky, few historians will. I thought of speculating a bit, of adding my stories in with theirs, but I held back. Literature, too, might have helped (it appears here and there in the following pages) but I decided to stick to documents, even if it meant I might miss "the history of what hadn't quite been said," what Raymond Williams called "structures of feeling."[1]

The potential problem with this approach I have chosen is, in a way, similar to that arising from the *alltagsgeschichte* approach to twentieth-century German history. Just as historians' quest to capture everyday life under the Nazis, or under Vichy or Stalin, ran the risk of normalizing people's choices and paths, a relativization that by reducing actions and inactions to their smallest component might be read as an apology, my approach perhaps runs the risk of minimizing the horror, of exaggerating order at the expense of disorder.[2] I recognize that the "disaster history" or "crisis studies" approach might feel more realistic to readers. I agree with the editors who wrote that disasters "reveal how societies operate – who wields power, how cultural and economic assumptions inform people's reactions, who is perceived as part of the community and thus worthy of rescue or protection, and how and to whom resources are allocated."[3] But too often, especially when the disaster being looked at is plague, the assumption is that things fall apart, and I would argue that such an approach, at least in the case of the great Castilian plague, does few favors to my subjects and the structures and challenges they had to deal with every day. Too often, even modern accounts assume pandemonium. This book, then, actually is not so much about the plague as it is about everything else surrounding the plague.[4] The argument is just that: that practices and assumptions continued working as they had for many years; since time immemorial, as people would say. By removing chaos from the scene, simply because I find it nowhere in the documents,

---

[1] Catherine Gallagher and Stephen Greenblatt, *Practicing New Historicism* (Chicago, IL: University of Chicago Press, 2000), 62–3. It is worth remarking, however, that contemporary literature is almost silent on the plague.

[2] For overviews of the historiographic debates see the special issues of *New German Critique* 44 (Spring/Summer 1988) and *The Russian Review* 45:4 (October 1986).

[3] Elinor Accampo and Jeffrey H. Jackson, "Introduction," *French Historical Studies* 36:2 (Spring 2013), 165 (special issue called *Disaster in French History*).

[4] A similar approach was taken by Stuart Schwartz, who used hurricanes as a meta-narrative to understand the Caribbean through its responses; Stuart B. Schwartz, *Sea of Storms: A History of Hurricanes in the Greater Caribbean from Columbus to Katrina* (Princeton, NJ: Princeton University Press, 2015).

I do not mean to say that villagers, townspeople, and even the well-born did not suffer excruciating loss and become undone with sorrow. As Camus wrote, "The plague was bound to leave traces … in people's hearts." But they kept on living. They did not lose their collective mind.[5]

The republic, a name given to the kingdom as a whole and to every piece of it, was a physical place where Castilians bought and sold and governed and survived and died, but it also was home to more abstract notions such as history, neighborliness, cowardice, and charity. One could also see this division as that of the particular and the universal, two intersecting planes. I have rearranged chronology and geography in my account because it seemed to me that splintering the narrative of the great Castilian plague and anchoring each moment to a place, as I have done, would allow me to understand better the significance of the experience for all the people who made their way through cities, towns, and villages. My point is the simultaneity of things. To quote Peter Burke: "The problem I should like to discuss here is that of making a narrative thick enough to deal not only with the sequence of events and the conscious inventions of the actors in these events, but also with structures – institutions, modes of thought, and so on – whether these structures act as a brake on events or as an accelerator. What would such a narrative be like?"[6]

In the case of this book, the narrative is structured around sites, key places in Castilian communities that not only fulfilled a purpose but provided a perspective. I wish to literally embed the plague and the responses to it throughout the Castilian polity. The seven sites are: Palace, Road, Wall, Market, Street, Town Hall, and Sickbed. From the vantage point of each of these places, whether physically or discursively, things took on a slightly different hue, with different priorities or foci, though similar situations or dilemmas were found everywhere. Whether to lie or tell the truth, how to get money, how to survive, or how to work together – these were choices or circumstances found everywhere, in

---

[5] Albert Camus, *The Plague*, trans. Stuart Gilbert (New York: The Modern Library, 1948), 251. As the *New York Times* only somewhat facetiously wrote in an appreciation (December 28, 2017) of the late disaster studies pioneer Enrico Quarantelli, "disasters bring out the best in us." Also along those lines, see Rebecca Solnit, *A Paradise Built in Hell: The Extraordinary Communities That Arise in Disaster* (New York: Penguin Books, 2009). In a different vein, a work that appeared just as this one was being finished and which similarly rejects a "trauma aesthetic" is Susan L. Einbinder's *After the Black Death: Plague and Commemoration among Iberian Jews* (Philadelphia, PA: University of Pennsylvania Press, 2018). Einbinder found continuity rather than collapse, as I did.

[6] Peter Burke, "History of events and the revival of narrative," in *New Perspectives on Historical Writing*, Peter Burke, ed., 2nd edn. (Cambridge, UK: Polity, 2001), 283–300, p. 291.

every town and at every site. Following the plague through communities offers us a way of understanding the meaning and variations of each site and the conflicts around it, on the one hand, and more universal practices and beliefs, on the other. But though I aim to embrace particular and universal at once, I do not wish to privilege the top at the expense of the bottom, or vice versa. Each choice – to obey, cooperate, flee, protest, succor – embodies both immediate circumstances and deep-seated customs and beliefs that slice vertically and horizontally. "The local and the global cannot be conceived along a series of hierarchically ordered concentric circles widening from small to large," wrote Francesca Trivellato in her excellent essay on microhistory, and the same is true in this study.[7] Nothing necessarily comes before or lies above anything else. Furthermore, nearly every choice could just as easily be manifested in one of my seven sites as in another. There are multiple (infinite) starting points, and each one, to quote Virginia Woolf, is an atom saturated, "to give the moment whole."[8] And, finally, each set of simultaneous and connected circumstances, each context, inevitably affects and suggests its neighboring contexts. Notions of justice and good government bend according to agency, convenience, temporality, and remembered precedent, they are acts that form part of what William Sewell called a sequence of actions "profoundly dependent upon [their] place in the sequence."[9] They are found at court, on the road, in the marketplace, and in the hospital. Perspective matters. So does chronology. Where and when one encountered plague or had to fix a problem, whether at a government meeting or on the road, whether alone or accompanied, determined one's understanding of it. The swallow from above might have thought of towns as units, but it might not have spotted the rips and convulsions as the republic battled to survive. My tour through the towns, with stops at each site, seeks out what the bird's-eye view can't perceive.

There was a political disposition to the relationships and events of the plague in part because there is always a political disposition, but also because this plague took place in Castile, where the common good was wrapped into every decision and every conflict. There was also, obviously, a medical disposition, but there, too, I hope to show that civic

[7] Francesca Trivellato, "Is there a future for Italian microhistory in the age of global history?" *California Italian Studies* 2:1 (2011), np available online at escholarship.org/uc/item/0z94n9hq, accessed January 2019.
[8] Virginia Woolf, *A Writer's Diary*, Leonard Woolf, ed. (New York: Harcourt Brace Jovanovich, 1954), 136; she was writing about *The Waves*.
[9] William H. Sewell, Jr., *Logics of History: Social Theory and Social Transformation* (Chicago, IL: University of Chicago Press, 2005), 7.

organization and news and a sense of history and time could help position the discourse of health. Disputes over quarantine, taxes, or guard
duty were not only matters of public health or policing but also statements about past political practices and the meaning of good government. They also were fought out during times of economic crisis and
dearth, which gives us another necessary field of analysis. In an entirely
different context, Emma Rothschild once wrote, "A social theory of
people who make these judgments ... must be a theory of people with
theories."[10] Acts of prohibition, distribution, publication, punishment,
or charity by official entities contained within them both memories of
past such experiences and the political and civic convictions that were
the foundation of Castilian life – plague or no plague. This is similar
to Rothschild's restatement of Adam Smith's thoughts on the writing of
history: "Events, in Smith's description, have both external and internal
causes, or causes to do with circumstances and causes to do with sentiments. It is the neglect of these internal causes, Smith says, which makes
the writings of modern historians 'for the most part so dull and life-
less'."[11] I am proposing that the events of the plague had circumstances
and sentiments or, to put it in words much older than Smith's, that
plague could be "naturally understood" and "morally understood."[12]

The symptoms described by physicians and other witnesses are mostly
those of bubonic plague, the disease known today to be caused by the
pathogen *Yersinia pestis*, though some deaths may have been due to other
causes. That said, I must make two things clear at the start: I am not
taking a firm stand on this question, as I honestly don't much care what
the exact disease was or was not, though bubonic plague seems the
obvious choice. Doctors at the time fussed over whether it was "true
plague" or just "*secas*" and sometimes used what might have been
euphemisms to avoid the deadly word.[13] I refer to the disease as plague
or peste or contagion, understanding these generic terms to more or less
mimic the terms contemporaries used. Second, I am fully aware that over
the past couple of decades there has been a fierce debate among historians of medicine regarding the nature of the pathogen that killed millions

[10] Emma Rothschild, *Economic Sentiments: Adam Smith, Condorcet, and the Enlightenment* (Cambridge, MA: Harvard University Press, 2001), 157.
[11] Rothschild, *Economic Sentiments*, 7, citing Smith's lectures.
[12] David Nirenberg, *Communities of Violence: Persecution of Minorities in the Middle Ages* (Princeton, NJ: Princeton University Press, 1996), 234, on Jacme d'Agramont, a fourteenth-century medical professor in Lérida who wrote a plague treatise.
[13] *Secas* could be sores or swellings, also a euphemism for buboes; Daniel Defoe called them tokens. They are often mentioned in conjunction with *carbuncos*, which has a similar meaning though it might also signify anthrax.

in what has come to be known as the Second Pandemic, running from the fourteenth-century Black Death through the eighteenth century. I will elaborate more on this debate in Chapter 3, where I discuss contagion, and in Chapter 7, but for the moment let me say simply that I have concluded from the scientific literature that diseases mutate and that the identity of hosts and vectors may also have varied over time. It was not as simple as the fleas and rats paradigm. Such a flexible, though admittedly not rigorous approach, allows us to account for anomalies in how the disease moved from town to town and from person to person. Most notably, contemporaries believed the epidemic was passed through direct physical contact with people or certain objects, and I have resolved to honor that belief.[14]

"The great Castilian plague of 1596–1602" arrived on a boat, the "*Rodamundo*," coming from Dunkirk and/or Calais which in November docked in Santander.[15] By the end of the plague's wanderings, perhaps half a million people were dead.[16] Some towns reported that they had lost one-third or one-half their population. This book mostly follows the destruction in the northern half of the Iberian Peninsula, though the death tolls in the south, especially Seville, were probably proportionately greater.[17] The first places affected were, obviously, Santander, and then the rest of the Cantabrian region. The disease moved west to Galicia

[14] Bibliographic citations are in subsequent chapters, but for now the best and most recent summation is Guido Alfani and Tommy E. Murphy, "Plague and lethal epidemics in the pre-industrial world," *The Journal of Economic History* 77:1 (March 2017), 314–43, esp. p. 321.

[15] The expression is from James Casey, *Early Modern Spain: A Social History* (London: Routledge, 1999), 37.

[16] That would represent around 10 percent of Castile's population. For a concise demographic synthesis see Vicente Pérez Moreda, "The plague in Castile at the end of the sixteenth century and its consequences," in *The Castilian Crisis of the Seventeenth Century: New Perspectives on the Economic and Social History of Seventeenth-Century Spain*, I. A. A. Thompson and Bartolomé Yun Casalilla, eds. (Past and Present Publications, Cambridge University Press, 1994), 32–59; this article is an abridged version of a chapter in his much broader *Las crisis de mortalidad en la Espana interior (Siglos XVI–XIX)* (Madrid: Siglo Veintiuno, 1980). See also the landmark Bartolomé Bennassar, *Recherches sur les grandes épidémies dans le nord de l'Espagne a la fin du XVIe siècle. Problèmes de documentation et de méthode* (Paris: SEVPEN, 1969). Both writers, along with Bernard Vincent, "La peste atlantica de 1596–1602," *Asclepio* 28 (1976), 5–25, p. 11; and Antonio Domínguez Ortiz, *The Golden Age of Spain, 1516–1659*, trans. James Casey (New York: Basic Books, 1971), 174, accept the half-million figure.

[17] Two recent books in English on plague in Seville are Kristy Wilson Bowers, *Plague and Public Health in Early Modern Seville* (Rochester, NY: University of Rochester Press, 2013); and Alexandra Parma Cook and Noble David Cook, *The Plague Files: Crisis Management in Sixteenth-Century Seville* (Baton Rouge, LA: Louisiana State University Press, 2009), which actually concerns an influenza epidemic. I occasionally wander south as well.

and east to the Basque Country, then down through Álava, La Rioja, Burgos, Valladolid, Segovia, Toledo, and Madrid. It jumped around, skipping some places altogether and making return visits to others. There was plague in Lisbon as well, probably taken there aboard another ship, and it was in Andalusia and Morocco, which also may have represented a separate wave.[18] Madrid was sick already in 1597, well before most other cities (except for Santander), another sign of atypical transmission, in this case because the city was a hub. Because this book is thematic, not chronological, it moves around from place to place. Each town had its own peculiarities, of course, but in general the story is the same.

Bartolomé Bennassar, in his 1969 study, *Recherches sur les grandes épidémies*, suggested that others follow his lead and together create a document-based history of the plague in Castile at the turn of the century. No one took him up on it, and it was upon reading his work that I decided to try, though my questions are different from his and I do not share some of his assessments. While Bennassar wished to tie Castile together geographically, I do so conceptually. I cannot pretend to assess the epidemic's overall demographic impact, though historians seem to agree that plague cannot be held primarily responsible for Spain's subsequent enormous economic difficulties. Nor, I'm afraid, do I offer conclusive economic or demographic data for any particular town or city. One final methodological clarification: this book is not a comparative study, and therefore there is no mention, except in passing, of France, Italy, or England. (I cannot imagine that any historian of France, Italy, or England has ever had to apologize for not comparing her material with that of Spain.) All these places suffered from various waves of epidemics and each had its own approach. My interest lies elsewhere, in the experience of plague in a particular political and civic setting.

Each of my seven sites, then, are anchors. I am beginning the plague's journey at a place I call Palace, a misnomer and possibly a problematic starting place, though one has to start somewhere. "Palace" means the court, the monarchy, the law, the discourse and ideology of political organization and loyalty. Even when the crown was not an active participant in the struggle to fend off or conquer the plague – and part of my argument is that the action took place not in the Palace but in the towns – still the king was an omnipresent interlocutor, albeit a theoretical or silent one. From there, this chronicle travels throughout the republic. It goes down Roads and meets a variety of travelers, obstacles, news, and goods.

---

[18] Pérez Moreda, "The plague in Castile," 34, says the Portuguese case might have been an independent epidemic, as it first appeared in Lisbon in 1597, part of a larger Atlantic port problem.

It comes up against the Wall, where it either gets in or it doesn't. It reaches the Market, where food, livestock, and money, all radically diminished, changed hands. It travels down town Streets, where the sounds and smells and sight of plague transformed ordinary landscapes. It walks into the Town Hall, where leaders debated what to do as they applied both punishment and indulgence to their distraught citizens. And, finally, it reaches what I am calling the Sickbed, where medicine and prayer were invoked to relieve patients unlucky enough to have been caught at the end of this tortuous odyssey.

In this world that I am attempting to recover, disease was not simply a metaphor. It was a problem and a calamity, or sometimes an opportunity, but not something that stood for sin or evil or otherness, though it is also true that for some observers epidemic and hardship spelled confirmation of the end of Spain's glory years. Death was certainly terrifying, but the disease as such was not categorized as a "demonic enemy" resulting in the scapegoating of its victims.[19] Nor did it necessarily set off collective madness or social disorder. Nor did the reaction mark a stark contrast with allegedly post-Enlightenment rational responses. Given what they had to work with, denizens of late sixteenth-century Castile were admirably responsible. Theirs was not a world without logic. Nor was there a particular outburst of religiosity that I can detect. There were processions, of course, and presumably people prayed for it to go away, but that is neither surprising nor excessive. Language blaming their sins for the debacle and praising God's mercy for its departure often sound formulaic, which is not to say the language was not taken seriously, only that it was brief and episodic.

I am aware, as I have said, that this approach marks a contrast to what one might expect. It certainly is not what literary sources have always told us. As Paul Slack wrote, "One can never be entirely sure about the extent to which chroniclers of epidemics concentrated on social dislocation, the failure of doctors, flights to and from religion, rumours of poisoned wells, and similar phenomena simply because Thucydides and later writers down to Defoe taught them to look for them."[20] Here is part of

---

[19] Susan Sontag's language has been reproduced widely, but these words come from her February 23, 1978 article in *The New York Review of Books*.

[20] Paul Slack, "Introduction," in *Epidemics and Ideas: Essays on the Historical Perception of Pestilence*, Terence Ranger and Paul Slack, eds. (Past and Present Publications, Cambridge University Press, 1992), 9. Slack says the first English translation of Thucydides appeared in 1667. In Spain it circulated in Latin already in the fifteenth century; the first Spanish-language version in the Biblioteca Nacional dates from 1564. Nicolás Bocángel [also Bocangelino], *Libro de las enfermedades malignas y pestilentes, causas, pronósticos, curación y preservación* (Madrid: Luis Sánchez, 1600), for example, cites him on pp. 65 and 87.

Thucydides's famous description of the collapse of Athenian society: "The catastrophe was so overwhelming that men, not knowing what would happen next to them, became indifferent to every rule of religion or of law... In other respects also Athens owed to the plague the beginnings of a state of unprecedented lawlessness. Seeing how quick and abrupt were the changes of fortune which came to the rich who suddenly died and to those who had previously been penniless but now inherited their wealth, people now began openly to venture on acts of self-indulgence which before then they used to keep dark... As for what is called honour, no one showed himself willing to abide by its laws... No fear of god or law of man had a restraining influence."[21] James Longrigg has noted that many subsequent writers paid Thucydides "the most sincere form of flattery" in essentially cribbing his terrible and moving description, and that was true during the great Castilian plague as well. But Longrigg makes the very important point that the Greek chronicler's theme was, precisely, "the disintegration of Greek society. He is describing the processes by which social and political violence can undermine reason. The plague serves as a catalyst which expedites these processes."[22] Thus there was purposefulness in his account, not mere description. The prospect of the destruction of political order in a society as steeped in the notions of good government and republicanism as Castile was bound to disturb and horrify readers. Boccaccio's plague also led to social collapse, the pathology of the body politic as well as of the human body. "In the face of so much affliction and misery, all respect for the laws of God and man had virtually broken down and been extinguished in our city," he wrote. "It was not merely a question of one citizen avoiding another, and of people almost invariably neglecting their neighbours and rarely or never visiting their relatives, addressing them only from a distance; this scourge had implanted so great a terror in the hearts of men and women that brothers abandoned brothers, uncles their nephews, sisters their brothers, and in many cases wives deserted their husbands. But even worse, and almost incredible, was the fact that fathers and mothers refused to nurse and assist their own children, as though they did not belong to them."[23] Contrast this with Virgil's image of Aeneas carrying his father and the hearth-gods out of the burning city of Troy: "So come, dear father, climb up onto my

---

[21] Thucydides, *History of the Peloponnesian War*, trans. Rex Warner (London: Penguin Books, 1972), 155 [II:52–3].

[22] James Longrigg, "Epidemic, ideas and classical Athenian society," in *Epidemics and Ideas*, Terence Ranger and Paul Slack, eds., 21–44, pp. 27, 33.

[23] Giovanni Boccaccio, *The Decameron*, trans. G. H. McWilliam (London: Penguin Books, 1972), 52–4.

shoulders!/I will carry you on my back. This labor of love/will never wear me down. Whatever falls to us now,/we both will share one peril, one path to safety."[24] That was more like it, and indeed the haunting image of fathers abandoning their sons, and vice versa, is a recurring one in Spanish plague accounts. A chronicler of the monarchs Isabel and Ferdinand described an early sixteenth-century plague in words repeated by virtually every historian of the era: The epidemic "entered throughout the Kingdom of Granada and throughout all of Castile ... and thus the pestilence was general and universal ... Fathers could not depend on their children nor children on their parents, and the living fled from the dead and the living fled from each other..."[25] The most famous treatise-writer during the plague at the end of the century, Luis Mercado, remarked in general of the plague: "It is a miserable turn of fortune for any city, town, or village to be touched or contaminated by any sort of pestilent affect, and if one does not speedily and carefully manage to cut it off, it will quickly grow with such furious cruelty that parents will abandon their children and women their husbands, and everyone will just look out for himself, leaving what they most love and what most pains them in the hands of the most cruel and fatal illness that can befall them ..."[26] Philip II (r. 1556–1598) also hired physician Miguel Martínez de Leyva to write a treatise, in the prologue of which Leyva wrote: "I decided to write down the proper regimen against pestilence, as it is a thing of such great disorder and causes so much terror and fear and great ruin among people." Rulers, ministers, and doctors are confused and vanish, he wrote, "and relatives shun one another, denying their blood and progeny." Later on, describing the disease and its causes, he wrote, "Parents flee from their children and children from their parents, and relatives and friends put distance between themselves."[27] In France, as well (and probably most everywhere else), the trope was powerful. "Plague, noted Isaac Quatroux in 1671, 'cuts and severs all ties of blood and friendship.' Mothers and fathers abandoned their stricken and children, children their stricken parents..."[28]

---

[24] Virgil, *The Aeneid*, trans. Robert Fagles (New York: Viking, 2006), 99 [lines 880–3].

[25] Andrés Bernaldez, *Historia de los Reyes Católicos Don Fernando y Doña Isabel* [Biblioteca de Autores Españoles, vol. 70.] (Madrid: Atlas, 1953), 567–773, pp. 728–30. The chronicle was published sometime before 1513.

[26] Luis Mercado, *El libro de la peste del Dr. Luis Mercado con un estudio preliminar acerca del autor y sus obras por el Dr. Nicasio Mariscal* [1598] [Biblioteca Clásica de la Medicina Española, vol. 1] (Madrid: Imp. de Cosano, 1921), 227–8.

[27] Miguel Martínez de Leyva, *Remedios preservativos y curativos para en tiempo de la peste; y otras curiosas experiencias* (Madrid 1597), prologue and 76v.

[28] Colin Jones, "Plague and its metaphors in early modern France," *Representations* 53 (Winter 1996), 97–127, p. 110.

As far as I can tell, at the turn of seventeenth-century Castile parents did not abandon their children, nor did people stop caring for each other, though they may have gone insane from grief and certainly took precautions. One survivor of a later plague in Barcelona, Miquel Parets, remembered, "One saw that whenever anyone fell sick he lost all touch with friends and relatives, as there was no one who would risk contact with him, just the person nursing him. And it would have to be someone very close or related to him who would dare to take care of him, like a wife to a husband or a mother to a son or a sister to a brother, and even among these many fled or did not want to stay, for the plague was so evil and of such a bad sort that everyone fled."[29] So abandonment did occur, but it cannot be a general way of describing what happened. The people in this book owed allegiance to their neighbors, their God (though He is mentioned less than one might expect), and their king and his laws. Admittedly, sometimes they demonstrated even greater allegiance to themselves, though they generally explained that preference by pointing to the good it inevitably would bring about for others. Theirs was a moral community, even if people sometimes misbehaved or left their post. This book happens to involve a massive episode of contagious disease, but my interest lies less in the exceptional than in the usual, my point being that if we watch how exhausted people took care of one another, or didn't, under exceptional circumstances, we can grasp the power of the rules and laws and customs that bound them. Society did not become unhinged; it was bound to church and government, in the broadest sense of both words. But people at all levels had to make choices, and those choices illuminate for us where they placed themselves in their community and how they measured themselves against their past.

My principal primary sources are city council minutes and related correspondence, accounts, and ledgers. I also read lawsuits that arose as a result of the plague. I did not look at parish records, as I decided early on that I could not reach demographic conclusions. Most cities had special ad hoc health commissions that dealt with plague matters, but almost all their records have disappeared; Burgos is an exception, which accounts for its frequent mentions in these pages.[30] There are very few contemporary narratives, but I have used all I could find, and I read widely among medical treatises.

As I've been writing this story of plague, I was often reminded of the work of Albert Hirschman, who began his extraordinary intellectual life

---

[29] James S. Amelang, ed. and trans., *A Journal of the Plague Year: The Diary of the Barcelona Tanner Miquel Parets, 1651* (New York: Oxford University Press, 1991), 59.
[30] Seville's plague commission papers also survived.

as an economist. He was often struck by the little things, the patches and experiments, the devices and small ideas put into practice by individuals and towns in underdeveloped areas that somehow managed to triumph over all the economists' models, theories, and structures. Unexpected and surprisingly positive effects, unintended consequences, and new opportunities might ensue as people adjusted, made do, showed their inventiveness and their resilience.[31] During the great Castilian plague, certainly nothing was as usual, but as Hirschman once wrote, "Development depends not so much on finding optimal combinations … as on calling forth and enlisting … resources and abilities that are hidden, scattered or badly utilized."[32] In Castilian communities, and probably in communities most anywhere, the contingent could outweigh the established order even while whatever actions were taken gestured to tradition, the past, to time immemorial. Sixteenth-century municipal documents are full of small, good things that put the lie to any of us who might think that things were always one way, or always another way, but never both.[33] I also, as I have been writing, imagined the scenes in Pieter Bruegel's great genre paintings of dozens and dozens of peasants or town-dwellers all together and simultaneously tending to their jobs, their neighbors, acting out, playing, wooing, stealing. In pestiferous Castile, to the extent that they could, people kept right on doing those things. Possibly a few hundred years earlier they would have behaved differently, and that change is worth thinking about. I will not advance a theory as to how and when that happened. I am simply saying that by the end of 1596, when the pestilent ship docked in Santander, that's how it was.

[31] On Hirschman see the magnificent biography by Jeremy Adelman, *Worldly Philosopher: The Odyssey of Albert O. Hirschman* (Princeton, NJ: Princeton University Press, 2013).

[32] In his *The Strategy of Economic Development* (1958), which he cites in his *Exit, Voice, and Loyalty: Responses to Decline in Firms, Organizations and States* (Cambridge, MA: Harvard University Press, 1970), 12.

[33] "A Small, Good Thing" is the title of a frequently anthologized story by Raymond Carver that first appeared in his *Cathedral* (New York: Alfred A. Knopf, 1984), 59–90.

Site 1: Palace

The aim of this book is to describe, in physical detail, how people in the kingdom of Castile moved, worked, suffered, competed, and starved during the years of pestilence at the turn of the sixteenth century. It begins with the monarchy because everything began with the monarchy, though in the years we are examining, the monarchy was suddenly not quite there. Yet the language and the expectations prevailed; small towns might be rent apart, but they knew themselves to be republics of a republic and they reacted as such, expecting help, petitioning, managing, and obeying, all as vassals of a king. The themes to be explored in this book – memory, custom, law, charity, duty, justice, knowledge, belief – will be found at every stop along the way, but by beginning in the palace, as it were, we can see more clearly how these all functioned in the context of political relationships and ideology. The following glimpses of royal intervention in plague matters concern the new reign of Philip III (r. 1598–1621) and then look specifically at shipbuilding, judicial jurisdiction, and taxes, all realms in which the monarchy had to continue exerting pressure on localities beset by disease. There is something necessarily fragmentary and anecdotal about these examples, but they provide different slants on the ways in which plague pushed the structures of an already pressured state, and how the state pushed back.

The scourge on board the Flemish ship *"Rodamundo"* had not quite made its slow, patient way to central Spain as Philip II lay dying in El Escorial, his palace-monastery in the mountains outside Madrid. But it would. This was the ship, the Cortes pointedly wrote, that had been carrying correspondence from Archduke Alberto in Brussels for his uncle the king, which could be taken as a veiled suggestion that it was the crown that bore responsibility.[1] In any case, two months after the king's

---

[1] ACC vol. 15, p. 561, December 1, 1597. There was plenty of criticism of Philip II during this long session of the Cortes, the Castilian representative assembly; see I. A. A. Thompson, "Oposición política y juicio del gobierno en las Cortes de 1592–98," *Studia Historica. Historia Moderna* 17 (1997), 37–62. Though I say here that

death, a funeral Mass was held in Valladolid, and the speaker left no doubt that the royal demise was just one more in a long string of catastrophes spelling the definitive *decadencia*, or decline, of Spain. Bad health and pestilence reigned everywhere, he said, and the land was dry and broken, "ruined like a bad merchant," an image all too familiar. This multitude of evils had simply moved in and set up housekeeping, bringing with them troubles like Spain had not seen since the times of the Patriarch Tubal.[2]

The new king was twenty years old. With his father recently buried and the plague devastating much of northern Castile, Philip III was guided through the peninsula and in the arts of kingship by his favorite, Francisco Gómez de Sandoval, the ambitious marquis of Denia and later first Duke of Lerma, the name by which he is known. The immediate reason for what would end up being a nine-month trip was for Philip III to greet his new bride, Margaret, daughter of Archduke Charles of Styria, upon her arrival in Valencia, Lerma's home territory. The royal progress lengthened, however, as the itinerant entourage skirted the contagion, waited for the Cortes of Castile to approve an outlay, and visited the Barcelona Corts so the new king could be sworn in. Lerma was in firm control of the journey, all the while making key political appointments, marrying off his children well, and accumulating great wealth. The king, surprisingly, showed some interest in government, and several of the royal councils that his micromanaging father had essentially ignored were bolstered, mostly with noblemen of Lerma's choosing, and they began meeting more often.[3]

The plan had been to go from Barcelona back to Zaragoza in July, but by then that would have taken them dangerously near plague country. So, instead, they returned to Tarragona, then Valencia, and thence to Lerma's own town of Denia, where they spent a pleasant and lavish summer. In the words of Patrick Williams, "The journey witnessed the

central Spain was still relatively healthy, below it will be clear that Madrid itself was affected at this point.

[2] Geoffrey Parker, *Felipe II: La biografía definitiva* (Barcelona: Planeta, 2013), 962, citing Juan Íñiguez de Lequerica, *Sermones funerales*, fols. 85v–6, November 15, 1598.

[3] In general on Lerma see Patrick Williams, *The Great Favourite: The Duke of Lerma and the Court and Government of Philip III of Spain, 1598–1621* (Manchester University Press, 2006); on Philip III's early reorganization of government see Patrick Williams, "Philip III and the restoration of Spanish Government, 1598–1603," *The English Historical Review* 88:349 (October 1973), 751–69, and Santiago Martínez Hernández, *El Marqués de Velada y la Corte en los Reinados de Felipe II y Felipe III: Nobleza cortesana y cultura política en la España del Siglo de Oro* (Salamanca: Junta de Castilla y León, 2004), part III. The funding the king was awaiting from the Cortes was probably the latest *millones* grant, the most important indirect tax of the era.

final transformation of a monachal into a baroque court..."[4] At long last, in late October the entourage returned to Madrid, but "only when Denia [i.e. Lerma] was satisfied that the plague had died out in the capital did Philip travel into the city."[5] A couple of months later, the marquis received the ducal title.

The Duke of Lerma was the great-grandson of Bernardo de Sandoval y Rojas, second marquis of Denia and Count of Lerma who, curiously enough, also had experience shepherding around royalty living at the edges of plague territory. He had been governor of the household of Queen Juana, the essentially imprisoned mother of Charles V (r. 1516–1556 as King of Spain), and he and Charles kept her absolutely under control in the town of Tordesillas (Valladolid). With the arrival of plague in August 1518 and again in May 1519 they lied to Juana about death tolls, going so far as to stage fake funerals to convince her she had to leave. In the end the plague receded, and evacuation was not necessary, though she was forced to flee on a mule when plague reached Tordesillas in 1534. It is interesting to speculate what the great-grandson knew of his ancestor as he followed in his footsteps, stage-managing an isolated and vulnerable monarch.[6]

Lerma was ruminating on where to move the capital, as he did not wish to stay in Madrid. His motives had more to do with his own political ambitions than with the plague, though the plague was convenient. These considerations were known in royal circles. The second marquis of Velada, Gómez Dávila y Toledo, a close adviser to both Philip II and his son, wrote from Barcelona to a friend in June 1599 that "most of Castile is affected by *secas*. They say the healthiest places are Toledo and Ávila, and also San Lorenzo [de El Escorial], and that in Madrid more than one thousand *secas* patients are in the hospital."[7] Indeed, there is

---

[4] Williams, "Philip III and the restoration," 758; on the celebrations see Elizabeth Wright, *Pilgrimage to Patronage: Lope de Vega and the Court of Philip III, 1598–1621* (Lewisburg, PA: Bucknell University Press, 2001), 52–6; several contemporary printed and manuscript accounts of entrances and festivities in Valencia are in BN ms 2346. The entourage had also been in Denia earlier on the progress.

[5] Williams, *The Great Favourite*, 62, citing BL Add 28.422, fol. 140, Denia to Juan de Borja, September 1599. Even then, Philip spent most of what remained of 1599 at his country houses of El Pardo and Aranjuez; see Martínez Hernández, *El Marqués de Velada*, 409.

[6] Bethany Aram, *Juana the Mad: Sovereignty and Dynasty in Renaissance Europe* (Baltimore, MD: Johns Hopkins University Press, 2005), 122–3. Juana is often referred to as Juana la Loca. Her husband, Philip, had died in September 1506, probably of typhus.

[7] Martínez Hernández, *El Marqués de Velada*, 406, citing Velada to Don Pedro de Toledo (Marqués de Villafranca), June 14, 1599, ADMS Villafranca leg. 4.392 (carta 104). Velada's numbers seem reasonable; documents in AGS-E leg. 183 indicate dozens of deaths weekly from April to early September.

plenty of indirect evidence that Madrid, the capital and court, may have had plague cases right from the start. Antonio de León Pinelo's chronicle of the city remarks that "the plague [*peste*] never ceased" that year, for which reason there were multiple religious invocations and processions, which he says were remarkably successful.[8] A group of doctors in Burgos noted in May 1599 that Dr. Luis Mercado, the royal *protomédico*, had written in his *quadernillo de peste* that "this disease" had entered Madrid already in 1597.[9] A doctor in the Basque province of Guipúzcoa judged that the disease that struck San Sebastián in August 1597 was not plague at all but simply the high fever (*causón*) "that many people in Madrid also died of, and there they did not believe it was plague."[10] According to one correspondent of Diego Sarmiento de Acuña, later the Count of Gondomar, "los de El Escorial" were removing supplies from Madrid up to Philip II's monastery dwelling in August 1597 "because they want to guard against Madrid. This has raised such a fuss that doctors and surgeons have met … This place has never been healthier, though it is true that *secas* are going around, but they don't seem to stick, and they are cured with bleeding, and few people die of them, mostly worn down and poor people and low-lifes." Another of Gondomar's acquaintances wrote, also in 1597, "They write that Madrid is in bad health and that more than four hundred people have died of *secas* in just a few days. They say the whole palace and its patio are washed every day with vinegar."[11]

[8] Antonio de León Pinelo, *Anales de Madrid (desde el año 447 al de 1658)*, Pedro Fernández Martín, ed. (Madrid: Instituto de Estudios Madrileños, 1971), 161.

[9] AGS-E leg. 183 doc. 223; the quote appears in Bartolomé Bennassar, *Recherches sur les grandes épidémies dans le nord de l'Espagne a la fin du XVIe siècle. Problèmes de documentation et de méthode* (Paris: SEVPEN, 1969), 132. However the 1599 version of Mercado's treatise does not seem to contain this reference. See Nicasio Mariscal's introduction to *El libro de la peste del Dr. Luis Mercado con un estudio preliminar acerca del autor y sus obras por el Dr. Nicasio Mariscal*. Biblioteca Clásica de la Medicina Española, vol. 1 (Madrid: Imp. de Cosano, 1921), 65–6. *Protomédicos* were crown-appointed physicians, usually very prominent, who had medical, administrative, and/or didactic responsibilities.

[10] José Ramón Cruz Mundet, *El mal que al presente corre: Gipuzkoa y la peste (1597–1600)* (San Sebastián: Kutxa Fundazioa, 2003), 33, citing AM Pasaia, sec. C, neg. 1, libro 1.

[11] RBP II-2147, doc. 12, Gaspar Pérez de Matallana (in Madrid) to Gondomar (in Toro), August 29, 1597; RBP II-2147, doc. 17, Francisco de Villapadierna (in Valladolid) to Gondomar, August 1597. Pérez de Matallana later became one of Philip III's secretaries; Villapadierna may be Francisco de Quiñones y Villapadierna, a military man who served throughout Europe, Chile, and Peru. Gondomar was appointed corregidor of Toro in 1597, where he was during the plague; in 1602 he became corregidor of Valladolid. Further Gondomar correspondence about the presence of plague in Madrid in 1597 can be found in RBP II-2116, doc. 170, Antonio Alvarez, in Madrid, August 27, 1597; and RBP II-2147, doc. 58, Lic. Villagutierre (one of Gondomar's agents), in Madrid, September 11, 1597.

But by 1599 Madrid certainly was in better shape than the rest of Castile, though in April of that year Burgos assured the royal council that whatever disease was beginning to kill people there was not plague but rather "the disease that at present is in Madrid ... and in Alcalá and in many other places."[12] Velada did not think moving the capital from there was a good idea (nor did the city of Madrid, and nor did the Cortes), especially not to Valladolid, which was Lerma's preferred option. To another correspondent Velada wrote that none other than Mercado, soon the author of a massively distributed treatise, had told him Valladolid was a sick place and that the court should not move there. "I don't know what the mood is now," he wrote. "The lack of health there and the many who have died is well known and commented upon here. Now I am seeing that less is being said [about this] than before; I don't know where things will go."[13] When Philip III, then in Martorell (Barcelona), asked Mercado to reissue his treatise in the vernacular, the monarch said: "Given that one understands there is great hardship in my kingdoms of Castile, with the peste occurring in such a widespread and pernicious manner, it seems necessary to write a treatise so that all provinces, cities, towns, and villages can understand and know with certainty which disease it is and how they should protect themselves ..."[14] It was certainty that was needed.

Some but not all the king's councilors traveled with him on his nine-month progress, along with aristocrats, servants, aides, and ambassadors. One of the latter was Francesco Soranzo, of Venice, who kept the Senate up to date on the news as he trudged from Madrid to Valencia to Barcelona to Tarragona to Valencia to Zaragoza and at long last back to Madrid. He complained of bad carriages and mules, the excessive heat, and the ever-present fear of plague, from which he prayed God to spare him so he could continue serving his Venetian lords. "I will take exquisite care as I travel to remain far away from all suspicious places and dangerous things," he promised from Tarragona. This peregrination showed no sign of coming to an end, he complained two days later from Valencia, as the epidemic, too, was migrating and advancing. He had received word from his house in Madrid that several of his servants had

---

[12] Francis Brumont, "La peste de 1599 en Burgos, una relación del regidor Andrés de Cañas," *BROCAR: Cuadernos de Investigación Histórica* 13 (1987), 155–66, p. 162, which, in turn, refers to a letter from the city to the council.

[13] Velada to Juan de Sosa, February 23, 1600, IVDJ envío 86, caja 120, doc. 10.

[14] June 14, 1599; the letter is widely reproduced. For example, Alfredo Alvar Ezquerra, "Madrid reflejo de los problemas sanitarios de la peninsula: La peste de 1596 vista por un galeno de la corte," *Anales del Instituto de Estudios Madrileños* 20 (1983), 203–18, p. 207.

died of plague, which both saddened and worried him, given that his belongings might now be infected.[15]

Thus during this early ambulatory period of the king's rule, the plague mattered principally because it was one of the determinants of how long the court would stay away from the palace that had had to be washed down with vinegar, and where it would finally settle. The stack of reports from local governors (*corregidores*) discovered and published decades ago by the French historian Bartolomé Bennassar were requested by the king in mid-April, probably to help him decide where to go. Most of the reports were full of bad news and seem to have had little bearing on the king's or Lerma's final decision. The finalist apparently was Toledo, as Velada had surmised, and the winner was Valladolid, which in the summer of 1599 in fact was suffering the full onslaught of the disease, though by the end of the year it was better. At least 6,000 people died there.[16] It was chosen in part, and most obviously, because it was close to Lerma's Castilian domains and would get the new king away from his father's once powerful advisers whom Lerma had sidelined. But it was also closer to Portugal; it had been a capital in the past; it was the site of the Chancillería (the royal appeals court) and a main tribunal of the Inquisition; and it had a river, so it was not an entirely unreasonable choice. The move may also have been inspired (and was thus sold to naysayers) by a wish to leave the over-crowded, chaotic, and dirty city of Madrid after a phenomenally bad stretch of years and to promote the change as a sign of a new beginning.[17]

At the same time as Dr. Mercado and his colleagues offered medical opinions, the Council of Castile, the most important of the king's advisory bodies, on April 13, 1599 gave the king a long report summing up the state of affairs in Madrid, which Philip made notes on. The day before, as Velada had written, physicians had met with the Council and told them that in fact this was not really plague, because if it were, then all or most

---

[15] ASV Senato, dispacci Spagna, filze 31, nos. 25–61, scattered.
[16] Bennassar, *Recherches*, 43. Bennassar transcribed many of the documents in this bundle; I have used the originals, though I also consulted his versions.
[17] Antonio Feros, *Kingship and Favoritism in the Spain of Philip III, 1598–1621* (Cambridge University Press, 2000), 86–7; Williams, *The Great Favourite*, 70–3. Estimates of Madrid's population vary; according to Alfredo Alvar Ezquerra, "Estructuras socioeconómicas de Madrid y su entorno en la segund mitad del siglo XVI," PhD diss., Universidad Complutense de Madrid, 1988, p. 536, Madrid had around 80,000 inhabitants at the time of the plague. Annie Molinié-Bertrand, *Au siècle d'or l'Espagne et ses Hommes. La Population du Royaume de Castille au XVI siècle* (Paris: Economica, 1985), 208, gives a lower number, 65,000, in the city's eleven parishes. According to her study of various censuses, Madrid had just 4,500 inhabitants in 1528 and around 20,000 when the capital was established there in 1561. There is no debate over the fact that Madrid grew extremely quickly in the second half of the sixteenth century.

of the people in an infected community would die. (*"No se pueden dar por peste las secas por faltarles las calidades principales della."*) Nonetheless, they opined that the matter was serious and merited full-time city guards in the capital. Clearly, the king should not return for the time being, advice with which he agreed. The Council of Castile proposed that corregidores, who presided over city councils, begin sending weekly plague reports, that the Council essentially take over plague management in Madrid (which is why plague is scarcely mentioned in the capital's city council minutes), and that the king and his councilors also consider Segovia, Granada, or Guadalajara as good places to go. The report then, rather sinisterly, seems to take advantage of Philip's inexperience by urging him to undo his father's momentous decision to fix the capital in Madrid after years of itinerancy. "We would like to remind Your Majesty that your ancestors did not live in just one place but traveled throughout all their kingdoms, and that is why the kingdoms and cities and towns were so prosperous and abundant then. Today they are poor and troubled because all their efforts and business and profits go to Madrid, leading not only to the depopulation of the rest of the kingdom, as we see in Toledo, Medina [del Campo], Valladolid, Burgos, and everywhere else, where farming and all things linked to the common good have ceased, but also to confusion in Madrid, where idle and ill-intentioned people can live as they wish, offending our Lord ..." To which the king replied, "I will try to do this, depending on the place." Four days later, letters were sent out to fourteen corregidores asking for weekly reports on the state of the plague and public health efforts.[18]

As the king's intentions to move became more apparent, the Cortes appointed commissioners to coordinate their campaign to stop him from leaving Madrid, insisting that Valladolid's notoriously bad health and the expense of moving were powerful reasons to stay. In an early January 1600 appeal to the king the assembly wrote, "[The king] would not be able to permanently stay anywhere he went, even in Valladolid, given that that city has been so unhealthy, and people who recently have come

---

[18] AGS-E leg. 183 doc. 11, April 13, 1599. The letters were sent to Albacete, Aranda de Duero, Arévalo, Ávila, Burgos, Madrid, Medina del Campo, Olmedo, Palencia, San Clemente, Segovia, Sepúlveda, Toledo, and Valladolid. Some of these places are obvious choices, others not so much, with some logical ones missing, and I do not know what the crown's criteria were. The series are also incomplete. On corregidores, a post created during the reign of Isabel and Ferdinand, see Benjamin González Alonso, *El corregidor castellano 1348–1808* (Madrid: Instituto de Estudios Administrativos, 1970) and Jerónimo Castillo de Bovadilla, *Política para corregidores y señores de vasallos*, 2 vols. (Madrid: Instituto de Estudios de Administración Local, 1978), [facs. of Antwerp: Juan Bautista Verdussen, 1704) [1597]. In 1597 there were sixty-eight *corregimientos*, a district that usually corresponded to a city or town and the area surrounding it.

here from there say that supplies and everything else are incomparably more expensive there, and after gathering up all the clothes and linens after the illnesses, now they will take them out and sell them, and there is much to be feared from the risk to the royal persons and to all the Councils..."[19] But in January 1601 the transfer nonetheless took place, and Valladolid remained the capital until early spring 1606, when the court moved back to Madrid.

For the crown, peste was a monstrous inconvenience, but not only that. It offered the occasion to perhaps assert control over some municipalities, though also an unfortunate occasion for other municipalities to miss tax payments. It was no less a monstrosity or an opportunity for everyone else, of course, but for the crown – for the palace – it brought into focus the often conflicting obligations to care for vassals and guide the ship of state. With luck, it could do both. What the crown did not do, however, was use the disease to increase its power, whether because at that point, as the throne changed occupants, it was incapable of doing so, whether because the balance of power between palace and town hall was such an unshakable tenet of the Castilian polity, or both.[20] There was no panopticon; indeed, at times one gets the sense no one was watching at all. The corregidores' weekly reports, irregular as they were, were a crown initiative; so, too, was Mercado's treatise, and in a few cases, which we will look at below, the crown, through its tribunals and councils, stepped in to supervise public health efforts. But for the most part knowledge and policy were being generated by the towns. To some extent, this may also have been true during past epidemics, but the hands-off approach during this case is nonetheless notable and somehow emblematic both of the disease being regarded as an administrative management problem best left to locals, which was especially true as notions of contagion began being refined, and of the temporary absence, in all senses of the word, of the king.

But though information-gathering seems to have been centered in town halls, the crown's insatiable need for revenue (in the 1590s Spain was at war, in one way or another, with France, England, and the Dutch) provoked a relentless assault on municipal coffers. In part this meant that

---

[19] ACC vol. 18, 571–86, p. 586. Madrid corregidor Mosén Rubí de Bracamonte and the physician and reformer Cristóbal Pérez de Herrera also wrote appeals to the king; on the latter's arguments against moving the capital see Michel Cavillac, "El Madrid 'utópico' (1597–1600) de Cristóbal Pérez de Herrera," *Bulletin Hispanique* 104:2 (2002), 627–44.

[20] Nükhet Varlik, *Plague and Empire in the Early Modern Mediterranean World: The Ottoman Experience, 1347–1600* (Cambridge University Press, 2015), chapter 8, suggests that certain administrative and legislative responses to the plague in the Ottoman Empire contributed to state-formation there.

cities' requests for funds with which to fight the plague do not seem to have prospered, the crown preferring that townspeople tax themselves or borrow from wealthy locals. This would have highly damaging long-run consequences.[21] Nor would the crown step back from its defense commitments, which brings us to the first example I will offer of the ways in which the plague affected palace initiatives and political relations throughout the kingdom. This nexus should be obvious throughout the rest of the book, but by starting at the center, as it were, I hope to establish the importance of the principle of kingship and the inextricable ties and knots that linked the monarch and his vassals. The king, according to medieval Castilian law, "must protect the common good more than his own, love and honor all according to their estate, take pleasure in the company of the wise and the learned, bring love and harmony to his people, be rigorous and grant to everyone their right, and trust his own people more than outsiders."[22] This was a tall order.

By late summer of 1597, during the last year of Philip II's reign, the peste had made its way eastward from Santander to the Basque Country, home to some of Spain's leading shipbuilding sites but also by then the site of serious economic problems. In the province of Guipúzcoa it would not only claim thousands of lives, it would wedge its way into long-running antagonism between the crown and local municipalities over where to get the wood to build ships, how to manage the labor, and what the political process for making these decisions should look like. In the opinion of those in charge of ensuring delivery of six contested galleons (following twenty-nine built since 1594), locals were just using the epidemic as an excuse for their usual Basque stubbornness.[23]

The trees for the twenty-nine galleons had been taken from the rich forests of the town of Rentería, with no payment in return.[24] So the next

---

[21] Municipal debt would become one of Spain's major economic ailments; for bibliography see José Ignacio Fortea Pérez, "Hacienda real y haciendas locales en la crisis del siglo XVII: el ejemplo de Castilla," in *Le crisi finanziarie: Gestione, implicazione e conseguenze nell'età preindustriale* (Florence: Firenze University Press, 2016), 109n1.

[22] Partida II, tit. 1, law 9.

[23] This conflict has been written about before: David Goodman, *Spanish Naval Power, 1589–1665: Reconstruction and Defeat* (Cambridge University Press, 1997), chapter 2, on which I rely for some of the background; and Cruz Mundet, *El mal que al presente corre,* chapter 8, a very detailed account that uses valuable sources from local Guipuzcoan archives.

[24] Goodman, *Spanish Naval Power,* 94. Cruz Mundet, *El mal que al presente corre,* 199, adds that the captain in charge of that project left town without paying workers or suppliers. The degree to which Spain was stripped of trees in order to build the Armada is somewhat of a myth, though clearly it took its toll, and "Spain was forced to import larger and larger amounts of shipbuilding materials and naval stores from northern and central Europe"; William D. Phillips, Jr., "Spain's northern shipping industry in the

round of shipbuilding was an opportunity to draw the line. Rentería refused to house the carpenters assembling the ships in nearby Lezo, where the twenty-nine galleons had been built, and ordered guards to halt all traffic between the two towns, allegedly blocking even the passage of nails. These guards quickly turned into plague guards, leading to the accusation that Rentería was exaggerating the disease for its own benefit. But massive casualties in the town next to Lezo, the port of Pasajes de San Juan, tell a different story.

Early modern Castile was no stranger to standoffs between municipalities and the crown over the relative weight and meaning of laws and customs that inevitably dated back to time immemorial. That was true too in the Basque Country, which, strictly speaking, was part of Castile, and therefore had corregidores, who reported to the crown. But the political mesh was more complex there, given the involvement of old representative and executive bodies that had been incorporated into the Spanish monarchic system though were still operating within the framework of the old Basque laws, the *fueros*, which furthermore gave the region important fiscal advantages. Also, corregidores along the north coast and the border with France had more military functions than those in the interior and were joined by captains general, part of a military chain of command that oversaw the defensive presidios along the coast.[25]

Three royal emissaries representing three interlocking strands of the monarchy were on the scene as plague moved through Guipúzcoa: the corregidor, Diego Fernández de Arteaga; the captain general, Juan de Velázquez; and the general in charge of building the six ships, Antonio de Urquiola. Or, in other words, the king, war, and shipping – which itself could be state, war, and empire or commerce.

Velázquez told the king on September 27, 1597 that there was peste in San Sebastián. France, Navarre, and Castile had slammed their doors shut and the city was isolated and would surely starve, he wrote, and those who governed the city bore much of the blame: "Despite the fact that its troubles are so public and notorious they have issued statements

sixteenth century," *The Journal of European Economic History* 17:2 (Fall 1988), 267–301, p. 298.

[25] Despite the added layer of Basque jurisdictions, it is important to note that the supposedly incessant confrontation between Madrid and the Basque Country over questions of rights and privilege is often overstated. The *fueros*, a form of which existed throughout Castile, were a matter of fluid negotiation and emerged as a stumbling block in the Basque Country only in the later seventeenth century. On this see the excellent article, Susana Truchuelo García, "La incidencia de las relaciones entre Guipúzcoa y el poder real en la conformación de los fueros durante los siglos XVI y XVII," *Manuscrits* 24 (2006), 73–93. Military jurisdictional quarrels in the 1590s, which she describes, undoubtedly affected the conflict being described here.

saying they are healthy, as a result of which all such testimony from villages, even healthy ones, have lost their credibility … They respect none of my orders," he said, adding that the city had not even stopped people from going to fairs, the first measure taken by all Castilian capitals. Without force he could get nothing accomplished, he warned the monarch. The deluded city would not even accept money.[26] Indeed, San Sebastián was "the best example of how a community can ignore the evidence"; descriptions of the disease were unanimous, but no one dared give it a name.[27]

In late September, Urquiola told the king that 120 craftsmen from Lezo had simply vanished for fear of peste.[28] Urquiola, whom Philip II had appointed to oversee the massive post-Armada shipbuilding campaign, somehow had managed to put together a list of their names, which he forwarded to the corregidor. The distance between the galleon construction site and the infected town of Pasajes, among the most important shipbuilding centers on the north coast, was no more than two shots of an arquebus, he said, which was why guards were in place day and night around the town. But, he added, "We need a squadron of soldiers because the galleons are in an unpopulated area with no guards at the entrance to the port and, God forbid, someone with evil intentions could set it on fire or inflict other damages…" He also worried about where to stash the cash he had managed to get out of San Sebastián, and he unwisely decided on Rentería. When his men appeared at the city gates with carts full of coins, the people essentially rioted, believing the coins were infected. As night fell he was figuring out how to load the money onto boats, until the town doctor and others arranged for him to store it in the church. Gradually the missing craftsmen were picked up, but Rentería still refused to house them, saying they actually were twice as numerous as Urquiola claimed. Both sides told the provincial assembly (the Juntas Generales, where all towns in Guipúzcoa were represented) that the other was lying, and the Guipúzcoan government (the Diputación) asked the king directly to shut down the Lezo shipyards or at the very least ensure that workers there stayed there. It also told Urquiola that Rentería must be paid for housing workers, which would seem to have been a concession by Rentería, and insisted again that it was unsafe for people or goods to travel between towns.[29]

[26] AGS-GyM leg. 489, doc. 253. Velázquez was in Fuenterrabia, having left San Sebastián to escape the epidemic. In the first half of the sixteenth century, Fuenterrabia had been the military headquarters.
[27] Cruz Mundet, *El mal que al presente corre*, 32.
[28] AGS-GyM leg. 489 doc. 208. There are two documents with the same number.
[29] AGS-GyM leg. 490, doc. 127.

On October 9 Urquiola brought the king up to date on his problems. Having rounded up the craftsmen who had fled, and billeting them in Rentería, he now admitted they had fled again, and Rentería continued refusing entry to anyone from the outside. "They are saying that because three people have died in two houses, each a ways from each other between the shipyards and Pasajes and in contact with both of them, and it is true that they're not far from the shipyard, but aside from the fact that contact is forbidden, I have placed guards along the coast and on the roads and, glory to God, the people here are still healthy," he wrote, but he confessed he did not know what to do and was living in fear that the people of Pasajes, who were sick and wandering about aimlessly, might invade the shipyard and take or infect all the supplies he had stored there. The crown was unimpressed with these problems, and the king's secretary wrote on the overleaf that the corregidor must be told that shipbuilding could not cease.[30] Perhaps with that order in mind, Fernández de Arteaga visited Rentería and Lezo and assured the king on October 23 that both were healthy, which was not entirely true. But, he added, "I can tell Your Majesty that [Pasajes] is momentous, and along the coast there are piles of beds left behind by the dead. I ordered that they be picked up with iron hooks and thrown into boats to be taken out to sea, so that when the tide shifts they go someplace else, because burning them would cause great infection."[31] More than two months later he told the king, "The people here are up in arms concerning this illness and I think that if I push any more they will come after me and shoot me. So as to better serve Your Majesty, I calmed them down and [now] there is a signed agreement between Rentería and General Urquiola."[32] The beds he saw lying on the beach were from the hospital, which had been set up that autumn in a three-story private home requisitioned by the town government.[33] Patients were to bring their own beds and then leave them there. In principle, during the plague city councils throughout Castile reimbursed private citizens for seized properties, but the trail of subsequent documentation shows that payment often was not made because the money was not there, neither for beds nor for anything else. Already on August 7, with no recourse to any sort of credit, the town of Pasajes had held an open meeting (*concejo abierto*) of its *vecinos* and decided to mortgage all the town's incomes and properties plus their own private property. From eighteen women,

[30] AGS-GyM leg. 490, doc. 123.   [31] AGS-GyM leg. 490, doc. 330.
[32] AGS-GyM leg. 511, doc. 76.   [33] Cruz Mundet, *El mal que al presente corre*, 72–3.

of whom twelve were widows, they raised a total of 7,000 ducats at no interest for the first four years.[34]

Juanes de Arizmendi was a doctor who worked in several towns in the area, but he refused to enter Pasajes. "I wouldn't go there for any amount of money, I won't go in, and far less would I visit people who are ill there, now or in the future," he said.[35] He was in good company, as no other doctor went there either. (Barber surgeons did, but from August 1597 to February 1598, four of six died.) Instead, he and his friend Miguel Villaviciosa, a priest in Pasajes, would meet on opposite sides of the river, where the priest would shout out the symptoms and the doctor shouted back the treatment.

At the end of the month Urquiola once again informed the king of the state of affairs, which had only gotten worse.[36] No one was working at the shipyards, and the galleons were no closer to being built. Six people in Lezo had died, some of them because (Urquiola said) they had carried sickbeds from Pasajes. He ordered their houses to be burned and the linens to be flung into the sea. Urquiola went on to tell the king about Arizmendi's ingenious suggestion to resolve matters by simply burning Pasajes to the ground. "That way," he explained, "the illness would cease and the port would be free of suspicion [of illness] ... And the doctor says that the few *vecinos* who remained alive could rebuild it, with Your Majesty giving them help ... And people with whom I've spoken think it would be a good idea if Your Majesty ordered this before any more of the district gets infected."

Informed of the proposal to burn the village in order to save it, the corregidor advised the king it was not a good idea. Infested houses were surrounded by healthy ones, making it nearly impossible to do the job well, not to mention that the Diputación would not like one of its own municipalities going up in flames. It would be far cheaper to clean the town, and Fernández de Arteaga suggested hiring some Bretons whom San Sebastián had contracted to go house to house, sanitizing the dwellings of the absent sick and the dead. One thousand ducats should get the job done, he said, and the king would be showing great generosity should he give that amount to Pasajes.[37]

Also in late October the prince, the future Philip III, became involved in the increasingly tangled affair by asking the provincial assembly, which

---

[34] Cruz Mundet, *El mal que al presente corre*, 159. *Vecino* is usually translated as citizen; these were tax-paying heads of households, including widows. The multiplier for vecinos-inhabitants is usually 4.5. For more on *concejos abiertos*, see chapter 6. A ducat was a gold coin worth 375 maravedies, the smallest unit of account, or 11 reales.

[35] Cruz Mundet, *El mal que al presente corre*, 95–9.   [36] AGS-GyM leg. 460, doc. 394.

[37] AGS-GyM leg. 530, doc. 27 and AGS-GyM leg. 511, doc. 76.

was meeting in Deva, to please ensure that construction of the ships continue and to please cooperate with the general and the corregidor.[38] As a result, an investigatory committee of the corregidor (whom both Urquiola and Velázquez considered a pawn in the hands of locals) and provincial and town officials (one of whom Urquiola vetoed as "hateful") was formed to find out what the real state of affairs was in Lezo. But both the committee and the junta insisted the shipbuilding must cease for the time being. Five reasons were given: proximity to Pasajes; the danger of transporting materials to Lezo; the inadvisability of gathering large numbers of people; the possibility that the French might attack the ship once it was launched; and the fact that large parts of Guipúzcoa were isolated from neighboring provinces.[39] Letters and accusations continued going back and forth among the towns, the corregidor, the military, and the crown, but the work was halted.

By January 1598, San Sebastián appeared to be better, though the improvement proved temporary, and Fernández de Arteaga described to the king how sensible health measures had finally been implemented, in part thanks to the Bretons and a constable (*alguacil*) he had hired who had been unafraid to carry the sick and the dead in his arms.[40] Those who fled were gradually returning. The corregidor summoned all town leaders, prominent citizens, and medical professionals to obtain their opinions, and all agreed the city was healthy. Around 650 people had died in San Sebastián, he wrote, 400 of them women.[41]

Throughout this book it will be seen that people throughout Castile often attributed the origin of the plague in their town to a particular woman, often one carrying cloth, but the Basques appear to have been unique in insisting that women altogether as a sex bore responsibility despite the fact that, at least in the case of Pasajes de San Juan, they were subsidizing health care and certainly tending to the sick. Pasajes's reclaimed hospital had eight female employees, all of whom died in September and October, and after they were replaced their successors died as well.[42] Fernández de Arteaga in the aftermath of plague in San Sebastián expelled all single women who had not been born there,

---

[38] Cruz Mundet, *El mal que al presente corre*, 139, citing Juntas y Diputaciones, November 17, 1597.

[39] AGS-GyM leg. 491, doc. 333.   [40] AGS-GyM leg. 511, doc. 76.

[41] According to the website of the Instituto Geográfico Vasco, which does not give sources, the population of San Sebastián in 1600 was around 4,000. www.ingeba.org/liburua/donostia/51pobl/51pobl.htm, accessed January 2019.

[42] Cruz Mundet, *El mal que al presente corre*, 167, citing Archivo Municipal de Pasajes sec. C, neg. 1, leg. 1, fol. 78.

a solution he did not even bother to try to link to contagion.[43] The city of Bilbao would do the same the following year.[44] In Mondragón (Guipúzcoa), doctors Francisco López de Garita y Vergara, age 72, and Pedro García de Oro, over 80, offered a statement saying the plague had started because healthy towns had allowed the entry of "insignificant people, and the infection did not start with people of quality but rather in *mujercillas* of little significance who bought things for two when they were worth twenty, and thus they destroyed these republics."[45] The mayor of Elgoibar (Guipúzcoa) wrote to the Diputación that the plague had reached Lequeitio (Vizcaya) because a young woman had opened a bundle of clothing accompanying a cadaver.[46] In Pamplona (traditionally part of the Basque region), a city official named Martín de Senosiain, who wrote a long chronicle about the epidemic there, said the plague reached nearby Estella after a certain woman had spoken to certain guards. He also mentioned women who had gone to Estella to sell garbanzos and lentils in exchange for two pieces of colored cloth and a curtain, which of course was pestilent; she, her daughter, and her grandson were the first victims.[47] Villaviciosa, the Pasajes priest, in November wrote to the Diputación, pleading for assistance and scolding the institution for not having provided it: "The peste began here in early August. From what I can tell, its origin was some fisherwomen from here who bought some sheets by the San Sebastián bridge which appeared to be good and cheap, though they turned out to be bad and costly, as they were from Castro Urdiales [Cantabria] and other infected places. There were many people who bought them, and their impact was such that no one in any of their houses has survived."[48] And a fellow

[43] AGS-GyM leg. 489, doc. 227.   [44] AFB libro 023, January 21, 1598.

[45] Cruz Mundet, *El mal que al presente corre*, 169, citing Archivo General de Guipuzkoa, sec. 1, neg. 19, leg. 6, December 16, 1598. Cruz Mundet 165–70 specifically addresses women as a target for blame. The 1734 *Diccionario de Autoridades* defines *mugercilla* as "la muger de poca estimación y porte. Tómase regularmente por la que se ha echado al mundo," which might mean a woman of loose morals, but not necessarily. Alison Weber, in her study of Teresa de Ávila, says the earliest use of the term she found was in a 1260 translation of the New Testament, and that in the early modern age and henceforth the term generally refers to sexual license: Alison Weber, *Teresa of Avila and the Rhetoric of Femininity* (Princeton, NJ: Princeton University Press, 1996), 33fn41.

[46] Luis Murugarren Zamora, "La peste en Guipuzcoa (1597–1599)," *Boletin de la Real Sociedad Bascongada de Amigos del Pais* 40:1–2 (1984), 247–69, p. 250; the author provides no footnotes but says the correspondence was on September 11, 1597.

[47] Ignacio Baleztena, "Relación de la Peste desta Ciudad de Pamplona del año 1599," *Príncipe de Viana* 22 (1946), 187, 190, 198. Senosiain was secretary to the city council; his account is in the Archivo Municipal de Pamplona.

[48] Cruz Mundet, *El mal que al presente corre*, 31–2, citing Archivo General de Guipuzkoa 1–19-6; Villaviciosa's letter is published in Murugarren Zamora, "La peste en Guipuzcoa," 265–9. The latter refers to fishermen, not women, a typographical or

Basque man of the cloth went a step further: In Fernández de Arteaga's letter to the king of January 7, 1598, he quoted master Aluisu, a San Sebastián priest and aide to the bishop, as saying the loss of the 400 women "was a gift from God to the city, because they were more infectious than the peste itself."[49]

By February 1598 Pasajes (which lost over 350 inhabitants to the plague, around a third of the population) was healthy enough to petition the Council of War for help.[50] The town asked for 1,000 ducats for cleaning, and the council told the king it thought he should do them that favor, possibly taking the money from English merchants. This probably was the same 1,000 ducats the corregidor had suggested to the king that he, the king, give to the town; the king had told Fernández Arteaga to ask Velázquez to pay him out of whatever he collected in fines for contraband, which Velázquez refused to do without a written order from the king. It is safe to think that Pasajes never saw the money.[51] The galleons were built and launched.[52]

Royal authority in Castile could be disorderly, and though laws and customs were on the lips of all political actors who argued that things should be one way and not another, the hierarchy showed itself to be opportunistically flexible. The monarchy could and did establish its

paleographic error; it is clear from the context that it was, indeed, women who bought the sheets.

[49] AGS-GyM leg. 511, doc. 76.

[50] AGS-GyM leg. 526, docs. 11 and 29. The death toll is from José María Imízcoz, "Hacia nuevos horizontes: 1516–1700," in *Historia de Donostia-San Sebastián*, Miguel Artola, ed. (San Sebastián: Nerea, 2004), 37–63, p. 60, no source given. Villaviciosa said in November that 307 people had died since August: 44 men, 147 women, 20 children from the ages of 10–13, and 96 children under the age of 7; cited in Murugarren Zamora, "La peste en Guipuzcoa," 266. Children aged 7–10 either were not tabulated or all survived, which is unlikely. Villaviciosa also notes the large number of orphans left behind. Finally, he says that at Easter of that year he counted 917 inhabitants, not counting outsiders and the men at sea. For a summary of the state of affairs in Guipúzcoa in March 1598 see the letter from a Pamplona envoy in José Joaquín Arazuri, "La peste en Pamplona en tiempos de Felipe II," *Príncipe de Viana* 35:134–5 (1974), 179–92, pp. 185–7.

[51] AGS-GyM leg. 512, doc. 173; AGS-GyM leg. 530, docs. 27–9.

[52] A list of ships built in Guipúzcoa and Vizcaya during these years indicates that in fact some forty ships were built during the plague years; Lourdes Odriozola Oyarbide, *Construcción naval en el Paris Vasco, siglos XVI–XIX: Evolución y análisis comparativo* (San Sebastián: Diputacion Foral de Gipuzkoa, 1997), 329. Urquiola, the superintendent of much of this shipbuilding, had troubles with towns all along the coast, and after his death in 1600 Guipúzcoan towns decided to no longer recognize the office of the superintendant at all; see John T. Wing, *Roots of Empire: Forests and State Power in Early Modern Spain, c. 1500–1750* (Leiden: Brill, 2015), 133–4; also on Urquiola see Ricardo Gómez-Rivero, "La superintendencia de construcción naval y fomento forestal en Guipúzcoa (1598–1611)," *Anuario de Historia del Derecho Español* 56 (1986), 591–636, p. 597.

physical presence throughout the kingdoms in a multitude of ways and at a multitude of levels. After the Council of Castile wrote its long memo to Philip III in April 1599 concerning the state of the plague, a health commission (*junta de salud*) was set up in Madrid which, unlike other cities' ad hoc juntas, answered not to the city council or to the corregidor but to the Council of Castile itself, and indeed it had members from the Council of Castile.[53] Because Madrid was home to the palace, its municipal affairs were always conditioned by its status as *villa* on the one hand and *casa y corte* on the other, and for that reason a version of this junta survived the capital's (temporary) move to Valladolid. The presence of the royal court in a particular city had financial advantages and disadvantages, but at times it meant the city council ceded control; for example, Madrid had its own law enforcement but also royal law enforcement, the Alcaldes de Casa y Corte, who furthermore had judicial powers. In the case of the plague, the Council of Castile at various points made decisions about payments to Madrid's guards and medical staff that appear in the city council minutes as dictates from above. On June 7, 1599, the city council protested the Council of Castile's decision to cut back the number of surgeons treating patients with *secas*. On July 21 the city again had to ask the Council of Castile to order all doctors and surgeons to treat *secas* patients, which clearly they were not doing. And on August 4, the city decided to lodge a protest with the Junta de Salud over the insulting manner in which city councilmen had been disciplined for alleged failure to do their duty.[54]

This ability of the crown to insert itself through any one of a multitude of advisory councils and bodies into matters of varied significance on various levels will be seen at several points during this chronicle of plague. One of the most beautiful and complete reports on the public health front was written by an unnamed envoy sent by the Council of Castile to Alcalá de Henares, the university town just to the east of Madrid.[55] A year earlier, in August 1598, Alcalá had requested permission from Philip II to raise a special sales tax (*sisa*) on certain foodstuffs

[53] In fact, this junta may have existed earlier. RAH Salazar leg. 23 carpeta 4 no. 11 is a very clear set of anti-plague instructions to cities, including Madrid, already in 1597, another indication that the capital was affected early on; "Memorial de advertencias que dio en la Junta de Salud…"

[54] AV Libros de Actas; also Alvar Ezquerra, "Estructuras socioeconómicas," 554–6. The city protested the Council of Castile's and the junta's decision to remove doctors, but by August 30 the city must have had a change of heart for it was advocating laying them off; now it was the junta that refused to let them go, and they were still working in November 1599.

[55] RAH Jesuitas 9–3662/182. This may be another example of scrambled jurisdictions; Alcalá de Henares had its own corregidor and city council, yet the Council of Castile was

to pay for increased guards during the town's fair of San Bartolomé.[56] The town may have escaped the plague then, but by August 1599 that was not the case. The subsequent report on plague abatement was printed, possibly because the modelic form both of the document itself and of the public health effort overseen by the author moved the Council to distribute it. The writer states that he entered the city on July 23, 1599. His account ends on October 8, by which time the plague had disappeared. In between, the man seemingly never slept. He started by counting the number of sick people (160, all of them in a hospital), the number of affected houses (all but twelve), and the number of people who had not been in contact with a sick person (zero). He praised the doctors and leading citizens who had stayed in town, including the Franciscan friars, the religious order that suffered the most deaths (twenty; in 1591 there had been a total of 126 Franciscans in the town).[57]

apparently managing its plague campaign (and also assumed responsibilities in a smaller Madrid town, San Martín de la Vega; see ARCM sig. 913598, carpeta 1776, June 1597). One odd thing about this report is that the town's famous university is never mentioned. It was its own jurisdiction, but one would think that the Council of Castile's emissary would be worried about infection there. By the end of the sixteenth century the university had a population of some 1,000 people; see Molinié-Bertrand, *Au siècle d'or l'Espagne*, 238. Previously, the university (along with those of Salamanca and Valladolid) had been under the judicial jurisdiction of the ecclesiastical courts, a situation Philip II remedied in 1593 by putting students, who apparently were out of control and going unpunished, under the jurisdiction of ordinary civil courts; on this see Ramón González Navarro, *Felipe II y las reformas constitucionales de la Universidad de Alcalá de Henares* (Madrid: Sociedad Estatal para la Conmemoración de los Centenarios de Felipe II y Carlos V, 1999), 77–8. On universities' judicial jurisdiction in general see José Luis de las Heras Santos, *La justicia penal de los Austrias en la Corona de Castilla* (Universidad de Salamanca, 1991), 131–5. See AHN Universidades, lib. 1101, no. 13 for a typically perverse jurisdictional fight about which entity, the university or the corregidor of Alcalá de Henares, was entitled to appoint plague guards in 1637.

[56] AMAH leg. 569/001. *Sisas* were the most common way for towns to pay for any extra expense, be it plague costs, special taxes owed to the crown, or raising soldiers. In the words of Felipe Ruiz Martín, they were "a magical resource drained to excess by the municipal authorities in the seventeenth century"; Felipe Ruiz Martin, "Credit procedures for the collection of taxes in the cities of Castile during the sixteenth and seventeenth centuries: the case of Valladolid," in *The Castilian Crisis of the Seventeenth Century: New Perspectives on the Economic and Social History of Seventeenth-Century Spain*, I. A. A. Thompson and Bartolomé Yun Casalilla, eds. (Past and Present Publications, Cambridge University Press, 1994), 169–81, p. 178.

[57] According to the 1591 census, Alcalá had 2,345 *vecinos*, plus 660 members of religious communities; González Navarro, *Felipe II y las reformas constitucionales*, 24. The town grew quickly in the sixteenth century. Throughout this book I give population figures for towns drawn from various censuses. The three primary sources are Eduardo García España, "Censos de población españoles," *Estadística española* 33:128 (1991), 441–500; Eduardo García España and Annie Molinié-Bertrand, *Censo de Castilla de 1591: Estudio analítico* (Madrid: Instituto Nacional de Estadística, 1986); and Molinié-Bertrand, *Au siècle d'or*. A shorter, more synthetic analysis is David S. Reher, "Castilla y la crisis del siglo XVII: Contextos demográficos para un ajuste de larga duración," in *Madrid, Felipe*

"As soon as I arrived, wishing to reduce confusion and separate the healthy from the sick, I managed to move all those suffering from *secas y carbuncos* outside the town," he wrote. "To that end, I extended the hospital by three passageways, with one large one so that even though there were 450 patients, along with many nurses and servants, the men could be separate from the women and the dangerously ill from those who were not so sick and convalescing, and by cleaning and burning [aromatic herbs] it was acceptable enough that doctors, surgeons, barbers, and nurses were not in danger." The hospital staff was fed "good meat, very good wine, and good bread." Ecclesiastical judges determined that fish was not required on eves of holy days. The dead were buried in a deep pit in a large corral lined with lime. The town was divided into eight districts, each led by a prominent citizen, each with a doctor and clergy and constables to take patients to the hospital if necessary. Linens were burned in a large oven a quarter-league away from the town. Already soon after his arrival, the author wrote, he could sense the improvement. Whereas when he arrived twenty-five or thirty people were dying every day, it had now gone down to four or five, "and today, September 20, there is no one in all of Alcalá who is dangerously ill with *secas*." By then the paid medical staff had mostly been laid off, and inhabitants who had fled were returning, though if they had been in diseased areas they were not allowed in. "We took great care with cleaning the streets and the town, and town criers announced that everyone who had a cart should help carry away the garbage, which they did with great love, and now the town is very clean." The poor were given food, medicine, clothing to replace what had been burned, and alms ("My lord the cardenal of Toledo gave 1,500 ducats," someone wrote by hand on the document's margin). "An honorable man [*un hombre honrado*] named Morales" helped the clergy in their good work, the author wrote, startling testimony of the goodness of someone whose name he did not know and who probably was no one in particular. He described the giving of last rites, the organization of guards, the expulsion of outsiders, the grand massacre of cats and dogs, and instructions to laundresses who worked down by the river. He ended with quick references to the plagues of Venice, Messina, Milan, and Trent, and by mentioning Alcalá de Henares's vows to Santa Ana and San Roque.

II y las ciudades de la Monarquía, Enrique Martínez Ruiz, ed., vol. 2 (Madrid: Actas, 2000), 347–74, which also has a useful bibliography. There were a multitude of censuses taken during the sixteenth century, generally for military or fiscal purposes, in different jurisdictions, by different levels of authority, and with different measurements. The aim of the survey might determine people's willingness to be counted.

In short, "Everything that Dr. Mercado ordered with such erudition and prudence was put into effect to the degree possible, and it was very helpful in this town that the executors were so distinguished [*tan principales*], as was said, because laws, orders, indications, orders cried aloud [*pregones*], and proclamations can do little if men do not attend to the public good."

This was government as it should be. The Council of Castile had entrusted someone obviously well equipped to visit Alcalá de Henares who had done the job thanks to the commitment of the religious communities and the town's civil population. They used common sense, exhibited charity, and made sacrifices. Similar examples abound of officials stepping into the breach. Both in theory and in practice, good government was inextricably institutionally and ideologically linked to justice, and there were a vast number of judicial jurisdictions in early modern Castile that all frequently fought one another over precedence.[58] The king always had the last word, a capacity granted to him by God, though perceived arbitrary rule based on something other than the ultimate good of the kingdom could be and was contested, successfully or not, by vassals up and down the social ladder. Corregidores themselves were first-instance judges (their lieutenants also could hear cases), towns without corregidores had a battery of other judges, there were two royal appeals tribunals (the Chancillerías, in Valladolid and Granada), and most of the royal councils and privileged corporations (universities, consulates, the sheep ranchers of the Mesta, etc.) had their own courts of justice. The Council of Castile, the apex of the conciliar system, was the court of highest appeal though, again, the king could follow its ruling with his own. Castilians were not shy about asserting their rights, and they had an endless number of forums in which to do so.

But once the plague arrived, they were threatened with having fewer. In April 1597 the Valladolid Chancillería allowed Castro Urdiales to cancel its local court sessions so as to minimize comings and goings for fear of contagion, and by August, after hearing from a Burgos official about how sick the region was, the cancelations had spread throughout northern Castile and the Basque Country.[59] This did not sit well with the court's criminal judges (*alcaldes de crimen*). They were in the minority

---

[58] In general on the Castilian judicial system, Richard Kagan, *Lawsuits and Litigants in Castile, 1500–1700* (Chapel Hill, NC: University of North Carolina Press, 1981).

[59] ARCV cédulas y pragmáticas 7–42 for this entire discussion about suspending court sessions. Castro Urdiales had a population of 1,500 families in 1595, which plummeted to 700 two years later and to just 300 families in 1609; see Pedro Andrés Porras Arboledas, "La práctica mercantil marítima en el Cantábrico Oriental (siglos XV–XIX). Primera parte," *Cuadernos de Historia del Derecho* 7 (2000), 13–127, p. 67,

compared to the civil judges (*oidores*), who tended to be hidalgos, men with noble status exempt from certain taxes. So when the majority voted to suspend sessions across the north, the criminal judges argued at considerable length that their jurisdiction had been violated and that the way in which the order had been issued undermined proper protocol. (The leader of the *alcaldes*, the irascible and quite brilliant Rodrigo de Santillán, himself broke all protocol on August 18 by marching into the chief judge's chambers with a notary by his side to protest the measure, though not much seems to have transpired.[60]) But aside from the terrible offense they had suffered, the *alcaldes* also pointed to some practical consequences of the *oidores*' decision such as the appearance of new lawsuits should incompetent judges intervene and difficulties in transporting and housing prisoners pending litigation.

The Council of Castile asked the Chancillería to write a report for Philip II about the matter. So the judges recounted what the emissary from Burgos had told them (in person or in writing, it is not clear) about how the once powerful commercial city was now hemmed in by pestilent towns. In one of them, Melgar de Fernamental, a visitor from Calahorra de Boedo had sought the advice of a local *letrado* (lawyer), and a day and a half later the man's wife, his sons, his daughters, and his servants were all dead. Nine people.[61] There had been talk with the Valladolid city council about setting up guards, but the *oidores* said there was no point in putting up guards unless litigation in pestilent towns and the villages near them was halted. According to what Valladolid Corregidor Garci López de Chaves had told the *oidores*, his sources were all confirming the rumors about peste in the outlying areas, but he "did not dare" order guard duty to commence unless the Chancillería would stand with him, surely because he did not want to discourage commerce. The *oidores* also told the Council about the standoff with the *alcaldes*, which included sending notaries back and forth between them, and they noted in passing that *alcaldes* were far better suited for guard duty than the *oidores* themselves. In short, they reassured the king that their only wish was to serve God and His Majesty and protect the public good and the health of Valladolid, to which end litigation in diseased areas must stop. In what was possibly a

citing unspecified documents in AHPC Protocolos. The use of families as a population measure is unusual.

[60] Santillán and the chief judge, Pedro Junco de Posada, had a history of mutual antipathy; see Ruth MacKay, *The Baker Who Pretended to Be King of Portugal* (Chicago, IL: University of Chicago Press, 2012).

[61] Report dated August 27, 1597, in ARCV cédulas y pragmáticas 7–42; this story also appears in AMB-HI 3653, July 25, 1597. It prompted a letter from Philip II to the corregidor of Burgos which was printed; BL Eg. 356, vol. 2, fol. 296.

cover letter or an addendum to the missive, the *oidores* and the chief judge expressed dismay that not only was the disease not under control but it had "multiplied," principally because poor people were not burning their clothes and linens or they coveted goods they anyway had no use for. More information was needed, to which end Valladolid was sending messengers out to the surrounding areas, and once their reports were collected another messenger would be sent to the king.

The Council of Castile was not happy with the *oidores*' report. Their order to suspend legal actions "appears to be a grave error and excess, and [the *alcaldes*'] condemnation of it seems just," it wrote, adding that they should have first consulted with the king and the Council itself. That said, Santillán had misbehaved, no doubt, and he must be told that next time the punishment, in Madrid, would be far different. Litigation thus did not cease in pestilent areas. Corregidores and local judges had their hands full over the next two years managing their cities' public health efforts, so possibly there was less litigation, which would also make sense as the population diminished. But plague-related cases from these dates do appear in the records when they were appealed. The docket probably thinned, and there appear to have been surprisingly few criminal cases arising out of quarantine, but there were some.

Two years after the preceding conflict, during Valladolid's terrible summer of 1599, the Chancillería sought permission to leave.[62] In the judges' opinion, city council members had been quite remiss, and, indeed, Valladolid had operated slowly and badly. Given the city's inadequate leadership (López de Chaves left the city in early June 1599 and was replaced by Antonio de Ulloa), Chief Judge Pedro Junco de Posada had decided, or had been asked by the king, to take matters into his own hands, probably in spring. This was a move similar to the executive role taken by the Council of Castile in Madrid and in Alcalá de Henares. There are many examples in the early modern era of the royal appeals courts edging into governmental terrain – often, precisely, into the Council of Castile's terrain, explaining their traditionally testy relationship. In Thompson's words, "The function of the lawyer in the restoration of royal authority at the end of the Middle Ages and in the maintenance of order and obedience was by no means lost on contemporaries."[63] Judges frequently acted as royal inspectors or enforcers on matters ranging from public order to secret inquests to military

---

[62] AGS-E leg. 184, docs. 287, 290, 291 for discussion of the court's departure.
[63] I. A. A. Thompson, "Absolutism, legalism and the law in Castile, 1500–1700," in *Der Absolutismus – ein Mythos? Strukturwandel monarchischer herrschaft*, Ronald G. Asch and Heinz Duchhardt, eds. (Cologne: Böhlau Verlag, 1996), 185–228, p. 203.

recruitment. These were entirely ad hoc appointments at the pleasure of the monarch and were nowhere codified or specified. In addition to these temporary individual appointments, the institution itself frequently could be found standing in for the monarchy, especially during civic disturbances, effectively supplanting municipal authorities. Assumption of such powers echoed neither the spirit nor the letter of the appeals courts' statutes, but rather than indicating any over-reaching by the courts, this merely indicates that the courts embodied royal authority in the same doubling way that Madrid (and then Valladolid) could be both *casa* and *corte*. It shows that statutes and jurisdiction were highly malleable. In the words of a historian of the Chancillerías, referring to a slightly earlier period, "It is very possible that the origin of the problem is precisely that it was no easy matter to define or delimit permissible actions in precise jurisdictional terms, especially if actions that were openly prohibited were easily authorized as soon as circumstances so required..."[64]

After having supervised the anti-plague efforts in Valladolid for probably several months, Junco de Posada decided they had done what they could but now it was time to go. In any case the court was doing hardly anything. There were neither lawyers nor litigants, and the courtrooms were closed, he said. Jurists themselves had been affected; staff members, including one *oidor*, had died, and Junco de Posada and his colleagues had lost relatives and servants. No other city would allow Valladolid court employees past their gates, statutes of limitation had become meaningless, and court appearances were not being enforced, as a result of which decisions might later be overturned for default. "Should the illness continue, Your Majesty could order the court to move to a healthy place, because Castile can no longer be without the force and authority of this tribunal," the court told the king, adding that such a measure would not contradict what they had done in similar occasions in the past. The request was passed on to the Council of Castile's president, the Count of Miranda, who must eventually have agreed, because the court's legal decisions soon state that it is in Medina del Campo.

---

[64] Carlos Garriga, *La audiencia y las chancillerías castellanas (1371–1525). Historia política, régimen jurídico y práctica institucional* (Madrid: Centro de Estudios Constitucionales, 1994), 241–4, p. 242. The Chancillería intervened during the 1640s uprisings in Granada (I. A. A. Thompson, "Las Alteraciones Granadinas de 1648–1652 a la luz de un nuevo testimonio presencial," in *Homenaje a Don Antonio Domínguez Ortiz*, Juan Luis Castellano, et al., eds. [Granada: Universidad de Granada, 2008], 3 vols., vol. 2, 779–812); to quell resistance to military recruitment (Ruth MacKay, *The Limits of Royal Authority: Resistance and Obedience in Seventeenth-Century Castile* [Cambridge University Press, 1999]); and in the case of other disorders. On the Chancillería in general see Heras Santos, *La justicia penal*, 65–79.

The loss of the court was always deeply felt. According to Bennassar, its crucial place in the city's economy was acknowledged indirectly in rental agreements, which stated that rent must be paid even if the court should leave town.[65] He also cites a document created when the court left the city in 1519 on account of the plague stating that between 2,000 and 3,000 people in Valladolid might have depended on the court for their living, so one can assume that the number had risen considerably in eighty years.[66] Already in 1561, a census reported that Valladolid had 404 inhabitants directly employed by the courts: notaries, lawyers of various sorts, magistrates, bailiffs, and so on.[67] The Chancillería had a constant stream of visitors, and the surrounding streets were full of inns that lodged litigants and their lawyers. Clerks, carpenters, shopkeepers, notaries, and moneylenders, not to mention lawyers, all lived off the business of litigation. In the words of the Valladolid city council on July 28, 1599, moving the court "would be the destruction of everything." On previous occasions, the crown had sometimes agreed with this assessment. Indeed, there were times when the court announced it was leaving because of plague, or simply halting operations, and the king told the judges to stay right where they were. It happened in 1530 and again in 1565–1566, when a terrible peste laid large parts of Castile to waste. In the latter case, Philip II told the court to stop blocking traffic into Valladolid, which was only serving to clog the court calendar and slow down litigation. Only when the guards were absolutely sure that people were actually dying in visitors' hometowns should their entry be denied, the Council of Castile said.[68] Nonetheless, on August 18, 1599, the city council minutes record the news that the Chancillería this time would leave for sixty days, "and if that happens this city is lost because it will depopulate and all business and commerce will end, which will greatly affect royal income and taxes," the city council told the king, none too subtly. The usual stream of petitions went out to the Council and the king, to no avail.[69]

One of the chief judge's alcaldes de crimen, Melchor de Teves, stayed behind with the title of Pest Commissioner. The previous year he had served in Galicia as one of Philip II's army of judicial officials collecting

---

[65] Bartolomé Bennassar Valladolid au siècle d'or: Une ville de Castille et sa campagne au XVI siècle (Paris: Mouton, 1967), 123, citing AHPV, leg. 37, fol. 216.
[66] Bennassar, Valladolid, 124.   [67] Bennassar, Valladolid, 118.
[68] ARCV Cédulas y pragmáticas, cajas 1,10; 4,35; and 15,34 for measures taken in 1565.
[69] AMVA sig. 22-0. A similar situation occurred in Pamplona, where the Royal Council of Navarre, the highest judicial court there, decided to leave because of the plague, disregarding the city's protests. It was gone for forty days; Santiago Lasaosa Villanua, El "Regimiento" municipal de Pamplona en el siglo XVI (Pamplona: CSIC, 1979), 257–8.

information, keeping the king up to date on the plague's slow departure from that important military zone. In his opinion, it was a disease of the poor, outsiders (*forasteros*), and single women (*mujercillas solteras*), showing he shared the outlook of some of his Basque colleagues.[70] After being Pest Commissioner he went on to greater things, perhaps as a reward. He was eventually a member of the councils of Portugal and Castile, and he married well. But first came Valladolid, "the most pestilent place in all of Spain," he wrote to his friend Diego Sarmiento de Acuña, the future Count of Gondomar.[71] The chief judge and the court "took over the government of this city, helping the corregidor, who works extraordinarily hard but it is impossible for him to do everything, and the city councilmen pay more attention to their expenses than to their duties, aside from which some of them are very, very afraid. After much giving and taking between the city and the court about who should take charge," the city had been divided into two parts, eight parishes apiece, and Teves got one of them. "I'm up to my elbows in it," he wrote, adding that he was unafraid and was taking precautions. There were still over 1,000 patients in the hospital; "there are so many they are practically crawling into my bed, and there is no solution in sight." A month later he finally could breathe and had left his post, giving up "four servants, three notaries, and lots of work." Since Sunday only five people had died of fever (*calenturas*) in his eight parishes, he wrote to his friend. It may be worth pointing out that another of Gondomar's correspondents differed with Teves, and they must have known each other: whatever you've heard about the health situation in Valladolid "is much ado about nothing," this man reassured Gondomar, adding the interesting information that the corregidor had gone to Palencia that very week to investigate the granting of an *hábito*, a membership in one of the military orders, which can hardly have been a priority at that moment, and the city of Palencia would not let him in, showing Palencia knew Valladolid was sick even if its own nobility did not.[72]

If the critical arenas of defense and justice, centered in the palace but utterly dependent on local cooperation, were forced to accommodate to the exigencies of the plague, the same was true of royal finance. There was nothing more critical to the crown than money. All these arenas, as well as others we shall see, were sites of encounter and negotiation that

[70] This episode of plague may have moved west from Santander or may have been independent; AGS-GyM leg. 515, doc. 177, June 13, 1598.
[71] RBP, II-2163, doc. 224, Teves to Gondomar, July 24, 1599.
[72] RBP, II-2138, doc. 196, Teves to Gondomar, September 29, 1599; RBP II-2138, doc. 50, Francisco de Villapadierna to Gondomar, sometime in August 1599, "*mayor el ruido que las nueces.*"

remained open for business even as the economy reeled. They all relied upon ceremonies of testimony. The language of justice and the language of information-gathering was one of witnessing. Criminal, civil, and Inquisitorial case files all include a section where the parties call witnesses who essentially recite the same story again and again. Plague survivors and their descendants were also witnesses, and as soon as towns were healthy, they began describing their ordeal to the crown in the hope that their taxes would be cut. Tax petitions in some ways resembled legal proceedings, which is only appropriate being that justice was at stake. They also exemplify the complications of jurisdiction. If towns were to receive compensation, as it were, for their suffering, they would have to be adept at picking their way through the thicket. The northern towns naturally came first, and the rest of Castile followed suit in 1600, most asking for a reduction in the general sales tax, or *alcabala*, arguing that as commerce and population had declined or collapsed, so too should taxes. They petitioned the king, royal treasury authorities, and the Cortes, whose interests did not always coincide and whose jurisdictions overlapped. Hearings were held, exhibits such as past tax rolls and plummeting baptismal registers were presented, and oral testimony was collected from residents and *vecinos* in neighboring towns who one after another certified that the town that had once been bustling was now moribund and therefore should pay less.

The *alcabala*, the most important of royal revenues, was effectively a regressive 10 percent tax on all sales and purchases, though far less than 10 percent was actually ever collected and certain products were exempt. The clergy was exempt from paying, but the nobility was not. At times it was paid directly to the crown through the work of a leasee (*arrendador*) who bid for the job or simply bought the rights. It was also sometimes paid to the ruling nobleman of a *señorío*, a practice in theory prohibited by the crown.[73] During the reign of Charles V the *alcabalas* began being sold; when the crown sold towns and other jurisdictions, usually to nobles but also to councilmen, towns, and religious and corporative entities (from whom they may previously have been bought), often in exchange for other valuable properties, *alcabalas* and other rents were included. Such sales increased during the reign of Philip II.[74]

But mostly the *alcabala* was subject to the *encabezamiento*, a fixed sum or ceiling, the result of the crown – institutionally incapable of managing

[73] Juan E. Gelabert, *La bolsa del rey: Rey, reino y fisco en Castilla (1598–1648)* (Barcelona: Crítica, 1997), 177–97. A *señorío* was a lordship, a seigneurial jurisdiction.
[74] Salvador Moxó y Ortiz de Villajos, "La venta de alcabalas en los reinados de Carlos I y Felipe II," *Anuario de historia del derecho español* 41 (1971), 487–554.

the tax – having temporarily, starting in 1536, granted the Cortes the right to collect the tax, the total sum of which was negotiated in a contract with the crown, and the Cortes having negotiated with local powers the amount to be collected according to a distribution, or *repartimiento*, among the forty districts of the eighteen provinces of the kingdom of Castile, along with all their subsidiary districts and municipalities, with smaller villages and towns sometimes being burdened with a disproportionate share.[75] This effective outsourcing meant that municipalities to a large degree controlled who was taxed and how, and that was true not just with the *alcabala* but with other taxes as well. They might choose to lease out portions to individuals or corporate entities, tax outside vendors and suppliers, tax *vecinos*, or establish exceptions. In the words of José Ignacio Fortea Pérez, the *encabezamiento* system "sanctioned a *decentralized* fiscal regime that allowed for broad tax *autonomy* at the local level, which reinforced the notable structural *heterogeneity* of the Castilian fiscal realm."[76] The period we are examining, including the plague years, was subject to the fourth general *encabezamiento*, implemented in 1578, which represented a substantial increase over the previous one. Philip II's heightened war obligations, which would only increase in the following two decades, and the collapse of the treasury forced him to accept continued nominal control by the Cortes in exchange for greater tax revenue and assured collection of a fixed amount.[77] The fixed amount also meant the treasury could not automatically take advantage of rising prices in the second half of the sixteenth century, which was why it was renegotiated upwards several times, often to the detriment of peasantry who lived in commercial territories but who themselves did not traffic.[78]

---

[75] Though not always; José Ignacio Fortea Pérez notes that the city of Burgos shifted onto itself (or claimed to have done so) its subject towns' tax burden; *Monarquía y Cortes en la Corona de Castilla: las ciudades ante la política fiscal de Felipe II* (Valladolid: Cortes de Castilla y León, 1990), 269, citing AGS-PR leg. 81.

[76] Fortea Pérez, *Monarquía y Cortes*, 467, emphasis in the original. See also Fortea Pérez, "Impuestos o Servicios? Las Cortes de Castilla y la política fiscal de Felipe II (1573–1598)," in his *Las Cortes de Castilla y León bajo los Austrias: una interpretación* (Valladolid: Junta de Castilla y León, 2008), 161–90.

[77] Miguel Artola, *La hacienda del Antiguo Régimen* (Madrid: Alianza Editorial, 1982), 37–52.

[78] Francisco Tomás y Valiente, "La Diputación de las Cortes de Castilla (1525–1601)," in his *Gobierno e instituciones en la España del Antiguo Régimen* (Madrid: Alianza Editorial, 1982), 91–2, p. 97; José Ignacio Fortea Pérez, "Entre dos servicios: La crisis de la Hacienda Real a fines del siglo XVI. Las alternativas fiscales de una opción política (1590–1601)," *Studia Historica. Historia Moderna* 17 (1997), 63–90, p. 76; this article provides a detailed analysis of the crown's financial straits at the turn of the century and includes several very interesting *memoriales* that circulated at that time.

Ultimately, no royal tax, regardless of how it was structured, was believed by the Cortes to be beyond its power to examine and control. Taxes embodied the relationship between king and kingdom.[79] The Cortes was called the kingdom (*reino*), or the *reino junto en Cortes*, and the critically important *rey-reino* relationship in the late sixteenth century was centered on continual negotiations over one tax or another that revealed the balance of power between the various political instances of Castile. The reign of Philip II from beginning to end was characterized by confrontations with the cities which together formed the Cortes, and the king did not always triumph. Indeed, he often had to give in. The Cortes in session during the plague, which had begun meeting in 1592, was the longest ever, ending in 1598. The representatives (*procuradores*) were not of one mind as to whether to continue supporting Philip II's ruinous foreign policy; some were even willing to think about letting go of the Netherlands. There were frequent references in the minutes to the fact that they were not getting paid. Their patience was nearly at an end.[80]

An example of an unsuccessful revenue request by the king that took place just before and then during the epidemic was the campaign for 500 cuentos.[81] The idea was to raise funds to facilitate negotiations with the state's creditors, who already were owed everything in the treasury. On November 29, 1596, Philip II declared his third bankruptcy, details of which were signed with creditors in February 1598. In early 1597 the king alerted his most reliable corregidores that they should be prepared to push their respective city councils to, in turn, authorize the cities' Cortes representatives to vote in favor. Nothing much seems to have transpired because a renewed effort by the crown, this time in the person of Prince Philip, took place on April 8, 1598. "I have written you several times that my finances are finished and consumed as a result of my having fulfilled my obligations to defend our holy Catholic faith, security, and peace in these kingdoms," he wrote. "Your delay has been such that the damage is nearly irreparable, which astonishes me, as it is so unlike the manner in which you have been accustomed to serve me in

[79] The bibliography on Spanish Hapsburg fiscal politics and the relationship between the crown and the Cortes is enormous; see all articles by José Ignacio Fortea Pérez in the bibliography; Pablo Fernández Albaladejo, *Fragmentos de Monarquía* (Madrid: Alianza Universidad, 1992); and I. A. A. Thompson, *Crown and Cortes: Government, Institutions and Representation in Early Modern Castile* (London: Variorum, 1993).
[80] The essential article on this point is Thompson, Oposición política, *Studia Historica. Historia Moderna*, 37–62.
[81] Five hundred cuentos was equivalent to around 1.3 million ducats; this campaign was supposed to be the continuation of the first *millones* tax, which expired in 1596.

the past.[82] The letter was written to the city council of Burgos, not to the corregidor this time, as well as to those of León, Granada, Jaén, Salamanca, Segovia, Valladolid, Soria, and Guadalajara. The city of Burgos that same week was dealing not only with a long list of pestiferous towns surrounding the city, where hundreds had already died, but also with grain shortages and requests from the crown to raise soldiers.[83] In response to the crown's insistence, cities began placing conditions on their vote. Segovia sent in thirty-one conditions, prompting the Junta de las Cortes, a consultative body, to advise Philip II to tell Corregidor Íñigo de Cárdenas y Zapata to just tighten the screws on his city council. Toledo and Cuenca were no better, but even if these three could be persuaded to relent just a bit, the remaining holdouts were impossible, the junta said.[84] By mid-1598, by which time the plague had reached most of the northern peninsula, including Madrid, only seven of the cities represented in the Cortes had agreed to support the 500 cuentos plan. Finally, the king and his son sought advice from their closest ecclesiastical advisers, García Loaysa y Girón, Fray Diego de Yepes, and Fray Gaspar de Córdoba. A few of the cities had assented voluntarily, they said, but the rest had assented only after being forced (*violentadas*) by the "powerful hand of the corregidores." Cities had been threatened and extorted and their arms had been twisted, they wrote, "and it is not that they are less loyal than others, or less willing to serve Your Majesty, but it is impossible for them to do so, which is obvious to everyone." As a result, the three clergymen reported, at the most recent junta meeting the members had voted ten to two in favor of dropping the effort to raise the 500 cuentos, a decision they said they agreed with.[85] In Fortea's words, "the consequences for the royal treasury could not have been more devastating."[86]

It was exactly then that towns en masse began requesting a reduction in their taxes because of the plague. The *encabezamiento* contract between the Cortes and the crown provided for the possibility that towns affected

---

[82] ACC vol. 16, 26–61 passim, also summaries in vol. 17, 309–10; the prince's letter, vol. 16, 59–61.

[83] In the city council minutes, also in AGS-GyM leg. 516, doc. 34, in which Corregidor Diego Vargas Manrique explains to the king that he will not allow a levy campaign ordered by Don Diego Brochero, who was in charge of the navy in La Coruña. Brochero himself, in letters in AGS-GyM leg. 515, told the king and the Council of Castile the following month of the devastating impact of the plague among his men in Galicia.

[84] ACC vol. 16, 534–56, passim. The Junta's consulta was dated May 14, 1598.

[85] ACC vol. 16, 568–70, letter from San Lorenzo, July 30, 1598.

[86] Fortea Pérez, "Entre dos servicios," 66. Loaysa was on the Council of State and adviser to the prince, Yepes was Philip II's confessor, and Córdoba was the prince's confessor.

by fire, disease, bad harvests, or general depopulation might not be able to pay their assigned amount.[87] Decisions on these cases would be made by the Contaduría Mayor de Hacienda, the central financial accounts office, taking into account the opinions of the Cortes ("*oyendo a los dichos Diputados del Reyno*"). If the request were granted, the resulting shortfall would be made up by funds called *sobras*, excess amounts from *alcabala* collections that sat in town coffers and which in theory, since 1560, could be spent by towns without having to request permission from the Cortes or the Diputación, its standing committee while not in session, or from the Contaduría Mayor de Hacienda; in fact, the royal treasury took an increasingly invasive attitude toward them. But if there were no *sobras* corresponding to the place requesting a reduction, the shortfall would be proportionately distributed among all districts to be paid by the towns and cities or by those appointed by the towns for that purpose.[88] A series of investigations during the reign of Philip II showed that far less than the 10 percent ever entered the Treasury.[89] Yet even so, perhaps testifying to the system's irregularities, by the turn of the century many towns had *sobras*. In 1590–1595, for example, 4.9 percent of the total collected in Castile (for *alcabalas* plus *tercias*, another tax) was considered *sobras*; in Burgos it was 6.9 percent, in Valladolid 7.4 percent, in Segovia 2.9 percent, and in Madrid, an extreme case, it was 25.7 percent.[90]

When towns requested discounts (*bajas*), which occurred more and more as the *encabezamiento* rose (regardless of the plague; Cádiz requested a reduction in 1596 after the British sack, Vigo did the same after corsair attacks, and districts whose commerce had shrank found they were better off paying the 10 percent than the fixed sum and thus they withdrew from the *encabezamiento* contract), the *sobras* came into view.[91] Santander was, logically, the first city to request a discount because of the plague, followed by Castro Urdiales. Actually, even before

---

[87] This was condition 15 of the contract: ACC vol. 5 (supp.), 639; the original condition 15 from the 1536 contract seems to have become condition 16 in the 1560 contract; on this see Tomás y Valiente, "La Diputación," 121.

[88] Fortea Pérez, *Monarquía y Cortes*, 462–3, and correspondence with the author; Tomás y Valiente, "La Diputación,"102.

[89] Ruiz Martín, "Credit procedures." The investigations, called *expedientes de hacienda*, are in AGS.

[90] Pilar Zabala Aguirre, *Las alcabalas y la hacienda real en Castilla* (Santander: Universidad de Cantabria, 2000), 315–18. She cites Bennassar's book on Valladolid as saying *sobras* were mostly used to buy grain to store in the *alhóndiga*, or *pósito*, the town granary.

[91] On Cádiz see ACC vol. 15, pp. 512–15, July 5, 1597; and pp. 543–5, August 26, 1597; also Ruiz Martín, "Credit procedures," 175. The clearest explanation I have found of the *sobras* is Tomás y Valiente, "La Diputación," where, on p. 122, he mentions requests for *bajas* by La Coruña, Carmona, Seville, and Salamanca. By the mid-seventeenth century, most cities had withdrawn from the *encabezamiento*.

Santander got around to presenting a petition to the Cortes, Burgos's representatives spoke up on behalf of the port town and its neighbors, saying the Santanderinos were unable to conduct commerce and were dying of hunger. Burgos – the first inland city in the epidemic's line of fire and therefore very keen to halt it immediately – asked that the assembly "help them in their need with some *sobras* from the general *encabezamiento*" and also that a physicians' commission be convoked in Madrid.[92] Two days later a majority of the representatives voted to ask the king that 4,000 ducats of *sobras* be given to the Archbishop of Burgos, "prelate for all the lands where there is peste," so that he could organize medical relief and food shipments.[93] Over a month later, correspondence between the king and his advisers indicates payment had not taken place, despite everyone's agreement that it was a good idea, and that furthermore plague had spread to the Burgos town of Melgar de Fernamental.[94]

On November 5, 1597, the Cortes heard a petition directly from Santander saying that "because of the peste there, more than five thousand people have died or left and most of the city's finances were used to cure the sick and care for them and bury the dead, and houses were torn down, and therefore the said town is in great need and in debt and cannot pay its debts or the price of its *encabezamiento*," for which reason it asked that its payment be reduced for ten years, "being that it is such an important port."[95] The minutes reveal that Santander had first appealed to the king, who sent the matter to the Council of Finance, which told the city to go the Reino, which was sympathetic given that "His Majesty has not given this town anything with which to alleviate its need," and a few days later Santander was given a six-year break, which was probably what the city wanted, having requested ten. But the Cortes attached the condition that a portion of the relief would come from money the city owed the king from 1596 when it had bought back city posts.[96]

The process of requesting *bajas* was, to say the least, convoluted. The change in kings coincided with reorganization of various financial bodies and an excruciating need for revenue accompanied by the towns' patent inability to oblige. The parties in question were the Cortes, represented

[92] Burgos always spoke for Cantabria in the Cortes. Representatives from Toledo opposed using the *sobras* for this purpose; ACC vol. 15, p. 501, June 17, 1597. It is unclear if Burgos wanted the *junta de médicos* in Madrid because the capital was affected or simply because it was the capital.

[93] ACC vol. 15, p. 508, June 19, 1597.　　[94] ACC vol. 16, 510–11, July 9 and 31, 1597.

[95] ACC vol. 15, p. 553.

[96] ACC vol. 15, pp. 557–9, November 10 and 14, 1597. My thanks to Tony Thompson for clarifying this operation, called *resumen de los oficios*. The Cortes forwarded its petition in this regard to the king on December 1, specifying that it thought the money should be used to build a hospital; ACC vol. 15, p. 561.

once the long session was finally over in 1598 by the Diputación, whose role grew in importance precisely because of the *encabezamiento* of the *alcabalas*; the powerful Contaduría Mayor de Hacienda; the Contaduría Mayor de Cuentas; the king's Council of Finance (established by Charles V but which, because the Contadurías did most of the work, became a council like all the rest only in 1593); and the king himself, along with his advisers. All had overlapping functions, if in fact their functions were even defined, and Juan E. Gelebart notes that jurisdictional battles were inevitably accompanied by complaints that everyone had far too much work.[97] As we saw, condition 15 of the *encabezamiento* contract said the Contaduría Mayor de Hacienda, with input from the Cortes, should make decisions regarding *bajas*. It also functioned as a court of law for *alcabalas* matters, superseding the corregidores, and furthermore, according to condition 66 of the 1560 contract, was in charge of resolving all conflicts regarding the *encabezamiento*.[98]

As the plague made its way through the peninsula, subsequent requests for relief grew more contentious as a result of jurisdictional squabbling, with the Cortes accusing the various financial bodies of improper interference. Philip II himself already in late December 1595 had told the Contaduría Mayor de Hacienda that while a new contract was being renegotiated, it should administer revenues on behalf of cities, a way of taking power away from the Cortes.[99] This did not sit well with the Reino, of course, which wanted (and was entitled) to administer both the *sobras* and the investigations into towns' financial status that would determine what they paid in *alcabalas*. In August 1596 the Cortes protested to the king that the Contaduría was acting autonomously, entirely overlooking the Cortes.[100] A few days later the Cortes launched an attack against the president of the Council of Finance, Francisco de Rojas, the marquis of Poza, for having violated the contract. The Reino's complaint to the president of the Council of Castile, Rodrigo Vazquez de Arce, suggested that he, too, was being undermined by the wily Poza.[101]

This all went back and forth as the new contract was being negotiated over the following few years, each side claiming precedence and writing

[97] On the limitations of the Council of Finance and the general jurisdictional confusion during this period, see Gelabert, *La bolsa del rey*, 273–9, this reference p. 278; also Tomás y Valiente, "La Diputación," 37–150 and Fortea Pérez, "Entre dos servicios."
[98] Tomás y Valiente, "La Diputación," 102–3, referring to condition 16, in ACC vol. 5 (supp.), 639.
[99] ACC vol. 16, p. 33 and 378–81, and 353–90 passim.
[100] ACC vol. 15, p. 125, August 13, 1596.
[101] ACC vol. 15, p. 131, August 17, 1596. For more alleged violations of the Diputación's authority with regard to the *sobras* see Tomás y Valiente, "La Diputación," 120. Arce was sacked in May 1599 and replaced by the Count of Miranda.

dozens of allegations, complaints, and arguments. Amidst it all, towns devastated by the plague did not seem to know where to turn for help: to the king, the council, the accounts offices, or the Cortes. And once they petitioned, it was unclear if the old contractual system of paying for *bajas* with *sobras* would even be continued. In fact in July 1597 – right after the two representatives for Burgos in the Cortes spoke up on behalf of Santander – Philip II ordered the Cortes to use *sobras* to pay his ministers 6,000 ducats; this was "something new that has never before been done," responded the dumbfounded Cortes, adding piously that those ducats "must be distributed among the poor and the needy."[102]

One of the next supplicants to appear in the Cortes minutes was Cogollos, a Burgos town that had been quarantined in late 1597, very sick in January and February (defying the usual bubonic plague pattern), and declared healthy in May 1598.[103] There is no indication that Cogollos delivered its petition to anyone other than the Cortes. Of its 120 *vecinos*, it told the assembly in late April, only forty had survived. More than 600 people had died. Because no one had been allowed to enter, commerce had collapsed and with it the town's *alcabalas*, so it asked for a four-year moratorium. The initial reaction by the procuradores was that they needed to study the matter further.[104] Two weeks later one of their members reported that he and his colleagues believed Cogollos deserved a fifty-percent reduction. However, Cogollos's case was now joined to that of the town of Aguayo, whose paperwork, the member said, should be forwarded to the Council of Finance, and the debate contained several references to unacceptable interference by the Contaduría.[105]

Of course, by the time most towns began petitioning, the king was Philip III, who was on the road and apparently also in the dark as to the *sobras*.[106] By December 1599 the Reino, the Contaduría, and the Council of Finance seemed to be finding some common ground, and *bajas* were being granted.[107] But the benevolence does not seem to have lasted long. On May 9, 1601, the Council of Finance sent Philip III a

---

[102] ACC vol. 16, 508–9, July 13, 1597.
[103] The declaration of health is in AMB-HI 3650, late May 1598 (fol. 63).
[104] ACC vol. 15, 586–7, April 28, 1598. Cogollos's numbers are a bit suspect if the *vecino*-inhabitant ratio is a generous 4.5.
[105] ACC vol. 15, 596–7, May 18, 1598.
[106] The king was only briefly in Madrid in 1600, then going to Toledo, Segovia, Ávila, Salamanca, and, finally Valladolid. On his itinerary, Santiago Martínez Hernández, *El Marqués de Velada y la Corte en los Reinados de Felipe II y Felipe III: Nobleza cortesana y cultura política en la España del Siglo de Oro* (Salamanca: Junta de Castilla y León, 2004), 410–11.
[107] ACC vol. 18, p. 387, October 13, 1599; ACC vol. 18, pp. 524–6, December 13, 1599; Tomás y Valiente, "La Diputación," 120–2.

memorandum instructing him how this business of the *sobras* was done and reminding the king of the content of previous memos, including one from April 25, 1600, from the Contaduría Mayor de Hacienda.[108] At that time, the Contaduría told the king that once-pestilent villages and towns throughout the kingdom were writing that their *encabezamiento* should be lowered because they had lost crops and spent all their money and that people had moved away and many had died. The Diputación of the Cortes was insisting the *bajas* be paid with *sobras*, but if there were no *sobras* (the Contaduría said) then the difference would have to be divvied up among all cities. And, the Contaduría reminded the king, the bond debt (*juros*) had to be paid off. The king replied that he was worried about "opening the door" to more requests from plague-stricken towns for tax breaks, but he said the Council (sic) surely knew best. The Council itself on May 9, 1601 explained the complicated procedure for *bajas* and *sobras* to the king, who was understandably mystified. The Council seems to have been arguing both that the Cortes's jurisdiction had to be respected and that the Contaduría was stepping onto Council territory. In any case, the two latter bodies finally were merged in 1602.

The Cortes did not much care if *bajas* were granted, as the total amount of the *encabezamiento* would remain the same and the treasury could make up the loss with the *sobras* in municipal coffers. But as time went on the Cortes's sympathy for the desolate towns appears to have waned, possibly because they were worried about how to pay outstanding bonds. On February 22, 1601, the Diputación explained to the Cortes that the reductions that had been approved on account of the plague added up to far more than the *sobras*. In response, the Cortes ordered new investigations into the actual damages suffered by towns, implicitly suggesting that the damages had been exaggerated, and that the reductions be reduced.[109]

A series of petitions from the present-day province of Ávila shows that on the local level people held a keen conviction that verifiable information was an essential tool of justice and government. Vadillo de la Sierra claimed that it had lost one-third of its population as a result of disease, hardship, and exodus. Therefore, the town's *procurador general*, an elected municipal official representing the interests of the commons in municipal councils, Juan Ximénez de Hernández Ximénez, asked the

---

[108] The April 25, 1600 memo is AGS-CJH leg. 403 exp. 3; the May 9, 1601 memo from the Council is AGS-CJH leg. 413 exp. 5.
[109] ACC vol. 19, 826–30; Tomás y Valiente, "La Diputación," 122–3. Tomás y Valiente remarks that the Cortes's attitude was "selfish and narrow; above all, they had to save the *sobras*." Contemporary critics of the monarchy often pointed to the damage that public debt was inflicting on the economy.

Ávila corregidor, Pedro Ortiz Ponce de León, to hold an inquest to
determine if its *alcabalas* could be reduced. Rather than have the townspeople testify, however, Ximénez asked that information be gathered
from surrounding villages because, he reasoned, it would be more fair
to hear from those who had no direct interest yet were still well informed.
On August 4, 1601, therefore, eight men from the area, all of them
vecinos, testified as to the appalling state of affairs in Vadillo. Marcos
Hernández, who was 66, lived in Villanueva de Campillo, one league
away from Vadillo. For more than forty years he had known most of the
inhabitants of Vadillo. "He knows the town was very rich and had many
vecinos, and in the last twenty years he saw and knew that the said town
has diminished greatly in wealth and the number of *vecinos* because many
people have left and died." So, it appears, the plague was not entirely to
blame for the collapse. Francisco de Pasarilla, age 44, a tax collector in
the village of Gamonal (also one league away), said he remembered when
Vadillo had 400 *vecinos*, some of whom were rich and had lots of cattle
and movable property. But for the past fourteen or fifteen years, he said,
he had seen how the town had diminished and fallen onto hard times as
people suffered from diseases sent by the Lord, and he knew it to be a
true fact that one-third of the *vecinos* had disappeared. And, he added,
that meant he was owed a large quantity of money that he had no way of
collecting. The notarized testimony on behalf of Vadillo was followed by
long tallies of past *alcabalas*, all of which was delivered to the corregidor
and, possibly, to the Cortes. It appears the town's request was denied,
possibly because, according to the witnesses themselves, the bad times
has preceded the plague. Nearly three years later, Vadillo seems to have
again asked for tax relief, and the Cortes said it had doubts as to the
independence of the witnesses.[110]

Burgos itself spent much of 1600 insisting that its payments should
decrease; it appears to have won this concession but could not get it
confirmed; Valladolid was in a similar situation.[111] Soto en Cameros (La
Rioja) said that in 1599 it had lost three-quarters of its inhabitants to plague
and was ruined.[112] Correspondence a year later indicates the town had been
granted a reduction that was not being respected.[113] Tordelaguna (present-
day Torrelaguna, province of Madrid) said it used to have 1,000 *vecinos* who
paid taxes of various sorts, but then hidalgos, who did not pay taxes, had

[110] AGS-CJH leg. 413, exp. 5.
[111] For Burgos, AGS-CJH leg. 404 exp. 4; for Valladolid, AGS-CJH leg. 403, exp. 3, also
leg. 404, unclear document no., June 1600.
[112] AGS-CJH leg. 404, unclear document no., May 10, 1600.
[113] AGS-CJH leg. 413, exp. 5.

obtained half the town posts, thus increasing the tax burden on the rest. That was followed in 1599 and 1600 by the loss to plague of more than half the *vecinos* who still paid.[114] Castro Urdiales, which began petitioning for relief already in June 1597 and which apparently won a two-thirds reduction, in 1601 reported that a salaried tax collector was in town and somehow had imprisoned town councilors "and is doing so many things that the favor you [probably the Council of Finance] did for us will come to nothing.[115] And, finally, Gabriel de Loarte wrote to the Council of Finance on behalf of his town of Burguillos (today called Burguillos de Toledo) saying that most of the town's *vecinos* had died in 1599 of the plague sent by the will of God. Because the catastrophe had occurred in August, he added, the harvest had been lost. In addition, the town's meager funds had all been spent on doctors and surgeons and supplies, so he asked that an inquest be undertaken. On February 10, 1601, the council wrote on the cover sheet, *"no ha lugar lo que pide."* What the town was requesting was inappropriate.[116]

Jurisdictional impediments and the growing hesitancy of the Cortes and the various treasury bodies did not dissuade towns and cities from appealing for relief once the plague had left. Aside from the widespread general suffering, as well as the occasional skulduggery (people moving to towns that had obtained tax reductions, collectors ignoring reductions and insisting on collecting the old, higher amount),[117] what stands out is this obstinacy in the face of an administrative labyrinth. The plague destroyed hundreds of thousands of lives and large swathes of the economy. It did not destroy Castilian reverence for the machinery of justice and politics. It was that machinery, with the crown as its fulcrum that would adjudicate claims.

By the time most of the *alcabalas* appeals reached the Cortes or the councils of Finance or Castile, Philip III had moved to Valladolid. The young monarch in his palace had plenty of reading material, if he chose to look at all the treatises being sent to him advising how to address the infinite number of domestic and foreign problems facing Spain. Like so many Castilians, Spain itself was sick, and these treatise-writers volunteered their diagnostic and curative services. "Just as with great illnesses one's greatest hope for health is to know the causes, because only then will the remedies be correct. That is also the case with the

[114] AGS-CJH leg. 424 exp. 8.
[115] ACC vol. 15, p. 501; AGS-CJH leg. 413, exp. 5. It is not obvious who hired him.
[116] AGS-CJH leg. 416, exp. 3. Toledo's corregidor reported that 103 people had died in Burguillos; AGS-E leg. 183, doc. 310, August 27, 1599. Already in mid-June 1599 the city decided to shut down the inns along the road to Burguillos; in AMT Libro de Salud, Libro 176, unfoliated but in chronological order.
[117] AGS-CJH leg. 413, exp. 5.

illness besetting the universal state of the kingdoms to which Your Majesty has succeeded," said one such writer. Some, whose tracts were presumably written with the knowledge or encouragement of Lerma, blamed it all on the king's father, Philip II, and his allegedly inept or corrupt advisers.[118] "The cities and large towns of these kingdoms are losing people, and the small towns are entirely depopulated, and there is hardly anyone left to work in the fields," wrote another author, Baltasar Álamos de Barrientos, who indeed had been punished and imprisoned by Philip II. Castile in particular was groaning under its excessive tax load, he said, "and if any more is added [taxpayers] will be able to pay only with their children and their wives." Far more wealth was leaving the country than coming in, he added, "and thus every day we labor like the spider with what we can extract from our own entrails, and this will continue until we destroy ourselves."[119]

Collectively, these treatise writers are often referred to as *arbitristas*, authors of advice pieces regarding the economy, finance, commerce, government, foreign affairs, morals, defense, engineering, public debt, agriculture, and just about anything else that could be improved upon as Spain lurched into the seventeenth century. Some were cranks or hucksters anxious to make some easy money; others were learned and practiced men who were deeply disturbed to see everything go wrong at once.[120] Begging, vagabondage, and poverty formed part of their repertoire of social ills. Villages were emptying out, spilling their impoverished populations onto Castile's roads.

[118] BN ms 2346, "Sucesos de los años 1598 a 1600," fol. 23, an anonymous treatise bound with the much longer and more important one analyzed by Fortea in "Entre Dos Servicios." The application of the language of illness and cure to politics was ubiquitous.

[119] Baltasar Álamos de Barrientos, *Discurso político al Rey Felipe III al comienzo de su reinado* (Barcelona: Anthropos, 1990), 27–9. Álamos, who was far more than a mere tract-writer – he was a lawyer, a scholar of Tacitus, and "one of the most important political thinkers of the first half of the seventeenth century," in the words of J. A. Fernández-Santamaría – probably co-wrote the *Discurso* with Philip II's disgraced former secretary, Antonio Pérez. Álamos himself was imprisoned for nearly a decade but eventually attained important positions under Philip IV; see J. A. Fernández-Santamaría, *Reason of State and Statecraft in Spanish Political Thought, 1595–1640* (Lanham, MD: University Press of America, 1983), chapter 5, this citation p. 194.

[120] For an overview of the arbitristas see Juan Ignacio Gutiérrez Nieto, "El pensamiento económico, político y social de los arbitristas," in *Historia de la Cultura Española "Menéndez Pidal,"* José María Jover Zamora, ed., vol. 1, *El Siglo del Quijote* (Madrid: Espasa Calpe, 1996), 329–465, and bibliography therein, esp. 394–5; Jean Vilar Berrogain, *Literatura y economía: La figura satírica del arbitrista en el Siglo de Oro,* trans. Francisco Bustelo and Gerónima del Real (Madrid: Revista de Occidente, 1973); J. H. Elliott, "Self-perception and decline in early seventeenth-century Spain," in *Spain and Its World, 1500–1700, Elliott,* ed. (New Haven, CT: Yale University Press, 1989), 241–61.

Site 2: Road

In April 1599 Philip III sent letters to Castilian corregidores asking for updates on the plague in their areas. His cover letter read,

Recently there have been rumors [*ha corrido la voz*] that [the recipient's city] does not enjoy the health that would be desirable, and therefore in order to understand the nature of the illness I ask that you give me news in this manner: that every week you send me a list of those ill with *secas* or similar contagion so that correct measures are taken and we overcome this problem of not understanding its basis.[1]

The men who carried these requests and the intermittent replies formed part of what was apparently a small army of envoys, messengers, and inspectors crowding the pestilent roads and paths of Castile, attempting to verify and quantify the alarming rumors and to "understand the nature of the illness." Valladolid, for example, sent one of its postmen (*correos*), Simón García, to deliver one of its reports "to wherever the King Our Lord may be." He was to leave Valladolid "today, Tuesday, May 18, at four in the afternoon." After García found the itinerant royal court in Barcelona and obtained certification from one of the king's secretaries, he told Valladolid that, "His Majesty has seen the letter and papers sent by the city," and García was paid 114 reales the following month after his return.[2]

At the same time as inhabitants of quarantined towns were supposedly prevented from traveling, local governments and the crown were desperate for information and had no choice but to authorize this multidirectional traffic. The roads of Castile were crowded not only with people leaving wherever it was they were but also with messengers. One small example among thousands is Pamplona, which in January 1597 sent four men, including a doctor, to inspect Santander, Castro Urdiales, Bilbao,

---

[1] AGS-E leg. 184, doc. 272.
[2] AMVA-CH 130 a-4 (ant. leg. 321), fols. 43–4. A real was a silver coin worth 34 maravedies.

Laredo, Vitoria, Portugalete, Salvatierra, San Sebastián, and France.[3]
If this did not spread the disease, a notion which contemporary notions
of contagion logically would have supported, it certainly spread common
understandings of its origins and paths, and it also spread lies, or at least
confusion, for the information the men gathered and delivered might not
be true. Few cities seem to have trusted anyone, and thus requests for
status reports from elsewhere often were followed by reports by one's
own envoys, men instructed to sniff out the number of dead, examine the
walls and gates, interview *vecinos*, inspect the port, listen to the gossip,
and deliver a reliable account back home. It is hard to imagine that these
men did not run into each other as each inspected the other, moving
along the well-traveled routes of news and commerce that bound the
peninsula together. The roads were familiar, and so, too, were the news
and questions they carried. They probably had the same marching orders
their predecessors had had in previous epidemics; certainly that was the
case in Burgos, which had been devastated in 1565, all too recently. Thus
their furrows and trails traced memories, underlined the things one
ought to do, the things one needed to know. And, it is worth repeating,
the decisions as to what they needed to know and how to get that information were almost all being made by towns themselves, not by the
crown, though the crown was informed and many of the investigative
assignments were probably formulaic and routine.

Roads brought information, but also uncertainty. There was a sense of
being surrounded, of little republics bracing themselves for what was
coming down the road. "The enemy approached with such slow steps,"
wrote one of the few chroniclers of the epidemic, the physician Valentín
de Andosilla, who wrote an account of his time curing plague patients in
Navarre, La Rioja, and Castile.[4] The good news was that slow steps

---

[3] Santiago Lasaosa Villanua, *El "Regimiento" municipal de Pamplona en el siglo XVI*
(Pamplona: CSIC, 1979), 348n90; also José Joaquín Arazuri, "La peste en Pamplona
en tiempos de Felipe II," *Príncipe de Viana* 35:134–5 (1974), pp. 179–92. Pamplona
reacted very quickly. The total cost for the trips was 110 ducats. Similarly, when plague
reached neighboring Aragon in 1564, the Pamplona city council sent investigators to
Tudela, Borja, and Tarazona "and other places to find out what is happening and to bring
back testimony," and later sent them as well to Huesca, Zaragoza, and Jaca; José Luis de
Orella y Unzué, "El Cardenal Diego de Espinosa, consejero de Felipe II, el monasterio de
Iranzu y la peste de Pamplona en 1566," *Príncipe de Viana* 36:140–1 (1975), 565–610,
p. 583, citing city council minutes.
[4] "Venía el enemigo con pasos tan lentos," in Valentín de Andosilla Salazar, *Libro en que se
prueba con claridad el mal que corre por España ser nuevo y nunca visto: su naturaleza, causas,
pronósticos, curacion, y la prouidencia que se deue tener con él ...* (Pamplona 1601), fol. 111v.
For additional information on Andosilla see Félix-Tomás López Gurpegui, "Valentín de
Andosilla Salazar: *El mal nuevo nunca visto. Año 1601*," *Berceo* 164 (2013), 41–68. Ann
G. Carmichael, in her study of Florence, suggests a very sensible reason why chronicles

meant there was time to prepare, appoint guards, summon the doctors, decide what was best for oneself and for one's town, whether to stay or to flee, and where to go. Towns knew what was coming not only because they were in touch with other towns, but because all this was horribly familiar. As early as the fourteenth century, Catalonia knew the plague was coming from the other side of the mountains, though it did not have the repertoire of health measures that late sixteenth-century Castile did.[5]

Even when roads were good, the Iberian Peninsula posed challenges to travelers, be they on foot, on mule or horseback, or in carriages, as the region is traversed by mountain ranges and rivers. And, of course, the roads and bridges were not always good. Repairs were often the subject of litigation among the crown, cities, towns, universities, merchant organizations, and other jurisdictions, meaning that repairs often did not get done.[6] Ferdinand and Isabel granted tax exemptions in exchange for road and bridge maintenance and in 1502 ordered the merchants of Burgos to pay three-quarters of the cost of repairs between their city and Laredo, a crucial connection for wool (and, later, plague).[7] But despite the uneven and winding roads, news traveled quickly on the Iberian Peninsula. There was an intricate communication network dating back to the Middle Ages and before that to the Romans, and it grew during the fifteenth century as Castile's famed wool needed to reach northern ports. The polygon of Burgos, Valladolid, Zamora, Salamanca, Ávila, Toledo, and Madrid – the heart of Castile – had some 4,000 kilometers of roads.[8]

are in short supply: the upper-class, literate population had fled and therefore did not witness the events: *Plague and the Poor in Renaissance Florence* (Cambridge University Press, 1986), 101.

[5] David Nirenberg, *Communities of Violence: Persecution of Minorities in the Middle Ages* (Princeton, NJ: Princeton University Press, 1996), 233.

[6] On disputes over payment of road and bridge repairs in this region during the early sixteenth century see Jean-Pierre Molénat, "Chemins et ponts du Nord de la Castille au temps des Rois Catholiques," *Mélanges de la Casa de Velázquez* 7 (1971), 115–62. Towns were generally held responsible, paying with their own funds (*propios*), raising *sisas*, or levying an assessment (*repartimiento*), but there were inevitable conflicts over which towns benefited from which roads and bridges. Bad roads were a fixture in foreigners' accounts of their travels in Spain, though they cannot be taken at face value; for an uncritical account with meaty quotes see Alfredo Alvar Ezquerra, "Viajes, posadas, caminos y viajeros," in *La vida cotidiana en la España de Velázquez*, José N. Alcalá-Zamora, ed. (Madrid: Temas de Hoy, 1989), 109–26; for a more complex understanding see J. N. Hillgarth, *The Mirror of Spain, 1500–1700: The Formation of a Myth* (Ann Arbor, MI: University of Michigan Press, 2000).

[7] Carla Rahn Phillips and William D. Phillips, Jr., *Spain's Golden Fleece: Wool Production and the Wool Trade from the Middle Ages to the Nineteenth Century* (Baltimore, MD: Johns Hopkins University Press, 1997), 211.

[8] This number is cited in chapter 8 of Maria Montáñez Matilla, *El Correo en la España de los Austrias* (Madrid: CSIC, 1953) and Bartolomé Bennassar, *Valladolid au siècle d'or: Une ville de Castille et sa campagne au XVI siècle* (Paris: Mouton, 1967), 80, who both rely on

Toledo, an international center for the production of woolens and silks, lay halfway between Burgos and Seville, but also between Lisbon and Valencia, a major silk-producing center.[9] The northern part of the peninsula also benefited from roads leading west to the great pilgrimage shrine of Santiago de Compostela. Couriers such as Simón García of Valladolid thus attested to the breadth and density of peninsular communications. In 1561, there were eighteen couriers in Valladolid and fourteen in Burgos, though just two in Segovia.[10] There were nine in the great market town of Medina del Campo, but by 1597 the number was also just two, along with the postmaster and one postman.[11] The drop reflects not only the economic crisis but also the establishment of a fixed capital city in Madrid, and of course the two are not unrelated. Before Philip II chose Madrid, news and products had to be easily and regularly delivered to other Castilian cities that functioned as temporary capitals and to industrial and commercial centers, with their hinterland. After 1561 the system was reoriented, but the flow of information and goods remained constant.[12]

The area from Santander east to the Basque Country and south to Burgos and Valladolid (and from there down to Seville) was the heart of Castilian commerce and also the heart of the plague. The "*Rodamundo*" docked in late November 1596, Santander fell sick in the first week of December, which Burgos first heard about on December 31, and by early January Valladolid had gotten wind of the bad tidings.[13]

"Today we had news," the Valladolid city council minutes read, "that in the city of Burgos and other places they are carefully protecting themselves against the *mal de peste* from the ports of Bilbao and Laredo, and in order to find out what is happening we agreed to write to the city

---

the 1546 map by Pero Juan Villuga in his *Reportorio de todos los caminos de España hasta ahora nunca visto en el que allará qualquier viaje que quiera andar muy aprovechoso para todos los caminantes* (Medina del Campo, 1546; facs., Hispanic Society of America, New York: De Vinne Press, 1902). Subsequent maps of Spain's roads were published in 1576 and 1608; Alvar Ezquerra, "Viajes, posadas, caminos y viajeros," 110.

[9] Michael R. Weisser, *The Peasants of the Montes: The Roots of Rural Rebellion in Spain* (Chicago, IL: University of Chicago Press, 1976), 59–60.

[10] David Vassberg, *The Village and the Outside World in Golden Age Castile: Mobility and Migration in Everyday Rural Life* (Cambridge University Press, 1996), 170.

[11] Alberto Marcos Martín, "Medina del Campo 1500–1800: an historical account of its decline," in *The Castilian Crisis of the Seventeenth Century: New Perspectives on the Economic and Social History of Seventeenth-Century Spain*, I. A. A. Thompson and Bartolomé Yun Casalilla, eds. (Past and Present Publications, Cambridge University Press, 1994), 220–48, p. 244.

[12] On the impact of Madrid becoming the capital, David Ringrose, *Madrid and the Spanish Economy, 1560–1850* (Berkeley, CA: University of California Press, 1983).

[13] The Burgos city council announced the news with a public proclamation prohibiting people from the Cantabrian towns from entering; BL Eg. 356, vol. 2, fol. 373r.

of Burgos asking that they advise us which places they are guarding against."[14] Burgos, which had always faced north to the port cities of Bilbao and Santander, had immediately sent its people out into surrounding jurisdictions to deliver orders and collect intelligence. On January 21, 1597, a messenger named Pedro was charged with going straight to Ampuero (Cantabria) and to "under no circumstances" enter an area suspected of being contagious.[15] He was carrying a letter for Juan de Espina, a *vecino* of Ampuero, who, in turn, would assign someone there to go out and visit smaller villages,

> with special attention to which places they are and their names and the people who die every day and the treatment they receive and if the Santander and Castro [illness] has moved on to other places, and if you can you should bring [written] testimony from every village and district [*merindad*] and valley and if you cannot then memorize it so we can understand what is happening.

From there he was to travel north to Laredo and deliver a letter to the corregidor there asking him to write to Burgos with news and to also tell him that Burgos was at Laredo's service to help in any way it could. While there, he should inquire about Santander, Castro Urdiales, Colindres, etc., and then return to Ampuero, from where he should send his report. Attached to his instructions was a list of towns that Burgos currently was guarding against, perhaps so he could match it up with the information he uncovered.

Cities often had permanent commercial or political agents in Madrid and other centers, who now passed on plague information as well, and cities also used their own council members (*regidores*) as envoys or they deputized constables or prominent *vecinos*. These men were paid for their troubles, at least in theory, and Castilian municipal records are full of invoices and calculations as to how much was owed to whom once it was all over. Valladolid hired one of its own notaries, Juan García de Juria, to travel fifteen leagues throughout the city's hinterland, for which he presented an invoice in April 1599.[16] In the same city, Alonso del Castillo complained he had gone to Dueñas, Palencia, Villa Martin, Mazariegos,

---

[14] AMVA sig. 21-0, January 8, 1597. Foreshadowing Bilbao's refusal to admit the truth to Burgos, described in detail in chapter 4, Valladolid continued to query Bilbao in 1597 and discovered in October that indeed it was pestilent and, in response, established quarantine rules. Bennassar thinks the rumor was false, as there is no trace of plague in the Bilbao city council minutes, though I'm inclined to believe that by then there were infected people in the city: Bartolomé Bennassar *Recherches sur les grandes épidémies dans le nord de l'Espagne a la fin du XVIe siècle. Problèmes de documentation et de méthode* (Paris: SEVPEN, 1969), 21–2.

[15] AMB-HI 3653, January 21, 1597. Pedro's last name is smudged.

[16] AMVA-CH 98-1 (ant. leg. 248), fols. 4–5.

and other places in Tierra de Campos and still had not gotten paid.[17] Francisco Palomino was owed 4,000 maravedies after spending ten days (at 400 a day) traveling around Tierra de Campos with a royal order to set up guards against affected towns.[18] Francisco Pérez, who, like Simón García of Valladolid, was a professional *correo* rather than deputized, and therefore probably was a person of means with horses and runners at his disposal, calculated after his trip north to León and La Coruña that there were seventy-three leagues between Valladolid and La Coruña, plus he had made a side trip to Astorga, so he was owed for eighty-three leagues at 5.5 reales per ten leagues, plus the return trip, plus he had stayed for two and a half days in León and La Coruña waiting for replies to his letters. He received 104 reales in the end.[19] There was money to be made.

The crown and city councils also deputized *alguaciles* to bear royal edicts instructing smaller towns to implement anti-plague procedures immediately. These envoys traveled holding high the staff of justice, *la vara alta de justicia*, making them the visible and rightful personification of royal authority. Local authorities, in the presence of a public notary, had to receive and acknowledge these orders and swear to uphold them and arrange for their own town criers (*pregoneros*) to publicize them. And in addition to the ad hoc messengers employed or reassigned during the epidemic, Castile also had a mail service, which is probably what the corregidores relied upon most, given the volume of correspondence they were producing.[20] The Burgos *correo mayor* asked for special keys to the city gate, suggesting he was very busy, which he received on condition he share them with no one.[21] Letters themselves were considered dangerous, and apparently the social rank of the remitter and recipient made no difference, as in the case of the corregidor of Aranda del Duero, who when he responded to Philip III's request for information excused the tardiness of the reply by pointing out that Madrid had twice refused to let his letter get through (which means the letters were going to the Council of Castile, not to the king, who was not in Madrid).[22]

The lists of towns to guard against, posted on wooden panels or posts at city gates and also publicized by the town crier, were the principal source of news. There were no public bills of mortality as in England, the ones diarist Samuel Pepys eagerly sought out each week during the

---

[17] AMVA-CH 99-19 (ant. leg. 249), fol. 61, also AMVA-CH 149–2.
[18] AMVA-CH 99-19 (ant. leg. 249), fol. 64.
[19] AMVA-CH 130 a-4 (ant. leg. 321), fols. 58–60, June 1599.
[20] The royal mail service for generations was run by the Tassio clan; its delivery men carried a cornet, a mail bag, and a royal seal, and inns often functioned as post offices; see Montáñez Matilla, *El Correo*.
[21] AMB-HI 3653, January 7, 1597.   [22] AGS-E leg. 183, doc. 315, May 11, 1599.

London plague of 1665 to see who was listed and if the numbers were diminishing. Some of these lists of towns were printed (and survived), so probably they were distributed and posted in town centers in addition to town gates. But printing might have been an impractical measure, judging from city council minutes, which are filled with updated lists and scratched-out names (Figure 2.1). This was a moving target, not only because the disease moved suddenly, unexpectedly, and then often halted during the cold months – "after having moved at the pace of a tortoise for more than ten months this omnivorous and insatiable disease attacked with inexorable fury and unheard-of impiety," Andosilla wrote – but also because at any given moment, the lists might not be reliable.[23] Cities exchanged sick lists, which was more efficient than all of them sending messengers to the same places, but it meant they relied upon each other's judgments and also ensured the lists would not match up as news trickled back to one place but not another.[24] Towns missing from the lists were probably good places to flee to. Those whose names appeared, however, at the very least suffered damaged reputations. Reflecting the possible harm that might come from unwarranted publicity, Burgos in July 1597 decided that guards should not tell people attempting to enter which names were on the list and which were not, so as to avoid travelers changing their stories according to what the lists said. Rather, guards "should carefully look at [the traveler's] testimony, and if they have come from pestilent places they should just tell them that they cannot enter." If the names on the list were known only to the guards, less mischief would be made, at least in theory.[25]

Some towns complained that their presence on lists was the result of malicious slander by those who wished them ill, and indeed some of the information was sketchy. When a line-up of witnesses testified regarding their knowledge of the state of health in Puebla de Montalban (Toledo), where "they say there is contagious illness," one witness (echoed by the rest) said he had been with

some people in the said town around twenty days ago, and later here, and before and continuously, they have told him that there is much illness in the said town and a great many people [*mucha multitud*] are dying, some days twenty people and other days thirty and some days fifty, and he has spoken of this in the

---

[23] Andosilla Salazar, *Libro en que se prueba con claridad el mal que corre*, 131r.
[24] Earlier we saw Valladolid asking Burgos for its list, and later, in July 1598, Burgos noted which Galician, Toledan, and Castilian towns Valladolid was guarding against; AMB-HI 3653, July 17, 1598.
[25] AMB-HI 3653, July 20, 1597.

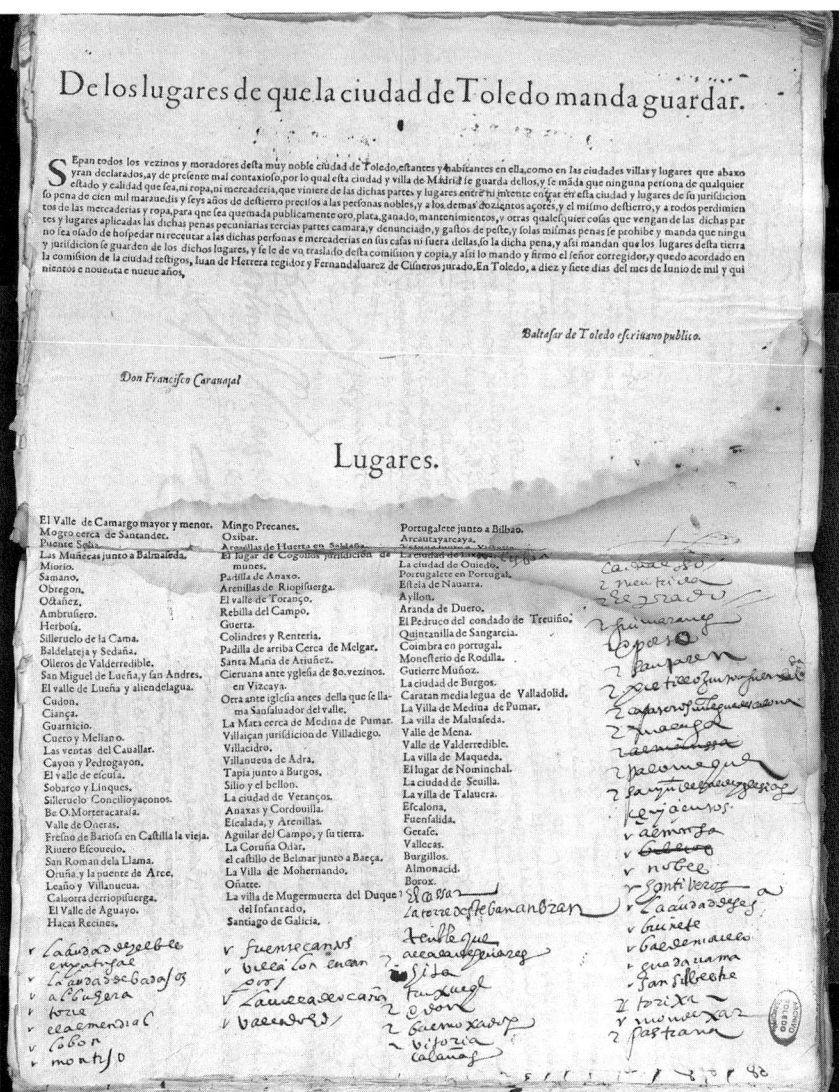

Figure 2.1 List of towns that were off-limits to Toledo because of the plague; 17 June 1599.

Source: Archivo Municipal de Toledo, Libros Manuscritos, Sección B, no. 176. Reproduced with permission from Archivo Municipal de Toledo.

fields [*el campo*] with people from the said town whom he met … and yesterday, Saturday, this witness … said that on the road to San Sebastián [he spoke with someone] who said that the week before 400 people had died in the said town.

Another witness confirmed the testimony, saying that "in this village and elsewhere it is public knowledge [*hay pública voz y fama*] that *mucha multitud* were dying in Puebla de Montalban."[26] The city of Estella (Navarre) prosecuted someone for having said it was sick when in fact, it claimed, it had never been healthier. The usual collection of *vecinos* and witnesses were called to testify, among them Madalena de Amezqueta, who was around thirty. She said she did not know for sure if Estella was sick or healthy, but she did know that around two weeks earlier when she was feeding barley to her horses some strangers told her that lots of people were dying in Estella, but they did not say of what. A tailor who was the brother-in-law of the vicar of San Miguel, and his wife, had died after eating sea bream and meat, leaving behind a baby girl, who also died, but later Madalena de Amezqueta had gone to Estella and she did not see anything amiss. She was asked why, then, she had told some *vecinos* of Artajona, the town where the defendant lived, that Estella was sick with plague, and she said she had done no such thing; she had simply asked where they were coming from, and when they replied Estella, she told them what she had been told and that it might be *peste*. "But she neither knew nor had heard anything for certain." The defendant, Salvador de Echaide, had reached the conclusion that Estella was sick when he learned that three houses had been shut, in two of which it was said that sixteen people had died. A tailor named Bernal de Igualde, a *natural vasco* who lived in Artajona, had been talking to Echaide in the home of Pedro de Sola, a shoemaker in the same town, along with two women, and Igualde said he had heard that in Estella two houses had been shut because of plague deaths, "and he did not say who told him this nor where, nor did he ask." So when Echaide returned to Pamplona and visited Carlos de Calva in his home and drank some wine with him, and Calva asked him after the general health of Estella, Echaide told him, and Calva promptly told the authorities. After Echaide was fined fifty pounds plus legal costs, he appealed. His lawyer argued that he had simply repeated what he had been told, was an honest upstanding man, and that other people were saying the same thing about Estella. Most important, "if my client were fined … that would strike fear not only in my client but in others who would not

---

[26] AMT Libros manuscritos sec. B no. 176, nf. The testimony might have been taken in the present-day town of Escalonilla or possibly a vanished village with a similar name.

dare to denounce and publicize news of suspicious illnesses in towns, which would be most harmful."[27]

Messengers who set out along Castile's roads to gather information had to weigh its merits, and gradually one sees town councils specifying exactly which questions they should ask and of whom, possibly reflecting exasperation with cheerful false reports by towns themselves, or excessively dire reports about neighboring towns. One city whose deception as to its health status brought tremendous suffering both to itself and the region was San Sebastián, in the province of Guipúzcoa. In January 1598, the Bilbao city council sent Martín de Aguirre there, as well as to nearby Lequeitio, to investigate; he spent sixteen days and earned 11,968 maravedies. In late July he was sent back to Guipúzcoa because of news that "the illness has returned." On August 7 he made yet another trip there: "Given that the city [of Bilbao] has received news that a man in the said city [of San Sebastián] when the contagious illness was afoot had sent to this city certain loads of linens collected in the time of the said disease," Aguirre was dispatched with a letter to the corregidor of Guipúzcoa to find out what was going on.[28] Bilbao itself would later deceive Burgos as to its own status. Even some of the reports sent to Philip III in 1599 at his request were, in fact, untrue or at least dangerously optimistic.

One example of improved specificity came when Burgos sent Cristóbal de Morales to visit the important and very troubled town of Melgar de Fernamental and its neighbors in April 1598. He was given a list of questions to ask; their tone, precision, and insistence are reminiscent of Philip II's famous surveys of Castile, the *Relaciones topográficas*, to which we will return. When did the disease arrive; what sort of disease was it; how many people got sick and died, what were their names and what sort of people were they; if the houses where they got sick and died had been closed up and if they were now open; if the houses had been reopened, how had they been reopened, and had they been cleaned with perfumed vinegar; had the clothing and linens been burned; and if the town or village was healthy, how long had it been healthy. For "each and every" item, Morales was to obtain testimony (meaning written and notarized) from witnesses who could give reasons for what they said and explain how they knew what they said and who could point to people, houses, and linens "so the truth can be determined." Once the questioning was over, Morales was to summon a variety of officials in every town he

---

[27] AGN TR Procesos 013291. The case took place in January–February 1603, when there were reappearances of the plague in some towns. Calva seems to have paid Echaide's bond, and Echaide was prohibited from leaving Pamplona during some time.

[28] AFB libro 023, minutes in chronological order.

visited, put them under oath, and then ask them if the town was healthy and free of contagion and peste and for how long it had been that way, "so that without endangering or harming health the said town may conduct business and communication with this city of Burgos and the other cities, towns, and villages in these kingdoms, warning them that if they should declare something other than the truth and if some hardship or harm should occur as a result, they will be severely punished ... And in the same manner you should summon the chapter of the clergy in the town and have them testify." Finally, Morales was told to be very careful about his own health, stay in each place as briefly as possible, and charge each town a prorated daily rate of 400 maravedies for his efforts.[29]

Messengers do not seem to have been sent by boat along rivers, but envoys and town councils with waterways were careful to include them in their quarantine efforts, as they posed as much danger as roads. (One of the reasons Madrid was relatively spared during epidemics may have been that it has no river to speak of.) An earlier example of this awareness came in July 1582, when the capital feared contagion from the south. A city council member from Madrid, Nicolás Suárez, was assigned the job of traveling through the Tagus and Jarama river valleys to ensure that no one from any of those towns entered Madrid.[30] His route included such important places as Aranjuez, Talavera de la Reina, and Toledo itself. Suárez was to inspect all river crossings, boatyards, and bridges to ensure they were well guarded, and in addition inspect gates and streets all along his journey. He was to secretly meet with doctors in Toledo and find out if someone who recently died in Aranjuez had earlier been in Córdoba. He was to determine if bridge guards were literate. In Colmenar de Oreja he tricked a boatman into taking him and his notary across the river without demanding to see their passes, which got the man in trouble. He worried about low water levels enabling people to ford rivers. Towns along the coast naturally had an even bigger problem, and fishing boats were sometimes ordered to be tied up, a decision with obvious economic consequences. Already in January 1597, just one month after the plague began, Bilbao prohibited boats within the city and its jurisdiction from taking people without proper passes across the Nervión River or across

---

[29] AMB-HI 3650, auto, April 11, 1598. Morales made this tour because the towns said they had recovered and should now be allowed to traffic with the outside; he was checking on their true status.

[30] AGS-CR leg. 115 no. 4. In the document he is referred to as Juárez, but Ana Guerrero Mayllo, *Familia y vida cotidiana de una élite de poder: Los regidores madrileños en tiempos de Felipe II* (Madrid: Siglo Veintiuno, 1993), passim, makes it clear he was Suárez. In 1573 he had had orders to accompany a priest who would exorcise a plague of caterpillars; Guerrero, *Familia*, 171.

the many inlets from the sea, and it ordered *vecinos* to organize guard duty across the bridges.[31] Violators would have their boats seized; a similar order two years later said the boats would be burned. When travelers arriving on foot were denied entry across bridges, the city council noted, they were solving the problem by simply going down to where the boatmen were, a practice that had to stop.[32] A similar situation in Valladolid near the Puente Mayor, over the Pisuerga River, could be fixed, a master builder successfully proposed, with a clay and wood contraption installed where fishermen worked by the shore that would bar passage; the project cost 200 reales (Figure 2.2).[33]

Back on the road, merchandise and food obviously had to keep moving, though there was much less of it as the months went by and goods from the coast were quarantined and harvests lost. Muleteers (*arrieros*) and carters were essential yet risky figures in this constellation. Already in the fourteenth century Burgos had a bustling business renting horses and mules to travelers and vendors.[34] Many farmers or peasants delivered goods as a sideline or in the off-season or even trafficked themselves, and if they were running their own business from the coast it is likely they bought their wares on credit, meaning they were ruined if they could not sell. In Burgos province, in the Bureba region, Francis Brumont found that nearly all the men worked as muleteers when they were not tending to their crops. There, in the village of Cantabrana in 1586, eight of the twelve male *vecinos* were *arrieros*, and in 1597 it was eleven of twenty-three, a rare sign of growth during these years. Villagers in Bentretea said they sent their seven muleteers to Burgos twice a week, and they traveled as well to Bilbao.[35] Muleteers also carried news, of course, just like the shepherds whose paths crisscrossed the heart of Castile. And because they or their cargo could also carry disease (wool was especially problematic), there are records of towns trying to keep track of where their muleteers were, so as to halt their return if they had visited suspicious areas. On his journey through the Tagus River valley in 1582, Nicolás Suárez stopped off in Sonseca, south of the city of Toledo, where he learned that *vecinos* who worked as *arrieros* were coming and going between Sonseca and Seville

---

[31] AFB libro 022, January 18, 1597.   [32] AFB libro 024, August 13, 1599.

[33] AMVA-CH 9-7 (ant. leg. 287), fols. 24–5. Valladolid had some six major bridges on the Duero and Pisuerga rivers; see Bennassar, *Valladolid*, 81–6 on the city council's incessant attention to the state of the bridges.

[34] Francisco José González-Prieto, *La ciudad menguada: Población y economía en Burgos S. XVI y XVII* (Santander: Universidad de Cantabria, 2005), 234–5.

[35] Francis Brumont, *Campo y campesinos de Castilla la Vieja en tiempos de Felipe II* (Madrid: Siglo Veintiuno, 1984), 166.

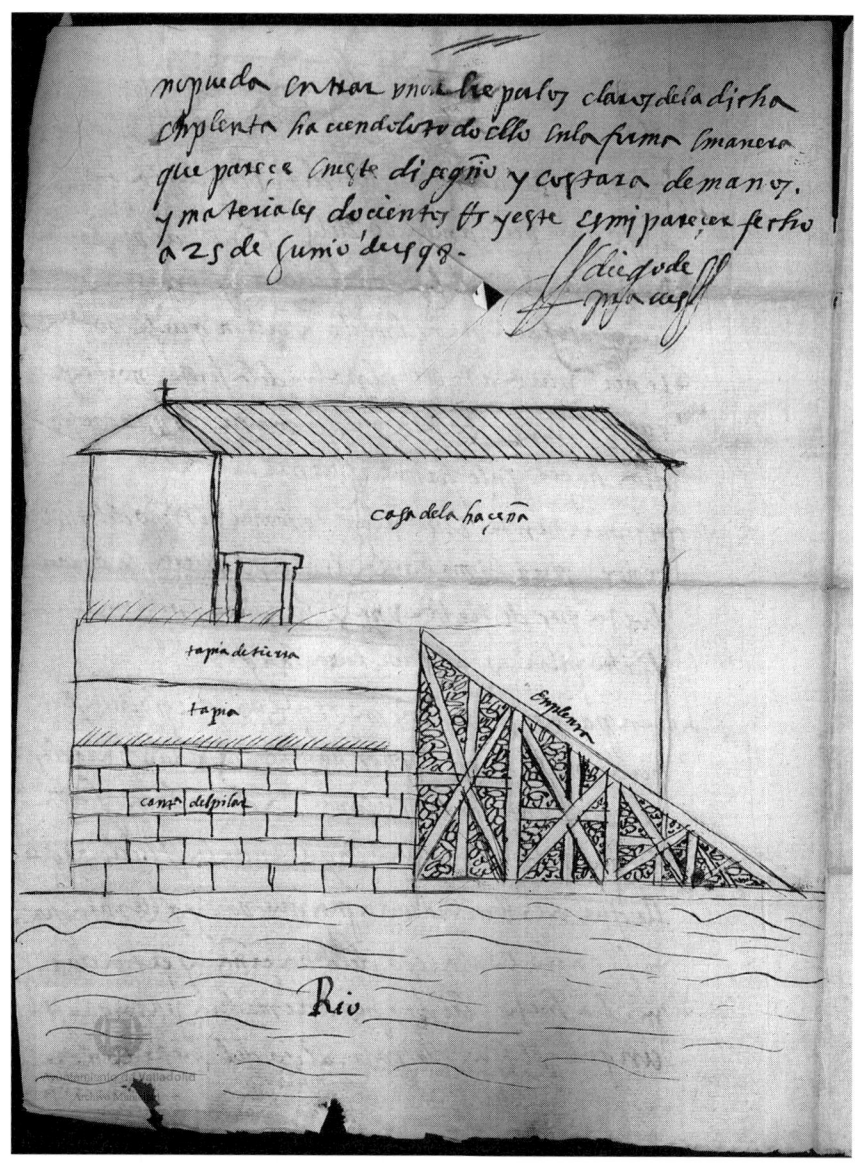

Figure 2.2 A device designed to impede foot traffic along river banks, and thus reduce contagion, submitted to the Valladolid city council.
Source: Archivo Municipal de Valladolid (AMVA), CH 9–7, fol. 24v.
Reproduced with permission from Archivo Municipal de Valladolid

and other places in Andalusia. He immediately put a stop to that and told the town to tell them via messenger to stay where they were until further instructions. No muleteers or their animals could enter Sonseca, he decreed, and if they did they would be fined 500 ducats, a huge amount they could not pay anyway, and "severely punished."[36] On June 28, the town produced a complete list of its muleteers and where they were right then and where they were going, information it collected from people in town: "I testify that Francisco G—, *arriero*, *vecino* of Sonseca, is gone from this town and he left four days ago for Medina del Campo, according to what was said, and [the witness knows] that other *arrieros* from here are also missing."[37] During our plague, as with so many other things, Burgos was first. It was ideally situated; not so close to the start of the chain as to be immediately infected, but close enough that measures had to be enacted quickly. In January 1597 authorities there ordered muleteers who had delivered sea bream (*besugo*, probably from Bilbao) to leave the city right away and also specifically prohibited muleteers Joan del Cerro, Joan de las Landeras, Bartolomé de Rojas, and a fourth man who had all been working in the mountains to the north from entering, probably meaning they could not return home.[38] Segovia was still allowing muleteers to enter in 1598, judging from gate records, though its liberal approach may have tightened up the following year.[39] Also in 1598, Burgos decided that muleteers could not enter Burgos with merchandise unloaded from ships in Laredo; rather, they would have to come from Bilbao, "a healthy port." But five months later, Bilbao, too, was sick and unreliable, so Burgos instructed muleteers carrying products unloaded from ships to go straight to Burgos, getting testimony at each healthy town they passed through. They would be punished "severely," in an unspecified way, if they opened up their sacks or bundles and removed anything; this was not an anti-theft measure, but rather an anti-contagion one.[40] In May 1601 Ávila instructed its commissioners in charge of guard duty (at that late date the city was worried about travelers from the south) to draw up a list of all the muleteers, along with every other *vecino* of the city who at present was missing, indicating where they were and when they were

---

[36] In the previous chapter we saw the Guipúzcoa corregidor estimating that it would cost 1,000 ducats to clean Pasajes, a large enough amount that neither the Basques nor the king could (or would) pay.

[37] AGS-CR leg. 115 no. 4, fols. 46–9. Francisco's last name is illegible.

[38] AMB-HI 3653, January 18, 1597. "Mountains" was the usual way of referring to Cantabria.

[39] AMS leg. 456/1.   [40] AMB-HI 3653, April 14 and September 16, 1598.

scheduled to return.[41] Limitations on their movements almost always appeared in lawsuits seeking compensation for reduced taxes levied on products coming into town. Plaintiffs inevitably argued that because they could not find muleteers, because so many town refused them entry, their revenue had plummeted.[42]

There was another reason why people might be on the road, someplace in-between: they were picking up supplies from what Ann Carmichael has called "the equivalent of a neutral zone."[43] Some of these included highly ingenious solutions for moving supplies from the sick to the well or vice versa. A tanner in Barcelona, Miquel Parets, who wrote a diary of the 1651 plague in his city, described a system whereby supplies could be transferred: city-dwellers with money stood on one side of a ditch and vendors with goods stood on the other. Planks were placed from one side to the other, with a lazy Susan device rigged up so goods and money (once a fair price had been determined by calling back and forth, and after the coins had been dipped in vinegar) could be placed on one side and spun to the other, a bit like the *torno* in cloistered convents.[44] Less elegantly, perhaps, the corregidor of Guipúzcoa, Diego Fernández de Arteaga, ordered that people in San Sebastián leave meals half-way to the hospital ("*en medio del camino*") so the staff could come and pick up the food.[45]

Most neutral zones in Castile, however, were shrines (*ermitas*), which also were used early on as refuges or interim hospitals for the sick. They had been constructed at some point in honor of some saint, but their use during the plague years had more to do with their geography outside towns than with any holy purpose, which, indeed, hardly was mentioned. The shrine operations launched by Burgos starting in September 1597 are a revelation of what people needed, where infection might come from, the relationship between Burgos and its towns, and which things people were afraid of. The view from the shrine was of largely empty

---

[41] AHMA Libros de Actas, libro 26, fols. 93r–4v. Ávila in February 1600 had 2,364 *vecinos*; Serafín de Tapia, "Las fuentes demográficas y el potencial humano de Ávila en el siglo XVI," *Cuadernos Abulenses* 2 (July–December 1984), 31–88, p. 74.

[42] A plaintiff in Navarre said that because muleteers were known to carry false travel documents, Tudela had outright prohibited them from entering, leading to his loss; however the case also includes the information that Pamplona allegedly allowed muleteers to be forced to carry goods; AGN TR Procesos 284021.

[43] Ann G. Carmichael, "Contagion theory and contagion practice in fifteenth-century Milan," *Renaissance Quarterly* 44:2 (Summer 1991), 213–56, p. 227, referring to fifteenth-century Milan.

[44] James S. Amelang, ed. and trans., *A Journal of the Plague Year: The Diary of the Barcelona Tanner Miquel Parets, 1651* (New York: Oxford University Press, 1991), 51–2.

[45] AGS-GyM leg. 489, doc. 227, September 20, 1597.

roads leading to towns one could no longer visit. They were places distant from one's own village, places where people might at least meet, chat, disobey, get sustenance.

Once the town of Revilla del Campo fell ill, Burgos's new corregidor, Diego de Vargas Manrique (on the job since just July, sent there expressly by the king to take charge of the anti-peste campaign), wrote to the town council there saying he had heard that the priest and the barber were afraid to enter houses ("which pains and troubles me"), so he was sending some sponges that he suggested be soaked in vinegar.[46] He advised Revilla to levy a sales tax (*sisa*) and told the council that as Burgos had sent a pharmacist (*boticario*), Francisco Ortuño, to Los Ausines, just a half-league away, with medicines and medical instructions, Revilla should write letters outlining its medical needs and leave them at the Santa Ana shrine between the two towns, where Ortuño would pick them up and leave his replies and medicines.[47] At the shrine there was a wooden barrier beyond which supplicants and messengers could not pass; next to that there was a box into which recipes (*recetas*) and medicines were carefully dropped. No bags or other potentially infected containers were to be used. But a few days later it transpired that Revilla's inhabitants had recklessly disobeyed Vargas and were entering Los Ausines itself rather than going just to the shrine. Not only that, but when they went to the shrine to get Ortuño's medicines they had gone inside carrying all sorts of jugs, boxes, sacks, bowls, and other implements that might be infectious. They were sharing the Santa Ana shrine with the town of Cogollos, whose people also had been instructed to get medicines there from Ortuño. Cogollos, on the road from Burgos to Madrid, was one of the very first towns away from the north coast to become infected and was also among the first to request that its *alcabalas*

---

[46] Vargas was a member of the Order of Alcántara and a *vecino* of Madrid who moved in lofty circles. He might have been a relative of poet Luis de Vargas Manrique, whose father was Philip II's secretary for Italian affairs, Diego de Vargas y Isla (d. 1577), and whose mother was Diego's second wife, Ana Manrique y Butrón. Our Vargas might also be the brother of Luis de Vargas Carvajal, yet another adviser to Philip II. A Vargas family tree (Guerrero Mayllo, *Familia y vida cotidiana*, 138) contains a reference to a Diego Vargas whose father was a Madrid regidor, Fadrique, and whose mother was Antonia Manrique; this also could be our man, though the tree does not give years or follow his particular line. A subsequent Diego Vargas Manrique was corregidor of Alcalá de Henares and a member of the Toledo city council under Philip IV, and there were a multitude of other Vargases in leadership positions in seventeenth-century Toledo. Our Vargas testified in the Inquisition case against Alonso de Mendoza, part of the case against Lucrecia de León, and told the court how well-acquainted he was with various Mendozas; AHN Inquisition 3713/4/11, fols. 153v–4v.

[47] Cogollos, Revilla del Campo, and Los Ausines are all still there, though the shrines appear not to be.

be reduced. Vargas's instructions to Cogollos were similar to those to Revilla, and, eventually, to all other neighboring towns, but they contain one of Vargas's occasional personal notes, for he suddenly interjected: "The twenty-four pairs of shoes that I sent should be distributed among the poor, that is my wish." Over the coming months Cogollos, Revilla, and the rest would get shipments of shoes, slippers, salt, melons, oil, vinegar, cheese, bread, wine, leather containers for the vinegar, onions, wax (tallow for candles grew scarce as cattle died off), sponges, baskets, juniper balls, horseshoes, locks, and keys, all of which would be left at the shrine.

The town that took up most of Vargas's time was Melgar de Fernamental, to the east, a wide open land of grain fields, though there may have been more trees then than now. Some 500 dwellings there were sick in September, leading Vargas to comment to the Council of Castile that if every town in the region were similarly affected and all their corresponding linens were burned, "then people would end up dying of the cold rather than of peste."[48] He took a more empathetic tone with the town, though he made clear to them that the toll of 500 could have been avoided had Melgar followed his quarantine and burning instructions to begin with. "This pains me infinitely," he wrote of the catastrophic situation, before moving on to discuss money laundering, Melgar's supply depot at the San Juan shrine, and information regarding the commissioner, Pedro del Castillo, whom he had dispatched to live in nearby Grijalba (along with a salaried doctor/surgeon), a few miles down a road today lined with sunflower fields. Castillo was to spend his days riding on horseback around the towns to make sure nobody was going in or out. "Under no circumstances" was he to enter Melgar, "but rather [he] must go to the usual nearby shrine where we leave messages and orders." There, if he needed to communicate with the town, he should hail the first passer-by and ask him to take the corregidor's message into town. He should wait for a reply and then ask the messenger to put the paper on the ground, sprinkle it with vinegar, and push it into a fire. The commissioner's job was not only to patrol the perimeter but to oversee the supply chain. He was the only person allowed to have a key

---

[48] The 1591 census conducted for tax purposes shows Melgar had 412 *pecheros* (taxpayers), so one can assume that virtually every household in the town was sick; Annie Molinié-Bertrand, *Au siècle d'or l'Espagne et ses Hommes. La Population du Royaume de Castille au XVI siècle* (Paris: Economica, 1985), 136. News of Melgar's illness reached Zamora in August thanks to news from a friar's parents, who lived there; José Carlos Rueda Fernández, "Aportación al estudio de la extensión geográfica de la epidemia de peste de los años 1596–1602: Un documento inédito del archivo municipal de Zamora," *Studia Historica. Historia Moderna* 2 (1984), 95–113, p. 98.

to the shrine, where he was to go every morning and every afternoon to see if anyone from Melgar had left requests. As in Revilla, requests should be left outside the shrine, and no one from Melgar was to enter or bring containers. On Monday and Friday evenings, the eve of market days in Burgos, the commissioner would send pack mules from the shrine to Burgos, where they would be loaded with the provisions requested by the town's inhabitants. The mule driver or someone with him would carry Melgar's list, which would say, in the corregidor's words, "The town of Melgar requests such and such things which should be delivered to the person carrying this letter, and the letter should be signed and taken to the markets in this city, which are on Tuesdays and Saturdays." The next day the laden mules would return to the shrine. Along with supplies, a notarized list of the purchased items and their prices would be attached. Payment would be made by carefully washing the money in a tub of vinegar that the delivery man would have brought with him. Letters between Melgar and Burgos should also be washed in vinegar. Like the people of Revilla, those of Melgar could leave messages for the doctor at the shrine, and if they were not happy with the *boticario* who lived in Melgar they also could leave requests for medicines there. "Under no circumstances" were they to enter the shrine, but rather they should ring a little bell hanging from a cord in front of the shrine, and the *boticario* would approach (it is unclear whether from inside the shrine or from nearby) to fill the prescription "on my account and at my expense" (*por mi quenta y crédito*).

The people of Cogollos, some of whose poorest residents now had shoes, were being referred to the shrine of San Juan as well as to Santa Ana. On October 2 the corregidor wrote Cogollos that he understood they needed a doctor. "I have tried to find a doctor to send to you, but even though I would pay him and give him a salary to tend to you in the San Juan shrine, no one dares go there," he wrote. "In the meantime, give your requests for medicines to Pedro del Castillo, and he will send them to me … Having understood your need, I am sending you sugar, jam, raisins, and wine." And, he added, he had heard that some people who lived in the butcher's house had died, "so I order that the butcher be removed and must not slaughter or sell meat, but rather someone else should do that." After consulting with physicians, the city of Burgos in September sent recommendations to Cogollos, Revilla del Campo, and other towns "where there is no doctor." These recommendations began with dietary suggestions, the elements of which were undoubtedly part of subsequent mule deliveries: people in areas affected by disease should eat "easily digestable food" such as fowl, mutton, chickens, goat, veal, partridge, fresh eggs, borage, lettuce, and very ripe plums. Moderate amounts of garlic and drops of bitter vinegar, lime, lemon, or orange could be added to broths and meals. It was better not to eat too much and not to get too tired. The wine should be good but watered down. Compresses soaked with vinegar should be carried on one's body.[49]

The shrine system continued functioning through at least 1598, with villagers throughout the infected portions of Castile going back and forth along the roads to pick up supplies and leave requests. Vargas died in January 1599 (I don't know the cause), and his successor during the subsequent catastrophe was less solicitous, though to be fair the situation by then had gotten much worse. In any case, the new corregidor did not show the same sort of personal attention to villagers in his jurisdiction who were hemmed in by disease, often deprived of their livelihood, and able to walk just that short distance to the shrine, from where they carted back foodstuffs and supplies purchased on their behalf by strangers.

Years ago David Vassberg wrote about what he called the "immobile village myth."[50] Migrant agricultural and domestic laborers, herders, shepherds, muleteers, and artisans may have thought of one particular town as home, but not necessarily, or not for long. Links to people and places were malleable, which becomes important when considering the displacements caused by plague, which possibly did not alter the social or psychological landscape as much as one might think. Traditionally, people from the northernmost provinces spent several months a year working in agriculture in La Rioja or Castile. Construction workers and artisans might also drift to the larger cities for spells. Lower-class people readily moved to other villages, towns, or cities in search of work and often stayed there if they found someone with whom to start a family. They may not have gone back; indeed, in a study of Inquisition defendants who were required to describe their life history for the court, only one-quarter returned, and then only because they had new employment possibilities, property holdings, or kinsmen to go back to. Of the 346 men and women whose cases were studied by Satoko Nakajima, only twenty-eight declared they had never left their hometowns.[51]

---

[49] This entire section on Melgar and the other towns is drawn from AMB-HI 3651, September 4 to October 2, 1597, fols. 20–80, scattered documents. Santa Ana was a plague saint, as it happens, but this does not seem to be relevant here; the shrine has disappeared. The two dozen pairs of shoes show up in accounts as costing 120 reales, which were paid to a shoemaker. To this day, Cogollos is populated by farmers of wheat, barley, and sunflowers, and it also is a bedroom community for Burgos.

[50] Vassberg, *The Village and the Outside World*, 1.

[51] Satoko Nakajima, "Breaking ties: marriage and migration in sixteenth-century Spain," PhD diss., University of Tokyo, 2011, chapter 1. See also Antonio Eiras Roel, "Migraciones internas y medium-distance en España en la Edad Moderna," in

During our plague, we have the example of a young Pamplona man whose wanderings were not exceptional but would end up changing his life. It's a long story, but one that encapsulates many of this book's themes: movement, entry, family, the law. After Bernart de Villadia, a 26-year-old hatter, was picked up for entering Pamplona's San Nicolás gate without papers, he was asked to describe his trip. He had left Logroño three days ago at 4:00 p.m., he told the court. He was French, but he had been working in Logroño for nine months in the home of master hatter Julio de Salinas. He had decided to go when people began leaving the city owing to "a certain disease" and he saw many sick people being taken to the hospital in the plaza of San Francisco.[52] As he started his journey on foot, he fell in with a young *boticario* who appeared to be eighteen years old, and when he asked him where he was going and the man, who was named Juan de Nagore, said Pamplona, which was where he was from, they decided to walk together. They did not enter a single village along the way because they had no travel papers indicating where they had come from, but people sold them bread and other things which they ate together off at a distance, he said.[53] They had no dealings with anyone on the road. When they arrived in Pamplona without papers, they wandered around to the San Nicolás gate, and there Juan de Nagore saw some students he knew, so they tagged along with the group and got in and no one stopped them. Somehow later they were caught. Nagore, meanwhile, testified that he had worked for an apothecary in Logroño and had left two days earlier than the Frenchman. He spent a couple of days down by the river, inviting a girl to eat with him, returned to hear Mass on Sunday at the Jesuit church, but then could not get out of the city. He waited until the guards at the gate were eating lunch and wandered back down to the river, where he started walking and soon ran into Villadia. He too said that they had entered no villages or towns along the way, and he repeated the story of how they managed to get into

---

Migraciones internas y medium-distance en la Península Ibérica, 1500–1900, Antonio Eiras Roel and Ofelia Rey Castelao, eds., vol. 2 (Santiago de Compostela: Xunta de Galicia, 1994), 37–84; the volumes in this 2-volume set each have a slightly different title. There are several articles of relevance to this book, including one by Vassberg on servants, who may have included young people orphaned by the plague: "Life-cycle service as a form of age-specific migration in the 16th and 17th centuries: rural Castile as a case study," in *Les migrations internes et a moyenne distance en Europe, 1500–1900*, Antonio Eiras Roel and Ofelia Rey Castelao, eds., vol. 1 (Santiago de Compostela: Xunta de Galicia, 1994), 385–402.

[52] For an account of the plague's arrival in Logroño and the city council's actions, see Fernando Pons Ibáñez, "Epidemia de peste en Logroño (Año 1599)," *Berceo* 73 (1964), 387–406.

[53] Travel papers are discussed more fully in the following chapter.

Pamplona with the students; he added that he recognized one of the guards as Lic. Miguel de Bayona. After the men were picked up, they were quickly jailed, and Juan's mother and sister, who had lodged them, were placed under house arrest as well. The women swore that they had admitted no other guests. They had given Juan and his friend bread and wine and a bed, which the men shared, saying that for the past three nights they had slept on the ground. They also washed the men's clothes in very hot water and then in the river. The Frenchman disappears from the record, but Juan, his mother, and possibly his sister all appear to have been sentenced to 100 lashes plus fines plus perpetual exile from the kingdom of Navarre, a monstrous punishment: "The sentences are arbitrary," the defendants' lawyer argued, "and my clients are honest members of a family who ask and beg you out of natural pity to show mercy, they are mother and child who naturally are obliged to help and assist one another in such cases." The two women were sent to a cabin or shrine outside the city, and the guard, Bayona, who was a lawyer in the royal tribunals, was also punished with house arrest, which he managed to avoid by paying a fine, as did two other guards, a shearer and a carder, referred to as *personas de poco discurso*; one of them spoke no Spanish. More than eighty days later the family, languishing in their nearby exile, asked that the punishment be lifted, pointing out that they had not gotten sick despite Juan having been in Logroño. The women were allowed to return to Pamplona but Juan was not. The sentence suggests he could have avoided banishment had he accepted an offer to go to the town of Viana, which must have been sick by then, and work there as a salaried *boticario*. Juan chose exile, a remarkable choice in some ways; it may be that he simply feared the plague in Viana, though possibly also it was a signal that he knew he had options, or wished to have an adventure.[54]

During the plague, then, the roads were not empty, even as towns closed in on themselves. There were people delivering messages, seeking information, gathering furtively at the shrines, driving mules, fetching wine from distant cellars, carrying merchandise, or simply illicitly getting out of their infected towns and into their fields or to the local grain mill or visiting friends in the next valley. They were fleeing to safety, both bereft refugees from the north ("Our experience is that most of these diseases come from the many poor who are traveling from Galicia and Asturias," wrote Alonso de Oquendo, corregidor of Arévalo) and well-to-do families and officials on their way to second homes.[55] They were sneaking out, like the young ironsmith Juan Sanz, who was forced to travel

---

[54] AGN TR Procesos 040255, June–September 1599.
[55] AGS-E leg. 183, doc. 303, April 26, 1599.

from Zúñiga to Salvatierra with his master in search of iron; his town punished his father, taking his grain, which a court later ordered to be returned to him.[56] They might have been young adults taking advantage of the crisis to move on. Or they were families hovering in place somewhere until receiving permission to continue their journey or return home. Residents of Bureba villages in Burgos province moved away for a few weeks in 1565, staying in makeshift dwellings until the danger had past, but in the meantime they were someplace else.[57] Their presence and passage offered new occasions for comment and fear; all these people were ambulatory warning signs. They were not to be given hospitality, that most sacred of civic duties and rights. They were outside their town walls but, unlike what Mack Walker describes for Germany in a later period, it was not true that "there and only there [i.e. inside the wall] he was a Burger. Outside he was nobody."[58] These people were not nobodies, but they were in limbo, what could be an informal yet cruel state of exile imposed by quarantine rules. It "smells more of inhumanity than of Christianity," remarked Andosilla, who went on to describe an apocryphal case of a "reasonably rich" man returning home late at night when his mule died, leaving him to walk down unfamiliar roads leading to towns that refused him entry, ending inevitably with the famished and exhausted man surrendering his soul to his Maker.[59]

Despite the extremity of all the cases mentioned until now, to some degree we can still say that these people were on the road by choice, either because they were carrying news or were working or had chosen to go somewhere or needed to get something. Perhaps they would have preferred to stay home, but up to a point the decision was theirs.

But others were on the road because they had been punished. Though a 1595 handbook defined banishment as "one of the worst calamities that exists," it was among the most frequent sanctions by civil, criminal, and Inquisitorial judges.[60] Juan de Nagore had plenty of company. As one small example, a study in Navarre found that of 150 cases of public disorders in the early modern period that reached sentencing, half involved banishment.[61] It was such an ordinary punishment, in fact, that,

---

[56] AGN TR Procesos 120790.   [57] Brumont, *Campo y campesinos*, 84–5.

[58] Mack Walker, *German Home Towns: Community, State, and General Estate, 1648–1871* (Ithaca, NY: Cornell University Press, 1971), 137.

[59] Andosilla Salazar, *Libro en que se prueba con claridad el mal que corre*, 116r–v.

[60] Juan de Aranda, *Lugares comunes de conceptos, dichos, y sentencias, en diversas materias* (Seville: Juan de León, 1595), fol. 25.

[61] Javier Ruiz Astiz, "El castigo de destierro en la Navarra moderna: el caso de los implicados en disórdenes públicos," *UNED: Espacio, Tiempo y Forma*, series IV, Historia moderna, 23 (2010), 129–51. Another little study of Navarre, Amaia Nausia Pimoulier, *Vírgenes o putas? 500 años de adoctrinamiento femenino (1512–2012)*

in a case unrelated to our plague but from the same period (1604), unmarried female stockingmakers in Valladolid were, in theory, punished with 100 lashes and four years' banishment if they plied their skills in public.[62] Nearly all the criminal cases I have seen emerging from the plague and nearly all edicts issued by the crown and municipalities specified that banishment would be the punishment for crimes that endangered the quarantine. Thus the two forms of isolation – banishment and quarantine – to some degree were opposite mechanisms yet both were used to control contagion. One was external exile, the other internal. Had the banishments been carried out, however, it would have been entirely counter-productive, putting people – disobedient people, at that – on the road precisely when they should stay home, like the tavernkeeper Antonio de Burgos, who left Burgos without permission to pick up belongings in Melgar de Fernamental and ended up unable to move in either direction.[63] Residents of Toledo with relatives in pestilent areas of Andalucia in 1582 were threatened with one year of banishment if they accepted letters from the south.[64] In fact, it is logical to think that banishment was hardly ever enforced, either because those with means chose to pay a fine instead, or they paid a border patrol (assuming there was one, which anyway is very unlikely) to say they had crossed over when in fact they hadn't, or they moved to the neighboring village, or they wandered off and later returned (possibly the case with Nagore), or they simply stayed put.[65] This is true not only concerning the plague but also throughout early modern times; it was of no interest whatsover to the Spanish crown to increase vagabondage – on the contrary, it was obsessed with ending it – making the punishment's longevity and ubiquity somewhat of a mystery.

Innkeepers obviously were a crucial component of the Iberian Peninsula's traffic in news and commodities. Brumont cites sources pointing to the frequency with which innkeepers along the Burgos-Miranda-Vitoria route got involved in lawsuits, a sure sign of profitability.[66] According to a 1561 census, in Burgos there were twenty-six innkeepers (*mesoneros*) and fifty tavern keepers (*taberneros*) who also probably had

(San Sebastián: Haran 7, 2012), 24, says women accused of prostitution or sexual crimes were also generally expelled.

[62] AHN CS Libro Alcaldes 1199, fol. 187.   [63] AMB-HI 3653, August 16, 1597.

[64] AGS-CR leg. 115, no. 4, fol. 45.

[65] On the irregularities of banishment see José Luis de las Heras Santos, *La justicia penal de los Austrias en la Corona de Castilla* (Salamanca: Universidad de Salamanca, 1991), 300–1. The crown was far more interested in making punishment useful, for example by sending men to row on the galleys or serve in fortresses.

[66] Brumont, *Campo y campesinos*, 165.

rooms to let; in Valladolid the numbers were twenty-five and twenty-nine, respectively; and in Segovia twenty-three and forty-four.[67] One would think that it would be important that they continue running their businesses, even in the case of bad behavior, but banishment was the preferred punishment. Innkeeper Juan de Buena, for example, was convicted of taking in guests in his town, Berlanga de Duero (Soria) in the autumn of 1599. Buena and his wife, said to have suffered from *secas*, were convicted, fined, made to pay legal costs, stripped of their profession for four years, and given four years of banishment. He appealed and obtained a reduction to two years' exclusion from the town and from the jurisdiction of the marquis of Berlanga, and the fine was reduced. He appealed again, insisting as he had earlier that by the time the alleged crime had taken place the plague had left town, but the Chancillería instead decided to expand the scope of the banishment to include Valladolid and its surroundings, though only for two years, with the other two years left to the discretion of the king, who by then, February 1600, was in Valladolid.[68] Every royal edict implementing plague rules made it clear that innkeepers could not take questionable guests; Madrid's health commission, for example, on May 4, 1601 ordered town criers to spread the word that no inn could take any guests without certification from the city gate testifying they had not been in pestilent areas; punishment for violators was 200 lashes and fines, and if they could not pay then they would get four years' banishment from Madrid and its surroundings.[69] One wonders where the banished innkeepers were supposed to go and how their expulsion could possibly benefit the city. In 1629, when Madrid was again protecting itself from plague, this time in Extremadura, town criers announced that innkeepers lodging guests without safe conducts would be fined, but by then the punishment would be *ten* years' banishment from the *kingdom*.[70] The rule survived at least until 1681, when Madrid innkeepers yet again were threatened with banishment if they lodged travelers from the pestilent south.[71]

But the number of banished individuals paled in comparison with the number of people expelled from their towns, not because of any crime

---

[67] Bennassar, *Valladolid*, 88; Manuel Fernández Álvarez has slightly different figures from the same census, in his "Burgos en el siglo XVI," in *La Ciudad de Burgos: Actas del Congreso de Historia de Burgos. MC Aniversario de la fundación de la ciudad, 884–1984* (León: Junta de Castilla y León, 1985), 221–32, pp. 222–5.

[68] ARCV Registro de Ejecutorías, Caja 1898, 69.

[69] AV Secretaría, 1-138-4, May 4, 1601.

[70] AV Secretaria 1-138-4, September 6, 1629. Butchers selling meat from infected areas were to receive the same punishment.

[71] RAH Jesuitas 9/3746/112. The proclamation was read aloud at all major intersections in the presence of "many people."

they had committed, but because of who they were. Women, for example; in the previous chapter we saw how San Sebastián and Bilbao expelled single women. Soria expelled Portuguese inhabitants because of the "great danger" they signified.[72] Burgos – not a university town but not for lack of trying – expelled students who had petitioned the corregidor about something already in February 1597, but clearly had not made their point, because they were kicked out again in June. This was before the city of Burgos was itself affected by the plague but was busy guarding against the north; the students may have been teenagers from one of many Latin secondary schools and colleges in the region, or possibly from the Universidad de Iratxe (Navarre) or the Universidad Sancti Spiritus in Oñate (Guipúzcoa), a town that six months later, in January 1598, was reported to have more than sixty dead, the result, it was said, of clothing being brought in from San Sebastián. Corregidor Vargas's order read: "Inasmuch as there are many students from the mountains and [other] pestilent places presently in this city and they are in touch with all the people from the other mountains ... [it is ordered] that [the town crier] publicly announce that the said students from the mountains leave the said city within one day and not return until they are allowed to do so ... and that no *vecino* of the said city accept them into their homes ... under penalty of 100 lashes and six years' banishment from this city and 50,000 maravedies ..." Two days later the city's health commission ordered someone to check "if some students have entered [the city] and if they were given lodging by a *vecino*, so they may be punished."[73] And though we cannot really speak of travelers being banished, the fact that in most of Castile, starting in 1597, inns and rooming houses, as well as private homes, were prohibited from taking in guests without airtight passports amounted to another way of ensuring that travelers slept on the road and that hospitality would be denied.

---

[72] Enrique Díez Sanz, *La Tierra de Soria: Un universo campesino en la Castilla oriental del siglo XVI* (Madrid: Siglo Veintiuno, 1995), 50.

[73] AMB-HI 3653. The Oñate information is in AHB-HI 3650, and sixty dead in the very cold month of January is striking. Burgos suggested to Philip II in 1592 that establishing a university there might spur the economy; Paul Hiltpold, "Política paternalista y orden social en la Castilla del Renacimiento," *Cuadernos de Investigación Histórica BROCAR* 13 (1987), 129–40, 136–7, citing city council minutes from September 23. See also Ana-María Carabias Torres, "Estudiantes burgaleses y colegios mayores (siglo XVI)," in *La ciudad de Burgos*, 343–60. On universities in general, see Richard L. Kagan, *Students and Society in Early Modern Spain* (Baltimore, MD: Johns Hopkins University Press, 1974), 42–64. In April 1564, a year before the arrival of a plague moving in from the east, Pamplona expelled a group of its own students who were studying at a secondary school in Huesca and had returned to their parents' homes, and the city threatened to expel the parents as well; Lasaosa Villanua, *El 'Regimiento' municipal*, 251, citing city council minutes.

The main story when it comes to expulsions, however, was the poor, which takes us to one of the most salient ways in which officials had to balance the fundamental tenets of good government in these grim times. The road became the terrain where needs and worth were sorted out and accommodated. To what degree did these expulsions violate rights accorded by natural law to citizens and inhabitants? To what degree did they violate Christian norms? Or simply custom? Charity, sociability, and hospitality are implicit or explicit in virtually all descriptions of how a municipality and the kingdom should function. But so are utility and the common good.

In general, sixteenth-century thinkers and political authorities agreed there was certainly no shame in being poor, a consensus revealed by the fact that every petitioner in the land used poverty as an argument for why their petition should be granted. Nor was there necessarily shame in begging, though sometimes there was. But the plethora of beggars and vagabonds toward the end of the century was among the most visible and disturbing indications that things were going seriously wrong in Spain, and what to do with them was the subject of a rash of treatises toward the end of the century. Most debated how to distinguish the true poor from the false, how to provide charity to the former and training to the latter, and to what degree begging and itineracy were licit. Among the first and certainly among the most important of these treatises was *Deliberación en la causa de los pobres*, by Domingo de Soto, a Dominican and one of the most famous of the Salamanca theologians.[74] Another outstanding figure among the reformers was Philip II's last galleys *proto-médico*, Cristóbal Pérez de Herrera. His ambitious proposal to construct homes or enlightened shelters for the poor and teach them useful skills (ideas already floated in the 1570s by Miguel de Giginta), to which the Cortes responded positively in 1595 and which was being implemented in some cities, did not stand a chance once the plague arrived and the old king died.[75]

---

[74] Domingo de Soto, *Deliberación en la causa de los pobres* (Salamanca: Editorial San Esteban, 2006) [Salamanca, 1545]; on political aspects of Soto see Annabel Brett, *Changes of State: Nature and the Limits of the City in Early Modern Natural Law* (Princeton, NJ: Princeton University Press, 2011), 25–9.

[75] Pérez de Herrera was involved in Madrid's anti-plague campaign and joined those protesting the new king's move to Valladolid. The finished version of his 1595 proposals, the *Discursos*, was published in 1598 and had been supported by the king's royal council. For a brief summary on him see Juan Ignacio Gutiérrez Nieto, "El pensamiento económico, político y social de los arbitristas," in *Historia de la Cultura Española 'Menéndez Pidal'*, José María Jover Zamora, ed., vol. 1, *El Siglo del Quijote* (Madrid: Espasa Calpe, 1996), 348–54. Giginta was a Catalonian cleric; Miguel de Giginta, *Tratado de remedio de pobres*, Féliz Santolaria Sierra, ed. (Barcelona: Ariel

There is never a good time for an epidemic, but this one came at the absolute worst time. The royal treasury had essentially collapsed, with the government continually shifting its dwindling resources around to finance its enormous war expenses, though Philip II finally withdrew in May 1598 from the French Wars of Religion. The towns and villages of Castile were not high on the dying king's list of priorities. Economic historians agree that by the 1590s Castile's population and wealth curves were definitely going downward and that the tendency had begun at least two decades earlier. Prices rose, and there was famine in much of the country. Sterile land and bad weather became commonplaces among treatise writers, and research has shown that their complaints had a basis in science, as it was much cooler that decade throughout Europe, including in Spain, where there was drought in the north and floods in the south.[76] To cite just one example, Burgos in October 1595 told the king that whereas supplies "used to be abundant," trade with the north had essentially come to a standstill, residents of the mountains being so poor that they could not afford to make the trip anymore; the mountain regions "are so destroyed and depopulated ... that they are almost finished," the city council wrote, adding that the plains and port towns were no better off.[77] Even without the plague, therefore, the roads were crowded with people trying to reach someplace where the living was just a bit easier, whether that be another town, a bigger city, an army where one might be fed, or America. The center was emptying out to the benefit of the coastal cities. Meanwhile, very soon after the *"Rodamundo"* docked, Philip II had declared bankruptcy, essentially a rescheduling mechanism to forestall creditors, and the debts had not gone away by the time Philip III ascended to the throne.[78]

Historia, 2000) [Coimbra 1579], a highlight of which is the dialogue on "Some differences between the rich and the poor," 155–7.

[76] Geoffrey Parker, "La crisis de la década de 1590 a debate: Felipe II, sus enemigos y el cambio climático," in *Hacer historia desde Simancas: Homenaje para José Luis Rodríguez de Diego*, Alberto Marcos Martín, ed. (Valladolid: Junta de Castilla y León, 2011), 643–70; also by Parker, *Global Crisis: War, Climate Change and Catastrophe in the Seventeenth Century* (New Haven, CT: Yale University Press, 2013), chapter 9.

[77] Paul Jacob Hiltpold, "Burgos in the Reign of Philip II: the Ayuntamiento, economic crisis, and social control, 1550–1600," PhD diss., University of Texas at Austin, 1981, pp. 310–12, citing Burgos city council minutes from October 30, 1595.

[78] The boat probably docked in the first week of November; bankruptcy was declared at the end of the month. There is an immense bibliography on the demographic crisis during these years, but for two examples from the region we are looking at: Bennassar, *Valladolid*, 199–207, which describes Valladolid towns that lost up to 10 percent of their population to hunger in the 1590s before the plague arrived; and Ramón Sánchez González, "Hambres, pestes y guerras. Elementos de desequilibrio demográfico en la comarca de La Sagra durante la época moderna," *Hispania* 51:2 (1991), 517–58, esp. 521–2, which looks at towns in Toledo. There is evidence that malnutrition and poor

That the poor suffered more than the rich from the plague (and from everything else) was obvious, but it was also obvious to contemporaries that that was not due to any inherent proclivity, other than the proclivity resulting from malnutrition, but rather the result of living conditions and simply because the poor often were the only ones left. As if confirming that assessment, Lic. Varahona wrote in May 1599 from Sepúlveda, "By God's mercy, no one well-nourished has been affected" by the plague.[79] The problem of what to do with the poor is possibly the subject that got the most ink in city council records. "There is no news in this city except fear," the Ávila corregidor wrote to Philip III, "over the great poverty and the miserable people here, among whom there are some who have *calenturas...*" The following month he added, "These are the poorest of the poor, and last year was so sterile, with no bread, and they had no work because the cloth industry is gone, so they are hungry and they fall sick in their houses and in the hospitals."[80] But the point is that they were, indeed, tended to in hospitals. Poverty might determine if someone fell ill, but it was his or her birthplace that would determine if they were allowed to stay. As the north became more and more pestilent, towns further south were faced with the influx; "For more than a year an infinite number of people have been coming down from Galicia and Asturias and the ports where there has been so much plague," wrote Valladolid's doctor, Antonio Ponce de Santa Cruz. "They are hungry and sick, and those who saved their lives have found the doors of pity open to them in Castile and they have mixed in, causing great harm to universal health, and sprinkling so many sick and contagious people in the cities is cause enough for peste right there, at least in Valladolid, where only the poor arrivals and the *pobres naturales* have died..."[81]

---

health increased individuals' risk of dying during a plague epidemic; see especially Andrew B. Appleby, "Disease or famine? Mortality in Cumberland and Westmorland 1580–1640," *The Economic History Review* 26:3 (1973), 403–32, and other articles by the same author; and Ann G. Carmichael, "Plague persistence in Western Europe: a hypothesis," *The Medieval Globe* 1 (2014), 159–92, p. 160. For an introduction to the economic crisis in general see the essays in Thompson and Yun Casalilla, eds., *The Castilian Crisis*; and James Casey, "Spain: a failed transition," in *The European Crisis of the 1590s*, Peter Clark, ed. (London: George Allen and Unwin, 1985), 209–28. On poverty see Linda Martz, *Poverty and Welfare in Habsburg Spain: The Example of Toledo* (Cambridge University Press, 1983); the excellent introduction by Michel Cavillac to Cristóbal Pérez de Herrera, *Amparo de Pobres* (Madrid: Espasa-Calpe, 1975), xcviii–cvi; and, in a different vein, Anne J. Cruz, *Discourses of Poverty: Social Reform and the Picaresque Novel in Early Modern Spain* (Toronto: University of Toronto Press, 1999).

[79] AGS-E leg. 183, doc. 254.

[80] AGS-E leg. 183, doc. 316, August, 18 1599; AGS-E leg. 183 doc. 311, September 1, 1599.

[81] Antonio Ponce de Santa Cruz, *Tractado de las causas y curacion de las fiebres con secas pestilenciales que han oprimido a Valladolid y otras ciudades de España* (Valladolid: Pedro de Merchan Calderón, 1600), 33r–4r.

The native poor, the *pobres naturales*, in theory were assured of health care. The poor from elsewhere, in contrast, the *pobres foresteros* who had plodded down the roads, should not have been there in the first place. Those already there were evicted, though usually towns gave them alms at the gate before sending them on their way and there was no guarantee they would not come back. From Segovia the lieutenant corregidor, Lic. Arce de Salazar told the king that poor people who were not from Segovia had been expelled.[82] (Arce de Salazar was taking the place of the corregidor, Íñigo de Cárdenas y Zapata, who had left or abandoned his post; just two months after Arce wrote these words, the city council rebelled against him for telling Madrid the truth about Segovia's bad health.[83]) Toledo also expelled poor outsiders.[84] In Bilbao, at the same time as the city expelled single and unemployed women who were not natives it also announced that non-native beggars (*pobres mendigantes*) had three days to leave.[85] And when Dr. Luis Mercado and his colleagues gave Philip III their assessments in April 1599, they were quite specific as to what Madrid should do with its poor: "We note the danger of this disease lasting a long time and growing as a result of the many newly arrived poor, be they sick or healthy vagabonds, and to prohibit and remedy this each parish should appoint six honorable and charitable people each month who visit every corner and house of each parish and discover who the *pobres naturales* are and give them alms from the said parish and help them so they do not fall ill, and outsiders [*forasteros*] should be given sufficient alms and then expelled, suffering enormous [*grandíssimas*] punishments if they return."[86]

Burgos moved quickly to deal with the problem. In late January 1597, one month after it learned about the plague in Santander, the city council or the health commission drew up a list of all the poor people to be thrown out. Each person was named along with the amount of maravedies they were being given (ranging from nothing to sixty-eight) and their birthplace. There were fifteen men and sixty-two women. There was no indication if they were married or had children. The

---

[82] AGS-E leg. 183, doc. 297, May 3, 1599.

[83] AGS-E leg. 183, doc. 322, July 24, 1599. Cárdenas y Zapata served simultaneously as Madrid's *alferez mayor*, or standard-bearer.

[84] Julián Montemayor, "Una ciudad frente a la peste: Toledo a fines del XVI," in *La ciudad hispánica durante los siglos XIII al XVI: actas del coloquio celebrado en La Rábida y Sevilla del 14 al 19 septiembre de 1981*, Emilio Sáez, et al., eds., 3 vols. (Madrid: Universidad Complutense, 1985), 1113–31, p. 1120, cites no source but probably AMT. Two examples from the present-day province of Madrid are Valdemoro, on March 4, 1598, AMVal Sig. 2547-1; and Chinchón in 1562, AGS-CR leg. 115, no. 4.

[85] AFB libro 023, January 21, 1598.   [86] AGS-E leg. 183, doc. 279.

corregidor, Gerónimo de Montalvo (Vargas's predecessor), in order to make sure they really did exit the city, ordered that they be accompanied outside the gates by *alguaciles* along with the inevitable notary to record the event.[87] In March 1599, by which time the plague had made its way inside the walls, the city council (now led by Francisco de Valencia, the deceased Vargas's lieutenant) agreed that the poor be divided up among the more prosperous residents (*vecinos de calidad*) to be fed. The city also decided to once again expel the poor from elsewhere, giving most of them each four reales – though some got up to twenty, depending on how far they had to go – a measure that even one of the regidores admitted three months later was useless: "Thus the city was cleaned of the poor although later they all came back, and today there is nearly as much disorder as before."[88] When he wrote these words, as the disease reached its peak, poor people were streaming into the city's extramuros hospital from all over the region. So many had arrived at the doors of its hospital in San Martín de la Bodega, today a district of the city, that they could not fit and were milling around the area set aside for convalescents. This prevented the city from carrying out its obligation to "cure the poor of the city who are sick here," the health commission noted, reiterating that no outsiders should be treated and that the native poor must possess signed certificates.[89] A year later, after Burgos had mistakenly concluded that all was safe only to see the disease return to some of its surrounding towns, the city revisited the matter of what to do with the poor, reaching an agreement to "cure the poor of the city suffering from buboes because of peste and then treat outsiders in the San Juan hospital." The majority voted "that the poor suffering from buboes in this city *who are vecinos and who were born here [naturales]* should be treated, and that those who came from elsewhere not be treated unless those of the city have been treated."[90]

The categories being invoked here are worth commenting upon. The poor who were not being expelled and who could receive medical treatment were referred to as *vecinos and naturales,* which in fact were different things, though definitions were hazy. Certainly one did not automatically imply the other. Generally, one requested to be a *vecino,* or citizen, which entailed a series of municipal, fiscal, and judicial privileges and obligations. It was a formal procedure and a legal status. A *natural,* on the other hand, was usually someone born in a specific place. There was no effort

---

[87] AMB-HI 3653.
[88] AMB-LA-130, March 2, 1599; Brumont, "La peste de 1599," 163.
[89] AMB-HI 3653, July 30, 1599.
[90] AMB-LA 131, fols. 228v–9r, July 13, 1600. My emphasis.

or merit involved, and birthplace did not necessarily entitle one to citizenship, though it might entitle one to better treatment or certain jobs. An outsider also could request to become a *natural*, even though this naturalization defies the very definition of the term. In the case of plague expulsions, two concepts seem to have been important for deciding who could stay and who would go: birthplace (though not every *natural* necessarily was born there, and someone born there who behaved badly might not be considered a *natural*) and citizenship (via *vecindad*). Thus towns were taking care of their own, weighing both passive and active virtues, and "vecino" assumed its modern definition of "neighbor." The poor were not being expelled because they constituted some shadowy threat or cosmic menace. Nor were they being moved as "an act of propitiation," as Brian Pullan wrote of Venice; officials there may have been appeasing God, but Castilians were satisfying law and custom.[91] The poor were not regarded as "the other," and in fact people whom one might think did fit that definition, such as gypsies or moriscos (Muslims or former Muslims), are rarely or never mentioned in the documents I handled. The official who led the clean-up of Alcalá de Henares, for example, reported that poor moriscos were said to be hiding bed linens or clothing and many had therefore died, but there was no animosity in the statement, and the same thing was said everywhere else about the poor in general. A sharper report from Ávila, where around 1,000 moriscos had been resettled after the Alpujarras uprising in 1570, remarked that some of the dead were moriscos "from Granada, and being that they are moriscos one can't find out the truth."[92] But the plague, as far as one can tell, was not a moment for scapegoating; indeed, Pamplona hired four moriscos to carry the sick and the dead.[93] The poor were sent away because or if they were outsiders, or possibly insiders whom no one wanted, but in any case a drain on the economy. It was not that they were different but that they were, in a way, a disappointment. As with all other social and taxonomic distinctions in early modern Castilian society,

[91] Brian Pullan, "Plague and perceptions of the poor in early modern Italy," in *Epidemics and Ideas: Essays on the Historical Perception of Pestilence*, Terence Ranger and Paul Slack, eds. (Past and Present Publications, Cambridge University Press, 1992), 101–23, p. 102. Italian historians also frequently comment on charitable treatment of the sick poor as a way for cities to expiate their sins; nothing like that appears in Spanish documents.
[92] The moriscos would, of course, all be expelled during the reign of Philip III. On Alcalá, RAH Jesuitas 9-3662/182; on Ávila, AGS-E leg. 183, doc. 311.
[93] José Ramón Cruz Mundet, *"El mal que al presente corre": Gipuzkoa y la peste (1597–1600)* (San Sebastián: Kutxa Fundazioa, 2003), 72, citing AMP Sanidad, ser. Epidemias, peste bubónica, leg. 1, no. 2.

dividing lines were blurred, though they were deployed by municipal authorities as if they were clear.[94]

Like Burgos, Valladolid began by making lists of the poor to be expelled onto the roads, or wherever, though it began later. The Council of Castile in mid-August 1597 had given the city instructions about the poorhouse, which may have been linked to the poor-reform efforts in the waning days of Philip II's reign, though it might also have been linked to plague preparations, as by then the north was seriously infected. In order to draw up a census of the *pobres mendigantes*, a town crier was dispatched to instruct everyone "to gather at the city mint on Thursday the 25th of [September] at one in the afternoon so a list can be made ... and the poor and beggars will be given a certificate [*señal*] and the rest shall be expelled from Valladolid as the [Council of Castile] orders." A week later the corregidor reported success. The poor who were truly *pobres mendigantes* could stay, but the rest, "who were fine and healthy and outsiders were expelled from this city." So the roll of the city's poor could now be revised. Another summons appears to have been issued for the poor to gather on a Sunday in late October under pain of exile (which was going to happen to them anyway, so it was not much of an incentive to show up) and the operation was repeated. According to Bennassar, 310 people were now recognized as being truly in need, and they received a certificate and their names were added to the parish and shelter lists. The rest were expelled.[95]

At that point, Valladolid was still healthy. By May 1599 that was not the case, and so the poor were expelled yet again. With the poor dying on city streets, the city council ordered that beds and linens be sent to hospitals so the sick poor at least would have a place to go.[96] On May 24 they met again "to discuss the hospitality which this city must give the poor sick who are here," deciding they should go to San Lázaro and San Bartolomé hospitals, where they would be given beds and assistance, all to be paid for with the 4,000 ducats that Philip III had said the city could collect through a *sisa* on wine and meat. But that was not enough, so once again the town crier was told to summon the poor. This time the

---

[94] Tamar Herzog, "Los Naturales de España: Entre el Viejo y Nuevo Mundo," in *De la Republica Hispaniae: Una vindicación de la cultura política en los reinos ibéricos en la primera modernidad*, Francisco José Aranda Pérez and José Damião Rodriguez, eds. (Madrid: Silex Universidad, 2008), 409–22; also her book, *Defining Nations: Immigrants and Citizens in Early Modern Spain and Spanish America* (New Haven, CT: Yale University Press, 2003).

[95] AMVA sig. 22-0, September 22, 1597, October 1, 1597, October 24, 1597; also Bennassar, *Valladolid*, 437.

[96] AMVA sig. 21-0, May 7, 1599, May 24, 1599.

gathering place was on the other side of the Rio Mayor bridge at eight in the morning. There, officials would separate the sick to be taken to hospital from the healthy, who were told to leave, with some "appropriate" pocket money. The following month the city asked the king if they could increase the *sisa* to 8,000 ducats, otherwise they would not be able to maintain the San Lázaro hospital.[97] This was the summer when the Chancillería took over the city council's administrative functions, and chief judge Junco de Posada wrote to Philip III on August 7, 1599 describing how poor and starving people from throughout Castile, Vizcaya, and Galicia had made their way into the city the previous summer and winter. He urged the city to expel the poor who could work, tend to those who were sick, and distribute the healthy poor unable to work, some 1,300 of them, among the city's citizens. Unlike Burgos, which distributed the poor among the comfortable to be fed, it appears Valladolid also intended for them to get lodging.[98]

A few months later, in late fall, the plague had subsided, but expulsions continued into 1600. Burgos decided that "beggar people who are not *vecinos* and *naturales*" [note the "and"] had three days in which to leave "to live and reside in other lands." Once again the poor were gathered, and somehow a determination was made as to those who were truly *vecinos* and *naturales*; those people were given a lead insignia showing where they were from, and the rest were given alms and sent off. Commissioner Pedro del Castillo, whom we last saw riding around small towns supervising the quarantine, now was charged with removing poor people who were not carrying the valuable insignia. That was in January; in April, long after the last plague victim had been buried, the campaign continued, with the city asking the prior at the Caridad confraternity, located in Nuestra Señora de Vejarrua, to stop giving shelter at night to everyone who was poor; instead, a selection should be made of those who were *vecinos* and *naturales*, and the rest should be expelled to join their brethren on the road. The messengers and envoys had long since gone home, but for the poor, at least for those from someplace else, the road still loomed.[99]

Almost by definition, nearly all stories about how the plague began in a given place involved someone coming from elsewhere. It was a traveler, a vendor, a vagabond, someone expelled from someplace else. Often it was a woman carrying cloth or a man seeking lodging. Travelers brought news and essential products, and they also brought disease. By tradition they were to be welcomed; now they were to be feared. We have a small, vivid example from Cogollos, the town that received shoes from the corregidor: Burgos authorities told Philip II on July 4, 1597 that "it is said that [the disease] reached Cogollos with some men who arrived there one afternoon from Santander, and in the inn where they stayed they said they had not slept in a bed all along their journey from Santander, and it is remarkable that in the inn where they stayed the illness did not stick, but it did in the tavern where they had lunch or dinner, where just a few days later three members of the same household died and two children who were there when they lunched also died because the men from Santander had given the children a bit of cake, and next in another nearby house three or four more people died, and so the illness passed to other *vecinos* in the said place, and since last Christmas until the end of June thirty-six people have died in Cogollos."[100] But during much of those six months of tenacious infection (before Vargas's arrival, it must be pointed out), Burgos, just a few miles up the road, apparently had been in the dark, though it immediately tried to make up for lost time. Cogollos had been deliberately secretive, Vargas told the king, which was why Burgos's attempts at information-gathering had been fruitless until the death toll reached such a point that there was no possibility anymore of hiding the dreadful truth. Churchmen were dispatched to order the town priest to open up his registry where the dead were listed. The churchmen were followed by a surgeon and, naturally, a notary. Until then, there had been rumors, sightings of houses where no one remained, suggestions in May not to tie up one's horses in a given spot, but the news was neither reliable nor were the city's orders obeyed. No one from Santander was supposed to enter Cogollos in the first place – or anywhere else, for that matter. Such a disaster could happen only if there were no guards at the town gates or if the guards were not doing their job properly. The cloth vendors, the refugees, the poor from elsewhere, the muleteers, and the messengers all had to talk their way through barriers, and it was at the gate, by the wall, where a traveler's right to enter was determined.

---

[100] AMB-HI 3653, July 4, 1597. As Cogollos is just south of the city of Burgos, it is likely that the infected travelers from the north also went through the larger town.

Site 3: Wall

One messenger who never made it past a city wall was Francisco de Nanclares, the chief city council notary from Burgos, who in late April 1599 knocked on Valladolid's Santa Clara gate with letters from his city about plague precautions there.[1] He remained outside for two days, during which time the Valladolid city council took care of him, spending fifty-nine reales on his upkeep. The man in charge of the gate was Diego de Caranda, a member of the city council. Nanclares and his servant ate two meals a day and slept in the home of a woman who lived in the nearby countryside. They rented two beds, which were transported from an inn to the woman's house. There was a load of hay and eight *celemines* of barley for their two horses. Rather than showing gratitude for this treatment, however, Burgos was shocked at the libel implicit in other cities' hasty conclusions about its state of health. "No one anywhere will take in [people from Burgos]. Instead, they receive them with spears, insolence, ferocity, and blind ignorance as if it were true that the city is pestilent," the aggrieved lieutenant corregidor, Francisco de Valencia, and his city's doctors wrote to the king. They admitted that "more than" eighty people had died in the past three months; that same week the figure was raised to 120. But the disease was not true peste ("people are dying there but it's not peste," a recipient wrote on the cover page), and thus it was unjust for Valladolid and other places to cut off communications.[2] Around a year earlier, in contrast, Valladolid had welcomed a messenger from Melgar de Fernamental, which had finally managed to be removed from the list of pestilent places. That man, named Diego González de Paredes, was allowed to enter all the towns on his route until reaching Madrid, where not only was he not allowed in, he was fined for insisting repeatedly that he had to give the Council of Castile a pile of papers about the alleged good health in his town.[3]

---

[1] AMVA sig. 21-0, April 30, 1599; also AMVA-CH 130 a-4 (ant. leg. 321), fol. 174.
[2] AGS-E leg. 183, doc. 223, May 4, 1599. A *celemin* was a dry measure of around 4.6 liters.
[3] AMB-HI 3650, July 29, 1598.

The Partidas proclaimed, "The walls and the gates of cities and of towns are called holy things."[4] But the walls surrounding, or almost surrounding, most Castilian towns and cities in the late sixteenth century bore little resemblance to the massive structures we see today around former fortress and border towns. Walls were often incomplete and they tended to crumble, as they were made of limestone and other shoddy materials. As decades went by, people built homes and shops within and atop the walls and then had to negotiate their rights of tenancy when plague arrived, as it inevitably did. The moats, if there were moats, or the space surrounding the barrier were sometimes filled with garbage. Many towns had no walls at all, or only in certain areas, making it easy to gain access. On June 9, 1597, a city as important as Valladolid sent city council members out to survey the city's boundaries to decide where to put up the barriers (*cercas*), which could have been fences or stone walls; judging from laborers' invoices, they were both.[5] Segovia in the 1650s placed or built a total of 1,065 *tapias* (walls or barriers) throughout the city along with sixteen doors or gates, some of them large, in order to "prevent peste in the city."[6] Ávila, today synonymous with its enormous and complete walls, also had to patch together a means of protection. In August 1597 the city approved a *sisa* "to build *tapias* to encircle the city and its outskirts" so as to defend itself from the Santander plague. Again, this "tapia" had little to do with today's "muro"; it was made of clay, was constantly being knocked down, and it encompassed not only the city but the surrounding towns, making it susceptible to widespread tinkering and damage.[7] Even Ávila's main wall itself was not secure, and there, as was often the case, it was the clergy who challenged barriers as a way of resisting the inconvenience of quarantine; during an earlier epidemic in 1518, after the city council had ordered small, unofficial doorways in the great wall to be blocked, the clergy protested and a door was burned down. The culprit must have been obvious, for the city straightaway called upon Charles V, the Council of Castile, and the archbishop of Santiago to excommunicate the Ávila cathedral chapter, a dispute that

---

[4] Partidas III, tit. 28, law 15, "Santas cosas son llamadas los muros et las puertas de las ciudades e de las villas."

[5] AMVA sigs. 22-1 and 22-0.

[6] Manuela Villalpando Martinez, "Un brote de peste en la Segovia de 1653," *Estudios Segovianos* 38 (1997), 17–26. The author cites AMS sig. J-2510, "Tapias para evitar la peste en la ciudad," from 1655; the project entailed payments for guards, laborers, wood, clothing, and rope-soled sandals (*alpargatas*).

[7] Serafin de Tapia, "Los factores de la evolución demográfica de Ávila en el Siglo XVI," *Cuadernos Abulenses* 5 (January–June 1986), 169, citing Libro 24 of the actas, now missing.

naturally lasted years.[8] In our plague, another man of the cloth else-where, Lic. Paez (who also was a professor of grammar), thrashed a guard with the man's own staff, prompting the corregidor to complain to the Council of Castile, which told the Burgos cathedral chapter to take appropriate measures and report back.[9]

Walls – I am calling them walls even if they might have been less imposing barriers – traditionally defined cities and protected them. In the words of James Tracy, a city wall "is almost of necessity a symbol of sovereign power, because no government of more than nominal authority will permit the massive mobilization of labor and capital that wall build-ing requires to proceed without its approval. At the same time, the well-ordered city is in many cultures the symbol of a larger cosmic order, and perfectly constructed walls can be the token of this earthly perfection that has meaning beyond itself."[10] But by the late sixteenth century in Castile, not only were they not as physically ubiquitous as before, their meaning had somewhat dissolved along with the limestone. Spain in general fought its wars elsewhere, a convenience that meant barriers were of more commercial than military concern.[11] They stood for security and peace, and also were a physical reminder of *vecindad*. The word generally is translated as citizenship, but etymologically it also refers to a place, in some ways a less stringent definition. As was seen with the expulsions of the non-native poor, inhabitants of a given town included *vecinos* (with privileges and obligations), *naturales* (who were born there), *moradores* (simple denizens), and *forasteros* (outsiders), but all these categories had slippage. There were people on the outside who were *vecinos*; maybe they were wealthy and had another house, or they were vendors or shepherds or farmers or envoys, but they still belonged to their place. Likewise, some inhabitants inside the walls were not truly members, though, if need be, they would use the language of community to demonstrate their deep attachment. Walls, even if they were not mighty stone structures,

---

[8] Gonzalo Martín García, "Las murallas en la Edad Moderna: obras de mantenimiento y nuevas construcciones," in *La Muralla de Ávila* (Madrid: Fundación Caja Madrid, 2003), 115–82, p. 139, citing August 1518 actas, today probably in AHMA.

[9] BL Eg. 356, vol. 2, fol. 391, November 17, 1597.

[10] James D. Tracy, introduction to his edited volume, *City Walls: The Urban Enceinte in Global Perspective* (Cambridge University Press, 2000), 5. Also in that volume see Richard L. Kagan, "A world without walls: city and town in colonial Spanish America," 117–52; elsewhere see Julio Valdeon Baruque, "Reflexiones sobre las murallas urbanas de la Castilla medieval," in *Estudios de historia medieval en homenaje a Luis Suarez Fernandez* (Valladolid: Universidad de Valladolid, 1991), 509–22.

[11] After the Christianization of the Muslim north, completed more or less in the eleventh century, there were aristocratic civil wars in the fifteenth century and the comuneros uprising in 1520. Not until the arrival of Napoleon's troops would the meseta see more warfare.

defined both those on the inside and those on the outside, but it is safe to say that the stark difference between those groups was diminishing as Castile entered the seventeenth century. A visible mark of this ambiguity during the epidemic was the area just outside the wall where Francisco de Nanclares of Burgos and Diego González de Paredes of Melgar waited to be heard and where poor, sick people streaming in from elsewhere hovered. During the plague, the area immediately outside the perimeter seems to have acquired its own identity as an intermediate, in-between place. The city council of Soria, tacitly acknowledging that the other side of the wall was a new fixture of the city's geography, in July 1599 ordered "that there always be bread and wine at the gate."[12] In many cities there were new marketplaces where those who could not get in could buy and sell; the city council of Burgos, alerted that hosiers and other enterprising craftsmen were doing business with migrants from the infected north just outside the wall, ordered them to stop immediately.[13] The space was also the site of religious ministrations and medical treatment, though one doctor stuck outside, Lic. Pérez, complained to Burgos that his contract with the city had not mentioned anything about not being able to enter. At least, he said, he should get a raise – which he did.[14]

Again and again and again, city council minutes during the years of epidemic record instructions and payments to city officials and laborers to repair walls. Caring for walls was an eloquent act of caring for one's community; it was also a perpetual task. Jerónimo Castillo de Bovadilla, whose massive guide for corregidores was published in 1597, said that, according to law, if a city did not have funds with which to pay for repairs, "*vecinos* and the clergy and the Churches and the villages and towns that find shelter there or use their fields and outsiders who have property there must all contribute. And in times of need, nobles and others with privileges must work with their hands in the building and repair of walls … Princes must oversee and exactly supervise [this work] and if they do not, great deformities will arise, with walls breached [*aportilladas*] and dismantled on the ground…"[15] There are no records during these years of noblemen rolling up their sleeves, though they

---

[12] Enrique Díez Sanz, *La Tierra de Soria: Un universo campesino en la Castilla oriental del siglo XVI* (Madrid: Siglo Veintiuno, 1995), 48–54; quote is from July 5, 1599 city council minutes. However Soria apparently was not too welcoming, as a Toledo cloth and silk merchant, Tomás de la Fuente, waited more than thirty days in Burgos for the Sorian corregidor to grant him entry; he must have gotten fed up and tried to enter anyway and was stopped on June 9, an event recorded in the minutes.

[13] AMB-HI 3653, August 13, 1597.   [14] AMB-HI 3653, March 13, 1599.

[15] Jerónimo Castillo de Bovadilla, *Política para corregidores y señores de vasallos*, vol. 2 (Madrid: Instituto de Estudios de Administración Local, 1978, facs. of Antwerp: Juan Bautista Verdussen, 1704), 314.

contributed in other ways. And the walls were a windfall for many. Locksmiths supplied locks; blacksmiths supplied hinges and bolts, masons and bricklayers built (and rebuilt) clay walls, painters painted. In Valladolid someone was hired to place a fourteen-foot wooden panel over a gate to ensure people would not sneak underneath; the panel cost three reales.[16] In the same city, Pedro del Aro, a master builder, submitted an invoice for four reales for wood for some gates, one real to the laborer who carried the wood, four iron braces, four pounds of fasteners, the labor of four journeymen craftsmen, plus two additional wooden panels.[17] A carpenter, Juan de la Fragua, then submitted a bill for repairing what would appear to be the same set of gates.[18] A laborer named Gabriel de Hermosilla built a fireplace in the guard house at one of the gates, and a mason said he had built no fewer than 185 tapias.[19]

If workers were repeatedly fixing the walls, that was because town inhabitants were repeatedly damaging them so as to avoid going the long way around, a practice uninhibited by threats of whipping. Once the plague and Philip III had left Madrid and the former capital was concerned only with guarding against the south, it began using fines for plague-related infractions to pay for repairs and guards. On May 23, 1602, city council member Silva de Torres noted at the council meeting that "the barriers of this city are being broken and ruined by the same people who live next to them so they can more easily reach their fields by not having to go around to the gates, and though this city is paying for closing and walling off the barriers, they break them again." The council decided to send a policeman accompanied by a notary to all the streets near the barrier, "and in each street six *vecinos* living closest to the barrier will be appointed to watch over it to ensure no one destroys it, and if it is destroyed, it will be restored at their expense."[20] A detailed thirteen-page ledger from early 1602 describes walls that were patched, keys replaced, and wooden panels installed so that lists of pestilent towns could be posted on them. All cities struggled with the incessant appearance of *portillos*, which also means back doors (also called *puertas falsas*), the impromptu gateways that allowed people to move around. The Madrid ledger mentions *portillos* on Calle de Embajadores, Santa Barbara, Calle de Lavapies, the Atocha walls, the Puerta de Alcalá, and by the Colegio de Doña María de Aragón (today the Senate); all the *portillos* were demolished and the walls rebuilt, and all expenses were paid from

[16] AMVA-CH 9-7 (ant. leg. 287), fol. 1.   [17] AMVA-CH 136-3 (ant. leg. 338).
[18] AMVA-CH 130 a-4 (ant. leg. 321), fol. 4.
[19] AMVA-CH 130 a-4 (ant. leg. 321), fols. 115, 154–7.
[20] AV Secretaría 1-138-4, May 23, 1602.

fines (*condenaciones*), the causes of which are not described.[21] Like carrying messages from one town to another, repairs were a potentially lucrative opportunity, a seller's market during lean times, and town leaders were aware of the potential for fraud. For that reason, the Ávila city council resolved in July 1601, when the city also was protecting itself against the south, that any work done on the barrier must be subject to open bids. The announcement of the job would be cried aloud by the town crier, with the bidding to take place nine days later, overseen by health commissioners and justice officials. This procedure would take place "with any job, no matter how small, and if it is done otherwise it will not count and the city will not pay."[22]

Walls were the physical embodiment of a town's limits, though not necessarily of its jurisdiction, but it was the guards who decided who would come in and who could go out. They also were paid, and at the very first news that plague had affected the north, cities throughout Castile set up shifts of guards and imposed *sisas* to cover the expense. But the taxes were never enough, and throughout the duration of the epidemic towns and cities repeatedly had to ask the crown for more money to pay them. Madrid's practice toward the end of paying them with fines obviously was an incentive to arrest and convict alleged wrongdoers. But aside from putting strains on municipal finance, the establishment and maintenance of a corps of guards raised important questions regarding privilege and obligation. Castillo de Bovadilla said the clergy was obliged to participate in guard duty if the city was in danger and must also contribute money to build and/or repair walls.[23] Long before that, the Partidas said the clergy had to guard if Moors or other enemies were besieging the town; though they were considered eligible, I have not found any doing rounds.[24] All city councilmen shared in guard duty, however, and so did some noblemen. A Madrid ledger of guard duty in 1598 listed parishes and their residents, including nobility; the Duke of Infantazgo, the count of Melgar, the marquis of Falces, the prince of Salerno, and several Mendozas show up, either because they themselves participated (doubtful in some cases) or because they were involved in the organization. In Madrid, as in most large places, some guards stood by gates while others circled on horseback. Shifts varied and could last for days if they slept in the guard huts.[25] Pamplona bought a

---

[21] AV Secretaría, 1-138-4.   [22] AHMA Libros de Actas, no. 26, f. 150r.

[23] Castillo de Bovadilla, *Política para corregidores*, vol. 1, 616–17.

[24] Partida 1, Tit. VI, law 52.

[25] AV Secretaría 1-138-1; Alfredo Alvar Ezquerra, "Estructuras socioeconómicas de Madrid y su entorno en la segund mitad del siglo XVI," PhD diss., Universidad Complutense de Madrid, 1988, 549–50.

horse which was shared by city council members who rode around the city's perimeter.[26] Toro also had guards on horseback; one of them, Diego de Medrano, was given orders on April 23, 1599 to rise at dawn and begin circling the city checking to make sure there were no *portillos* or other anomalies, and he was to continue on horseback until nightfall when the gates were closed, ensuring that no one enter on a path or over the wall or in some other manner. If he caught anyone, he had authority to arrest them and take them to jail.[27] Burgos appointed four of its city council members to each be in charge of two or more of the city's gates, which we saw above was also the practice in Valladolid.[28] The Valladolid city council, however, in June 1598 appears to have had trouble persuading all its members to guard and, as a result, it agreed that one of its more voluntarist members should ask Don Diego de Enríquez, presumably part of the clan of the mighty Dukes of Medina de Rioseco, and the other titled nobility in the city to help with guard duty, "because once the *caballeros* [councilors] see them guarding, everyone will do it, and [the city] will be well guarded."[29] Two months later the council minutes state that everyone was at last doing guard duty, but now the councilors were going home to sleep, leaving keys in the hands of the less distinguished members of the guard corps, resulting in "many improprieties," to which end the council resolved that "in the four gates through which people enter and leave this city there must be four gentlemen from this *ayuntamiento* in each one, starting tomorrow, Tuesday the 18th of this month of August, and they must remain at the said doors day and night and sleep there."[30] Gabriel de Hermosilla's fireplace would have to keep them warm, though in August that probably was not necessary.

Guards in all towns and cities had pretty much the same tasks. The nine-point instructions approved by Valladolid in September 1597 are among the clearest, though there are contradictions. Guards should not admit travelers on foot or on horseback or clothing or merchandise from towns on the list; they should not admit pilgrims (*romeros*) or poor people or anyone else suspicious, even if they had a safe-conduct, unless they were a known *vecino* and had not been gone more than two days; they

---

[26] Santiago Lasaosa Villanua, *El 'Regimiento' municipal de Pamplona en el siglo XVI* (Pamplona: CSIC, 1979), 348n90.

[27] RBP II-2163 doc. 241, "Ordenanza de las funciones a desempeñar…"

[28] BL Eg. 356, vol. 2, fol. 337, "Papel tocante a lo que se aze en Burgos…" an 8-page report by regidor Andrés de Cañas, one of the regidores on guard duty and the subsequent chronicler of the Burgos health efforts, transcribed in Francis Brumont, "La peste de 1599 en Burgos, una relación del regidor Andrés de Cañas," *BROCAR: Cuadernos de Investigación Histórica* 13 (1987), 155–66.

[29] AMVA sig. 21-0, June 23, 1598.

[30] AMVA sig. 21-0, August 17, 1598; a longer version appears in sig. 22-0.

must request a safe-conduct or clean bill of health from all travelers on foot and horseback showing where they had been, and if the travelers did not have notarized testimony they could not enter, and if they had testimony they should be asked if they had been someplace on the list, and if they replied that they had then they could not enter; guards should start their shift at noon and not leave until 10 p.m., when the gate was closed, and they should keep the key and not give it to anyone except the commissioner in charge of that gate. (This rule also states that city councilmen should start their shifts at 5 a.m.). Travelers with a proper pass book should have it stamped so they could find lodging; in case of dubious testimony, the traveler should not be allowed in until the gate commissioner or corregidor was consulted and the traveler's papers further scrutinized. Guards, be they city council members or ordinary residents, along with an *alguacil*, could arrest anyone violating gate orders, but the culprits would not be held in Valladolid; rather, they were to be sent back to their own town, or the town they came from. (The mechanics of this operation are unclear.) Anyone trying to enter with eggs or fowl or fish must bring notarized testimony of where the products were bought; and people with testimony lacking a statement from a notary that the person had lived twenty days or longer in the town he or she was coming from could not enter.[31]

The word most often used for what we would call a passport or safe-conduct was *testimonio*, a way of evoking the fact that someone had essentially spoken on behalf of someone, authenticating that they had been in a certain place and had come from a certain other place. The word echoes the role of orality, albeit virtual, in Castilian political life. These papers were not called *documentos* or *salvaconductas*. Though it is hard to believe that someone was not making good money with bad papers, the fact is that no such case has emerged in the archives I worked in, nor were there instances of people pretending to be someone else or showing papers with fraudulent stamps. Most often, controversies at the gate came from discussions over whether the town(s) listed were healthy or pestilent, disagreements which put to test the quality of information in the hands of the guards and their interest in abusing their own power. Guards cared less about the identity of the person than about where he, or occasionally she, had been.

Keeping track of gate keys was obviously crucial and apparently not easy. Castillo de Bovadilla included detailed instructions on the handling of keys in besieged cities, which is relevant inasmuch as more than one

---

[31] AMVA-CH 99-19 (ant. leg. 249), September 4, 1597.

person during these years spoke of the plague as an outside enemy. Keys should be in the hands of the corregidor, the castle governor, or the most senior city council member, "according to custom," he wrote. But in cases of squabbles, as many locks should be used as there were squabblers, all of the locks being attached to the same large latch which would encompass all the other locks with yet another lock and key, which would be guarded by the highest-ranking person, who would be the first to open it. And in the case of further jealousy or opposition, "it is a good idea to give the main key to someone different every night so that uncertainty puts an end to these thoughts."[32] Faulty security was a recurring issue. In Burgos someone named Pedro de Torrequemada who lived outside the city asked for copies of the keys, which he was given along with instructions not to share them with anyone and to not open the gate for anyone outside his household.[33] Nine months later, probably because the honor system was not working, Burgos decided to remove keys from the gates altogether, presumably keeping them with trusted officials, and to not make any more keys. It was then that the city also decided to use stone or clay, rather than wood, for the *tapias*.[34] In a long and complicated lawsuit in Bilbao filed by two sisters claiming they did not have to participate in a city-wide assessment to pay plague expenses, among the dozens of accusations aired was that a city council member had changed the locks (or the keys) of one of the city gates, to which the aggrieved councilor replied that he had that duty because private citizens had somehow obtained their own keys.[35] And in Valladolid, a problem developed in the summer of 1598 with individuals charged with collecting certain taxes; they possessed copies of the keys and were sharing them liberally without proper authorization from the gate commissioners, as a result of which merchandise and wine had entered the city without testimony of provenance. So the city decided to change the locks and keys and to add a new lock, the keys for which would be held only by town councilors, who would take them home with them at night. The guards had to sleep at their posts and anyone violating this rule would be fired. But given the excruciating need for guards, one has to assume that they were not, in fact, dismissed, but simply fined, the better with which to offset plague expenses.[36]

In Segovia one of the log books kept by guards during the plague has survived.[37] It lists those who entered the city through the Cal de Gascos

[32] Castillo de Bovadilla, *Política para corregidores*, book 4, chapter 2, no. 19.
[33] AMB-HI 3653, January 7, 1597.   [34] AMB-HI 3653, September 3, 1597.
[35] ARCV Registro de Ejecutorías, Caja 1990, 6. We will return to this lawsuit.
[36] AMVA sig. 22-0, July 20, 1598.   [37] AMS leg. 456/1.

gate in 1598, though not those who were turned away. Possibly the absence of the latter means no one was refused entry, but that is unlikely. The book opens with instructions from the corregidor, Íñigo de Cárdenas y Zapata, who soon left the city, more or less echoing the Valladolid instructions above, stipulating that guards were to work in pairs from 4 a.m. to 10 p.m. and that violations would be punished "rigorously." The book also includes ever-changing lists of off-limits towns that the guards consulted as people appeared at the gate. Some came alone, others came in groups. On June 28, for example, guards Juan Navarro (a *boticario*) and Juan de Montoya recorded around thirty individuals or groups entering the city, including Juan de Piedra, a *vecino* from Pedraza carrying testimony from the Pedraza notary; Juan de Baeza, Francisco López, and Juan García de Andrés, *vecinos* from a village near Pedraza, who were carrying three loads of wool certified by the notary in Collado; two more *vecinos* from the same place with ten cartloads of wool who explained that they had obtained testimony from the Collado notary only because they had passed through there; Alonso Martínez, a *vecino* from Tudela de Duero with notarized testimony from Tudela; Francisco Sastre Capón, a Segovia *vecino*, who was coming home with wine from Tudela de Duero; and María, a priest's servant, who had testimony from the notary of Sotosalbos, Alonso del Cauto. On July 6 two women from Navafría arrived. They were *vecinas* and "said their names were" Juana Álvarez, fifty years old, and María García, twenty, daughter of Juana. They were short, the guard wrote. They swore their testimony was true. A boy around fifteen years old dressed in black also entered, coming from Collado. On July 17 a man named Lucas García came in from Sepúlveda in search of his master. These travelers and many more came from throughout the province of Segovia and the surrounding provinces; they were farmers, vendors, servants, muleteers, clerics. On the busiest day, July 23, there were seventy-four individuals or groups, though that was unusual.

Travellers' safe conducts, both in Segovia and elsewhere, were signed by priests and notaries, the two classes of people with unquestioned access to truth. I have not uncovered printed forms with blanks for names, places, and dates, but it would stand to reason that notaries and priests did not start from scratch each time and must have had some sort of template (Figure 3.1). Vendors might have a collection of these papers by the end of their journey testifying as to their route through allegedly healthy towns and to the cleanliness of all the merchandise they were carrying. The documents also certified where he or she was from. So even when they were on the road, they still belonged somewhere. The notary of Venialbo (Zamora) on May 15, 1599, for example,

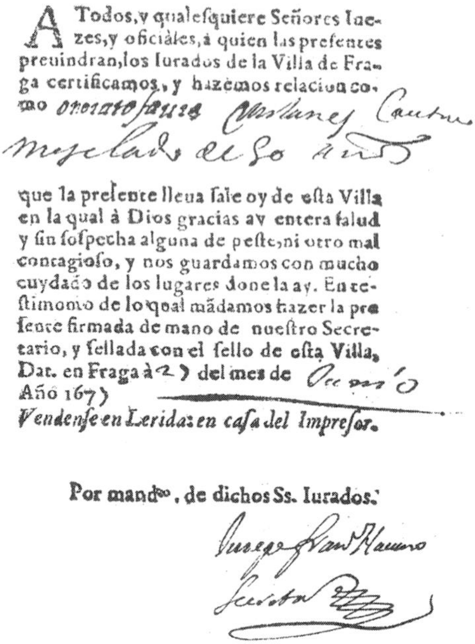

Figure 3.1 Safe-conduct from Fraga (Huesca), 1677.
Source: Manuel Camps i Surroca and Manuel Camps i Clemente, *La pesta de meitats del S. XVII a Catalunya* (Lleida: Seminari Pere Mates, Facultat de Medicina, Universitat de Barcelona, 1985), p. 229.

wrote, "I, Joan de Pezuelo … certify and confirm for anyone whom it may concern that thanks to the goodness of God, our Lord, this town, to our knowledge and understanding, is healthy and free of deadly peste and other contagious illness and it guards carefully against those areas where they say [there is illness]."[38] Travelers from Venialbo would carry this document to show they were not carrying infection. Similarly, in Burgos in September 1601 a certificate read: "I, Francisco Nanclares [the same man who was stuck outside Valladolid's gate] … certify and attest that in this city of Burgos by the mercy of God our Lord there is health and no illness of peste or other contagion and that the city is being guarded from those areas where it appears there is illness, and that this certificate comes at the request of Juan Gómez de Angulo, a *vecino* of this city, who is around fifty-six years old with a scar on his head and a grey beard and of medium height, and of Andrés de Angulo, his son, a handsome [*de buen gesto*] boy of around fourteen years of age whom

[38] RBP, II-2163, doc. 249.

I swear I know, and I have seen them reside in this city continuously for more than two months, and the said Juan Gómez de Angulo is going from this city to Valladolid and Medina del Campo on business for the said city by order of the city council."[39]

Perhaps the Segovia guards were overly welcoming, or perhaps travelers denied access were recorded in another book, we do not know. But not all guards were as undiscriminating. Guards everywhere at times ignored evidence of good health and turned travelers away (their actions inhuman rather than Christian, the physician Valentín de Andosilla had said), presumably because in so doing the guards had something to gain, be it seized merchandise or money or vengeance for whatever reason, or simply the enthusiasm of their own authority. In Burgos the corregidor demanded that towns under his jurisdiction immediately stop placing such obstacles in the way of commerce: "I order that all people carrying notarized testimony of the health of the place they come from, with a list of distinguishing characteristics of the person, his animals, and all things he is carrying, and testimony of having resided at least forty days in the place where he received the testimony … and the testimony's date not being old, and it carrying stamps from the healthy and unsuspicious places through which he has passed … be allowed to lodge and pass freely…"[40] The opposite problem occurred in Toledo, according to Agustín de Piedrahita Cueto, a *vecino* doing guard duty who snitched on a city police officer for opening a gate "and telling his friends that he was happy to open up for them any time they wanted." Piedrahita suggested that the city pay police to secretly guard the guards.[41] And there were cases in which the guard tried to do his duty but was undermined by arrogant officials, such as in Tafalla (Navarre), where guard Miguel de Góngora tried to stop an official from riding out to a nearby town, saying he was not going to let him back in again. The official paid no heed, rode off, and the following day returned through an "extraordinary" gate next to the town offices, compounding his actions by insulting the guard. "*Ruido, alboroto y escándalo*" ensued in the town, along with a personal injury suit which the guard appears to have won.[42]

---

[39] AMB-HI 687, September 28, 1601. As I was finishing this book I read Alexandra Bamji's very interesting study, "Health passes, print and public health in early modern Europe," *Social History of Medicine* (December 2017), https://doi.org/10.1093/shm/hkx104 (accessed January 2019).

[40] AMB-HI 3651, fol. 90, October 1, 1597.

[41] AMT Libro de Salud 176, unfoliated, loose petition tucked in back pocket of book. The town of Valdemoro (Madrid) in fact hired sobreguardas; AMVal 2547-1, June 15, 1598, fol. 31r.

[42] AGN TR Procesos 029357.

A town's walls or gates thus became places where the commercial and physical health of two communities, that of the traveler and that of the guard, or that of the guards and that of everyone else, along with the interests of each, were weighed against one another.

In June 1599, when Madrid hospitals were reporting dozens of new patients suffering from *secas*, the start of a long summer at the end of which some 3,500 people died there, Pedro Gómez was arrested at Madrid's Puerta de Segovia.[43] He was a *vecino* of Madrid, though he was also described as *portugués*. The arrest happened after the guards had watched him go in and out several times that day. The guard Alonso Nino grew suspicious, he told the corregidor of Madrid, Mosen Rubi de Bracamonte, when he saw him entering yet again at nightfall, this time accompanied by some washerwomen laden with bundles. A colleague testified that Nino had remarked, upon watching the comings and goings, that he had a bad feeling about Gómez (*le daba mala espina*), and a third said Nino had followed the women into the city a bit and then ordered them to show what they had. The women said it was laundry, but the laundry concealed linen belonging to Gómez. The culprit explained to the guard that a cloth vendor who had been unable to enter Madrid had later sold the cloth to Gómez thirty leagues away from the capital, and he was arrested.

In his trial testimony later, he said the cloth belonged to his brother, Francisco Gómez, a traveling salesman in Ávila who had bought a large amount of linen near the Portuguese border, probably in Vila Flor (Portugal). The bolt of cloth in question was extra, so Francisco gave it to Pedro to sell. Customs declarations backed up the cloth's itinerary, Pedro said, and when asked why he had tried to sneak it into Madrid he said he didn't want it taken from him. It may also have been the case that Francisco had tried to get the cloth in earlier and had been thwarted. Possibly Pedro tried to smuggle it in with a water vendor; he certainly admitted that he had spent an entire day trying to get it in. When he was asked if he was aware that town criers had publicized the king's order that anyone (except nobles) caught smuggling would lose their merchandise and get 200 lashes and six years in the galleys, he said he knew nothing.[44]

---

[43] The Gómez case is AGS-CC Memoriales leg. 813 no. 9. Madrid death toll is from AGS-E leg. 183, scattered documents on Madrid, tabulated by Bartolomé Bennassar in his *Recherches sur les grandes épidémies dans le nord de l'Espagne a la fin du XVIe siècle. Problèmes de documentation et de méthode* (Paris: SEVPEN, 1969); and from Michel Cavillac's introduction to Cristóbal Pérez de Herrera, *Amparo de Pobres* (Madrid: Espasa-Calpe, 1975), lii.

[44] This is an extraordinarily harsh punishment and may well have been fictitious, as no such royal order was included in the case file.

Then came the testimony that actually concerned peste, the presumed though never stated cause of the arrest in the first place. Not entirely truthful evidence was found from April by a royal notary saying Madrid was "clean of peste and other contagious diseases and is being guarded against the areas and towns where it is present" and furthermore that he, the notary, knew Francisco Gómez, a Portuguese merchant who had been living in Madrid for "many days," a man about twenty-eight years old with a chestnut-colored beard who had left for Ávila that day. This was Francisco's safe-conduct. He had another one from Ávila, also dated in April, also claiming that the city was free of plague, and another from Pajares, in Ávila. But these papers apparently did not do him much good in Madrid, because the guards also testified that they had stopped a Portuguese vendor the day of the arrest, berating him for not having proper testimony about the cloth, though clearly he had proof of where he had traveled, and they closed the gate on him. This was presumably also Francisco.

Pedro called his witnesses. Did they know that the cloth did not come from an infected area? Did they know that Francisco had bought it more than two months ago to sell in Ávila and furthermore that Vila Flor then and now was free of disease? Did they know that Pedro was a good, God-fearing Christian who, had he known the cloth came from a pestilent area (it was never stated that that was the case), would never have tried to smuggle it into Madrid or anywhere else? His witnesses could not only answer the questions, they had witnessed the purchase of the cloth in the first place. Another Portuguese cloth vendor from Vila Flor, who lived in Madrid, said the buyer was Pedro's brother-in-law Gaspar Correa, Francisco's business partner. He also saw the cloth being transported to Ávila, he said, and knew the leftover had been sent to Madrid. He verified that customs were in order and that the towns in question were all healthy. Another Portuguese cloth vendor, also living in Madrid, said he had known Pedro since he was born and that he, too, had witnessed the purchase in Vila Flor. And a third one said the same. And a fourth, and a fifth, who explained that the extra cloth was to be sold in Madrid to pay customs charges.

And yet, Pedro on June 19 was sentenced to six years of exile from Madrid and its jurisdiction and loss of the cloth, whose cash proceeds were to be split three ways, as usual, among court costs, the royal chamber, and the denouncer, which would explain Alonso Nino's tickle of suspicion.[45] Exile was certainly better than lashes or the galleys. But for a merchant it could be fatal, and Pedro appealed.

---

[45] In 1615 the Cortes complained about the practice of the three-way split, an invitation to misbehavior, and Philip III himself criticized it in 1604: Benjamin González Alonso, *El*

Alonso Nino, in Madrid, and the fifty-one pairs of men listed in Segovia's log book, and the rest of the untold thousands of men watching gates and walls during these years were probably common residents, not town councilors or other officials. A timesheet for Valladolid guards in 1597 lists *boticario* (we already saw another one), shoemaker, weaver, miller, and tailor.[46] Towns with smaller populations might get help from cities, which was the case with Burgos during the tenure of Diego de Vargas Manrique, who sent men out to help with (or supervise) guard duty: "Diego del Villar, *residente* [either yet another imprecise category for town-dweller or possibly an indication he was a city employee] of this city, [I order that you] depart with the raised staff of justice for the villages of Ausines and Valdorros, where you will stay for as long as I order to ensure that neither within nor outside the villages of Revilla del Campo or Cogollos anyone sell or buy animals or merchandise and that the *vecinos* of the said villages do not leave their town limits to buy or sell..."[47] Santander, Laredo, and Castro Urdiales, which had had no time to prepare anti-plague measures and therefore were devastated, asked Philip II to send soldiers to help guard because there were not enough inhabitants left to do the job.[48] Madrid seems also to have used soldiers along with civilians; in 1598 it had six guards on horseback and twenty-nine on foot who worked seven shifts in a row, and the heads of the contingents were called captains.[49] As time went on, neighborhoods were told to organize guard duty among themselves; in Madrid in 1602 the neighborhood around the present-day Senate building was given the choice of doing its own guard duty or having the gate there walled up.[50] Actually, by then one gets the impression that Madrid, abandoned and impoverished by the court, was paying more attention to catching interlopers in inns and rooming houses than at the sparsely watched city barriers that were being outsourced. That said, there does not appear to have been any real opposition to doing guard duty, though there were plenty of cases of men just slacking off. For one thing, guards were paid, no small thing in these terrible years. (When the future count of Gondomar was corregidor of Valladolid in 1602 he received a petition on behalf of Lorenzo López, who said he had been pushed out of his guard job by jealous competitors; he was poor, could not support his four children, and had a sick wife, he said, and he begged Gondomar to grant

corregidor castellano 1348–1808 (Madrid: Instituto de Estudios Administrativos, 1970), 173 and 178.

[46] BL Eg. 356, vol. 1, fols. 306r–24r.   [47] AMB-HI 3650, January 1598.

[48] AGS-GyM leg. 514, doc. 112, April 21, 1598.   [49] AV Secretaría 1-138-1.

[50] AV Secretaría 1-138-4, May 20, 1602.

him the favor of restoring his job, which would be of great service to our Lord.[51]) For another thing, just about everyone did it, including town leaders and the local nobility. It was certainly tiresome, but not something people were willing to fight.

However, there were some who argued they were exempt from this duty whose guidelines had existed in Castilian law for centuries. Castilian jurisprudence was a minefield of privileges, often perfectly legitimate ones. Individuals and towns could and did declare themselves unaffected by obligations to pay certain taxes or raise or billet soldiers, these being the principal ways the state entered the lives of the king's vassals. Exceptions were not exceptional, in other words, but in cases of dire circumstance the challenge for both sides was to prove that the circumstance did or did not outweigh the privilege and custom in question.

Two examples indicate the sort of situation that warranted (or not) an exception. Juan López de Unceta (or Unzueta), a vecino of Eibar (Vizcaya), argued in 1598 that he was not liable for guard duty because in previous lawsuits he had obtained rulings from the king, which he presented, saying he did not have to pay the same taxes and assessments as other hidalgos in town, and furthermore that his family had always been exempt from guard duty. "It is well known," he said, "that the said house and lineage of the Unceta and its owners, lords, and possessors have been and are free and exempt of all and any assessments and duties of any sort ... by immemorial custom." In the first round of arguments, the town said Unceta's claims "violate what all the *vecinos* of the said town, and each one of them without distinction, are obligated to do," and he was told to be at the Hurquicia gate at 5 p.m. the next day. At 5 p.m. the next day a local judge and town councilor and the inevitable notary appeared at the gate. There they found Cristóbal de Carranza, the other *vecino* assigned guard duty at that time, but not Unceta, though they waited until 7 p.m. The following morning the municipal crew returned at 8 a.m., and Unceta was still not there. So the town ordered that "valuable" goods be taken from him as a lien up to the amount of 1,000 maravedies. The items were sold in the town square, with the proceeds going to pay the guards who actually showed up. Unceta sued and lost and appealed to the Chancillería, which at that point was in Medina del Campo.[52] A second case of claimed exemption took place in Medina de Pomar, north of Burgos around halfway to Laredo and hence

[51] RBP II-2154-143.
[52] ARCV Registro de Ejecutorías 1946–88; ARCV Pleitos civiles Alonso Rodriguez (F) 895-1, 896-1. The case file, comprising some 5,000 folios, covers at least four years. There is an Unzueta Palace in the town today.

right on the plague's predictable route. Here the plaintiff was Francisco de Valdivieso, administrator of the Vera Cruz hospital outside the town walls, who argued in March 1597 that he was already guarding the hospital and therefore could not also guard the town. He lost the suit and appealed to the Chancillería (still in Valladolid), where he eventually prevailed. When news first reached Medina de Pomar that the region to its north was sick, town officials ordered all those holding offices and privileges to participate in guard duty and/or supervise ordinary guards. All the other hospital administrators received the same order, but only Valdivieso and one other, it appears, refused. Valdivieso lived in the hospital with his family, he said, tending to the poor and the pilgrims who showed up, and he also was guarding it against the plague, acts which were of utility and the common good not only for the hospital but for the entire town. In response, the town council pointed out that deaths had been reported just one league away, that the utility would be far greater if he would do his duty, and that "it would not be just for [vecinos] to enjoy the privileges and honors of the town, as they had enjoyed and continued enjoying them, while at the same time being excused from guarding." It would set a dangerous example. In retaliation for the administrators' obstinance, the town ordered that their respective hospitals' doors remain closed except to the poor seeking alms and (possibly) that the town itself bar entry to people from the hospitals. In addition, arrest orders seem to have been issued. Lots of briefs and arguments and testimony were passed back and forth at various lower levels until the Chancillería sensibly ruled that if Valdivieso found someone else to perform his duty to the town that would suffice.[53] Medina de Pomar did, eventually, succumb to the disease, possibly twice; in April 1599 Burgos was guarding against it, in July 1599 Toledo was, and in May 1600 there were new reports of illness there.[54]

Looking back to how it all began, townspeople and memoirists depicted an entry, a moment, something that crossed the wall and

---

[53] ARCV Pl. Civiles, Alonso Rodriguez (Olv.) 1428-15; Registro de Ejecutorias 1871/10. The case ran from March 1597 to July 1598. Medina de Pomar belonged to the Constable of Castile, the highest-ranking titled nobleman in Spain, and was governed by the Marquis of Berlanga.

[54] AMB-LA-130, April 1599; AMB-HI 3653, May 1600; Julian Montemayor, "Una ciudad frente a la peste: Toledo a fines del XVI," in *La ciudad hispánica durante los siglos XIII al XVI: actas del coloquio celebrado en La Rábida y Sevilla del 14 al 19 septiembre de 1981*, Emilio Sáez, et al., eds., 3 vols. (Madrid: Universidad Complutense, 1985), 1115. A survey in 1591 conducted by the crown for tax purposes, whose numbers therefore may be inflated, showed Medina de Pomar had 172 *pecheros*, or taxpayers; Annie Molinié-Bertrand, *Au siècle d'or l'Espagne et ses Hommes. La Population du Royaume de Castille au XVI siècle* (Paris: Economica, 1985), 147.

destroyed the world inside. Few accounts are as memorable as that
of Martín González de Cellorigo, a jurist, lawyer, town councilor of
Pancorbo, and author of one of the best-known commentaries on contemporary political, moral, and economic affairs. Valladolid had been
"entirely healthy," he wrote, and observing the festivity of the Holy Spirit
(Pentecost) when "this disease entered so deceitfully" (a traición). On
June 10, "whether because the constellation had arrived, or the contagion
had grown, or the Lord chose to act thusly with the multitude, many
people began feeling ill, and with the illness so evident our city was
disrupted, and little by little it began to be set afire. It was as if the illness
were a spirit that discerned things, that naturally took on the burden of
seeking out all corners of all homes, waiting for the cautious and
wounding the curious, removing some while dissimulating with others,
abandoning the abandoned and grabbing the most careful, seizing the
strongest and ignoring the weakest, healing the sick and killing the
healthy..."[55] The guards were there to prevent towns from letting in that
one person, that one untrustworthy traveler who might turn everything
upside down and visit death upon them all. They stood there to prevent it
from starting. When corregidores corresponded with Philip III in
1599 and when towns later requested that their taxes be reduced, it
was important for them to be able to identify that first case in order to
tell the story right, to draw a dividing line between before, when things
were good, and after.

That first link in a chain is of obvious epidemiological interest but its
weight was of a more narrative nature here. One ordinary person who
wore something in particular or sought lodging or sold something and
who was, deliberately or not, hiding his or her disease, spoke for the
insidious everyday nature of the calamity. It was a "disguised young
woman" (una moza disimulada) who broke the peace and quiet of the
town in La Rioja where Dr. Andosilla lived, arriving from "a place of sick
people" and surely entering the town freely, as the need for guards had
not yet been recognized. She died almost immediately, with a burning
fever, and then things went back to normal for two months. But later the
weather changed and a girl died, and then more people died, and little by

---

[55] Martín González de Cellorigo, *Memorial de la política necesaria y util restauración a la
República de España* (Madrid: Instituto de Cooperación Iberoamericana, 1991) [1600],
23. I do not know to which constellation he was referring. On Cellorigo see Juan Ignacio
Gutiérrez Nieto, "El pensamiento económico, político y social de los arbitristas," in
Historia de la Cultura Española 'Menéndez Pidal', José María Jover Zamora, ed., vol. 1, *El
Siglo del Quijote* (Madrid: Espasa Calpe, 1996), 344–8. J. H. Elliott described Cellórigo
as "perhaps the most acute of all the *arbitristas*": "The Decline of Spain," in *Spain and Its
World, 1500–1700*, Elliott (New Haven, CT: Yale University Press, 1989), 219.

little the town was engulfed.[56] But there was a starting point, the disguised young woman. During the spring of 1599, when Old Castile was keeping close track as the plague was closing in, such cautionary tales must have been on the minds of all authorities and guards, who did not want the disaster to happen on their watch. Earlier we saw that Melgar de Fernamental (and, with it, Burgos) believed the disease had arrived from Calahorra de Boedo with the man seeking legal advice whose overnight stay led to the death of nine people. (That story, Burgos authorities told the king, "shows clearly that this disease is acquired through contact."[57]) The corregidor of Ávila concealed from the king the presence of the epidemic in his city but was able to recount how twice he had barred its entry: On Sunday, July 18, a man arrived from Valladolid with an oozing sore (*seca escupida*) and was expelled, and the next day a local man fleeing peste in Cebreros was turned back and quickly died. That man's father buried him, along with his linens, far away from the city, and then both the father and the mother were expelled.[58] A friar from Valladolid arrived in Toledo with a fever and took eighteen days to die in the San Bartolomé de la Vega monastery, after which he was buried at a distance along with his bedclothes and clothing and covered with lime, "and all of this was done with great secrecy so as not to cause a disturbance in the city."[59] Likewise, Toledo corregidor Francisco de Carbajal told the king in July 1599 that the previous month a *forastero* carrying notarized testimony had been allowed to enter the city on the San Martín bridge and then went off to a *casa de vecindad* (probably a simple boarding house) near the San Agustín convent, where he stayed for one day. Then, the telepathic corregidor went on, "he left, afraid that it would be discovered that he was sick and was carrying fraudulent testimony, and a few days later a man in that same *casa de vecindad* got sick with a *carbunco*, and he died shortly, and before his death he told this story, and having learned all this I ordered the house cleaned of the filth that had been there for a long time and it was closed and locked." The outsider was buried outside the city, "with neither commotion nor fuss, modestly and in great silence."[60] Another first case dodged. Of course, the first link of them all was the arrival of the "*Rodamundo*" in Santander after its journey from Flanders. Later on, this ominous and singular event showed up in a

---

[56] Valentín de Andosilla Salazar, *Libro en que se prueba con claridad el mal que corre por España ser nuevo y nunca visto: su naturaleza, causas, pronósticos, curacion, y la prouidencia que se deue tener con el ...* (Pamplona, 1601), chapter 24, 111r.
[57] AMB-HI 3653, July 25, 1597.   [58] AGS-E leg. 183, docs. 327 and 328, July 21, 1599.
[59] AGS-E leg. 183, doc. 256, May 27, 1599. The eighteen days indicates the man probably had something other than bubonic plague.
[60] AGS-E leg. 183, doc. 321, July 5, 1599.

chronicle of the plague in Pamplona, and probably in similar accounts elsewhere, as an obvious way of starting the tale: "In the year of Our Lord Jesus Christ 1596, on the fifth day of the month of November, there arrived in the town of Santander, one of the Cuatro Villas de la Mar [the collective name given to Santander, Laredo, Castro Urdiales, and San Vicente de la Barquera] a vessel called Rodamundo, and Captain Terente … who had loaded his cargo of linens in Dunkirk, the port of Flanders, where there was peste at that time …; and when they unloaded it they began selling the linens, and immediately the illness was detected, and because of carelessness the illness swept over Santander in particular, which was nearly emptied."[61]

In Valladolid, the first case arrived from Covarrubias. On April 23, 1599, Dr. Antonio Ponce de Santa Cruz, the city's physician and a professor of medicine at the University of Valladolid, told the city's health commission that he had treated a man with a *seca* who had died after three days, and Santa Cruz believed he had peste. The city chose not to believe the doctor. A policeman, accompanied by a notary, immediately set off for the boarding house or inn where the man had been staying, next to the San Juan gate, where they asked two women where the man had come from, if he had arrived sick or healthy, and who had buried him. His linens and clothes, it transpired, had been taken by a messenger working for the confraternity of the Ánimas de la Magdalena, who, once he was found, was ordered to immediately take off the man's brown cape, which he had kept and was wearing, and to burn the whole lot. The following day the lieutenant corregidor went to the inn, which was owned or run by Francisco González, a stonemason, and proceeded to question everyone involved in the man's death. González's wife, Beatriz Casada, said the deceased, Tomás García, had arrived from Covarrubias on April 18 riding a large horse and was apparently healthy, though he complained he was hurting after riding hard for some 100 miles. So a surgeon or barber was summoned. He said García had a fever and that a doctor should be called, but at that point the wife of Gaspar de Lienzes, María de Villa, for some reason appeared and said the patient should go to her house, which he did, and he soon died. The surgeon testified that he had not wanted to bleed the man, who he said was in very bad shape. The next witness was another barber, named Juan de Valdivieso, who had been summoned to the Lienzes household to bleed García. He did so (right arm), noted that the man had a fever, and told

---

[61] Ignacio Baleztena, "Relación de la peste desta ciudad de Pamplona del año 1599," transcribed in *Príncipe de Viana* 22 and 23 (1946), 186–201 and 377–94; here see no. 22, p. 187.

a woman and a student there that they must not let García fall asleep. He bled him again the following day (left arm), and that afternoon the people in the house asked Valdivieso for *ventosas* (suction pads or a glass used as a vacuum over wounds), ordered by Dr. Santa Cruz, at which point the man died. The second barber testified he had treated him because the patient said his leg hurt, but he had nothing wrong in his groin, though on his right thigh he had a small white swelling the same color as his skin. Next was María de Villa, who said García, a *vecino* of Covarrubias, had arrived a week earlier in the company of a university man (*licenciado*, a clue no one investigated) and that they had stayed in the stonemason's home, where he fell ill with a fever. According to her, García said his stomach hurt and that he had eaten something bad. The barber bled the man in both arms. The following day, still according to María de Villa, the patient apparently told Santa Cruz that he had a *seca* on his thigh, but Santa Cruz said that if it wasn't in the groin it was not important. Finally, the doctor himself testified that on the 21st he had visited the patient and found him with a high fever and bloodshot eyes and delirious. He had a *seca* just below the groin, which the patient complained about on the 22nd, though he said he had gotten it after he got the fever, and the man died on the third day. Asked if he thought the deceased had had *mal contagioso*, Santa Cruz answered in the affirmative. On April 24, the day after all these inquiries, the city summoned five doctors who all agreed it was neither peste nor *mal contagioso*, "and they declared that mercifully this city is very healthy … and [the illnesses the city has] can be easily cured and are not *males contagiosos* but rather common and light illnesses."[62]

But Santa Cruz was right, and that autumn he published a plague treatise to prove it. In addition to broader medical considerations, the treatise recounts the sad events of late April when he treated the man who arrived on a large horse. "It was only a few days later that the contagion lit up the whole neighborhood around Calle Ruy Hernández, spreading throughout the city and emptying houses, and still they did not believe it was peste," he wrote. "Later I learned from Fray Luis de Covarrubias, who is from there and is a member of the Order of San Jerónimo, that the man who arrived sick had left a pestilent household, and that was the start of all the harm to that town."[63] It was also the start of Valladolid's terrible

---

[62] AGS-E leg. 183, doc. 302, April 23, 1599. This story does not appear in the city council minutes. It was transcribed into the lieutenant corregidor's letter to the king from health commission minutes which must later have been destroyed. Bennassar did not include doc. 302 in his transcriptions of AGS-E leg. 183.

[63] Antonio Ponce de Santa Cruz, *Tractado de las causas y curacion de las fiebres con secas pestilenciales que han oprimido a Valladolid y otras ciudades de España* (Valladolid: Pedro de Merchan Calderón, 1600), fols. 3r–v. It is worth noting, however, that when University

summer. While no town wished to admit it was sick, at some point it had no choice but to recognize that the epidemic had breached the walls and to assume the narrative, assigning a starting date and a carrier. Possibly Valladolid failed in this respect because its leadership was lacking; the fact that it was a lieutenant corregidor who took charge of the Covarrubias case and that a new corregidor, Antonio de Ulloa, arrived in mid-June, makes that a likely scenario, as does the subsequent appointment of Melchor de Teves as Pest Commissioner. In August 1599, at the height of the epidemic, members of the city council had to be warned that they would be fined if they missed meetings.[64] What is surprising about all this is that Valladolid had plague guards in place already in June 1597, nearly two years earlier, though the Chancillería that summer reported that the corregidor had said he did not dare order the establishment of a corps of guards without the court's assistance. Authorities knew that sooner or later there would be a first case, and as a result some sort of quarantine had certainly existed since Valladolid first received news from the north, or possibly from Madrid itself in 1597.

Authorities, including in Valladolid, at times showed considerable common sense and flexibility regarding the quarantine, recognizing that people had to be fed and had to move around. Farmers and peasants appear to have been in an especially awkward situation when quarantine was declared, and naturally their hardship affected everyone who wished to eat. Urban and rural were not separate worlds; plenty of peasants worked as artisans in the off-season; people in villages for generations had worked for the wool and linen industries; and almost all townspeople tended crops outside, whether as owners or laborers. A multitude of examples bear witness to authorities' recognition that rules had to be bent if anyone was to survive. At each gate in Pamplona, male and female servants and field workers left a note indicating the date they were leaving and when they would return, and upon returning they had to hand over their copy of the same, and the guards notified overseers how many laborers had left through the gate and how many were expected to return.[65] Wheat farmers living in Valladolid's San Juan neighborhood petitioned the city in July 1597 saying their fields were on the other side of the San Juan gate, by the Esgueva River. Given that all the streets and paths they used to use had been closed off (the humans might have passed muster, but their animals and foodstuffs and hay would not), they

of Valladolid medical professors signed a bill of good health for the city on May 15, Santa Cruz was one of the signatories, barely two weeks after this case; their statement is in Bennassar, *Recherches sur les grandes épidémies*, 181.
[64] AMVA sig. 22-0, August 27, 1599.   [65] Baleztena, ed., "Relación de la peste," 189.

now had to use the Tudela gate and the Tudela bridge in the southeast, crossing twice with all their mules and carts and personnel, which was very dangerous. Some sort of financial arrangement appears to have been worked out with the city.[66] Similarly, along his grand tour of the Tagus and Jarama river valleys to inspect anti-plague procedures, royal envoy Nicolás Suárez in 1562 had agreed that in Chinchón allowances could be made for farmers and peasants who had to reap wheat, and he determined that one gate – just one – would be kept open for them, under strict control.[67] To the north, the little town of Villasandino, under quarantine, sent a petition to Burgos explaining that inhabitants needed oxen to work in their fields, but that they would have to leave their town to buy them. They begged permission for three or four *vecinos* to be able to leave town and undertake the purchases on behalf of the rest. They also had wine stored in nearby cellars, they wrote, but being that their village had been declared pestilent they could not go out to the cellars to sell it, so they asked that the corregidor arrange that someone be given the key to the cellars and sell the wine on their behalf.[68] A certain *vecino* of Cogollos had fields that abutted onto the village of Valdorros, so the always solicitous Burgos corregidor (who had sent the town shoes the previous month) told his health commission, "it seems to me it is less disruptive for the Cogollos *vecino* to cease working that land near Valdorros and that people from Valdorros work the land instead and deduct [for the owner] the income they make, because otherwise there might be problems … So order the people of Valdorros to sow and cultivate these lands and tell the man from Cogollos not to…"[69] It was not just farmers and peasants who needed open gates: in Seville in 1600, by which time the plague had moved south, friars whose monasteries lay outside the city's barrier wanted the gates open because their houses "had seen a precipitous drop in the offerings brought in by city residents who routinely visited… In his petition, the prior of Nuestra Señora de los Remedios offered the city councilmen the choice of either opening the gate or providing financial support for the monastery." Gates were opened for limited hours.[70] The San Esteban district of Burgos also begged for flexibility, and there, too, churchmen were the protagonists. Already in January 1599, before the city fell ill, Lt. Corregidor Francisco de

---

[66] AMVA sig. 21-0, July 23, 1597.   [67] AGS-CR leg. 115 no. 4, July 9, 1562, fol. 8.

[68] AMB-HI 3650, March 9, 1598. If they were using oxen, then obviously they were leaving town to go into their fields, though maybe just the fields closest to the town.

[69] AMB-HI 3651, October 24, 1597.

[70] Kristy Wilson Bowers, "Balancing individual and communal needs: plague and public health in early modern Seville," *Bulletin of the History of Medicine* 81:2 (Summer 2007), 335–58, p. 346.

Valencia had written Philip III that there had been seven or eight deaths in San Esteban, one of Burgos's poorest areas.[71] One of the busiest and most articulate of Burgos's council members during these years, Andrés de Cañas, sometime later in 1599 wrote a brief report outlining "the reasons why the gate from the city to the neighborhood of San Esteban should be open." First, he said, the people who lived there "are parishioners of the San Esteban church, and it is very difficult for the priests of the said church to administer the sacraments because of the long road there, and people there have died without receiving the sacraments, or they might die, which would be greatly harmful." Second, vendors and merchants from elsewhere used to unload their wares in San Esteban, but they were not doing that anymore because there was no access to the city, a situation Cañas said violated "the royal privileges and *ejecutorias* granted to the said neighborhood for its preservation" which he implied had led to lawsuits by San Esteban, which depended for its survival on transactions with outsiders. With the gate closed, inhabitants would be forced to leave altogether; houses would be abandoned, income would decline, and taxes would go unpaid. And, finally, most inhabitants worked in the fields, which was now very difficult because of the long road they had to take to get there. I do not know if San Esteban prevailed, but the fact that Cañas – and, apparently, the clergy – was on their side suggests that it did.[72]

This balancing of needs, this occasional ingenuity and experimentation, is a reminder that in Castilian communities (and probably in communities almost anywhere), the contingent could outweigh the established order. The measure of people's relative claims, authorities' duties to both the small and the large, meant that sometimes individual remedies could prevail. Leaving a gate open thus was a significant gesture toward the efficacy of argument and the health of the political arena even as it was hemmed in by pestilence. People never stopped explaining or protesting, and sometimes they were heard. The open gate is also a moment when, though no one says this, private pursuits and public well-being were being assessed against each other.

---

[71] AGS-E leg. 183, doc. 267. By April 22 some eighty people had died. These are very cold months in Burgos, lending some credence to the Burgos doctors' earlier insistence that the disease was not plague.

[72] BL Eg. 356, vol. 2, fols. 344r–v. Priests in Seville similarly petitioned during a 1582 epidemic that gates be opened for them to administer last rites to the inhabitants of the San Vicente parish, which had been divided by the wall; Alexandra Parma Cook and Noble David Cook, *The Plague Files: Crisis Management in Sixteenth-Century Seville* (Baton Rouge, LA: Louisiana State University Press, 2009), 170.

The clergy frequently complained about quarantine, which is not surprising, though nothing like Ávila's door-burning episode in 1518 seems to have occurred at the end of the century. Carlo Cipolla has written that confrontations between state and church during epidemics tended to center on three issues: quarantine; requisitioning of monasteries and other church properties for hospitals; and the prohibition against large gatherings. To this I would add the clergy's occasional refusal to pay special taxes to offset plague expenses.[73] As in the San Esteban case in Burgos, the clergy worried that the quarantine prevented them from tending to the sick and prevented the healthy from attending services (though Cipolla's third issue comes into play here), or at least that was the argument generally used. Avoiding inconvenience was invariably linked to doing God's work. Two cases from Madrid are illustrative: in August 1599, when Madrid was quarantined, the Monastery of Our Lady of Atocha had ended up outside the quarantine barrier, making it impossible for people inside the city to honor the virgin. So the monastery wanted another, wider wall to be built that would include the monastery but that would cost more than 1,400 ducats. There appears to have been an agreement that the amount would be split between the city and the monastery, but the prior wrote to the king asking that he also contribute to the monastery's part, as the institution "is so poor and indebted that it cannot pay its share except by begging."[74] Another venerable religious institution in Madrid, the Descalzas Convent, in 1601 complained that its friars had to use the Fuencarral gate, quite a distance away. The more direct route would have been along Leganitos road. So they asked the city's health commission if a special little side door could be built in the barrier to be used just by them and for which they would have a key. The commissioners agreed to the request, emphasizing that no one else could use the door, even if they were *naturales* and well known in the city, and that churchmen from elsewhere would still have to use the normal city gates and present their credentials to guards.[75] The Toledo priest Luis de Vinuesa took matters one step further by saying that if the city council allowed him to come and go through the Puerta Nueva, which was closed, so he could administer last rites, he would pay the city whatever it wanted.[76]

[73] Carlos M. Cipolla, *Faith, Reason, and the Plague in Seventeenth-Century Tuscany* (New York: W. W. Norton & Company, 1979), 6. See chapter 7 for more on church disputes.
[74] AGS-CJH leg. 390-24, nd.   [75] AV Secretaría, 1-138-4, June 22, 1601.
[76] AMT Libro de Salud 176, unfoliated, August 1598.

Walls obviously also blocked products, not just the people transporting them. (The Pamplona city council, and probably others, had a storage facility outside the city where it kept goods seized at the gate.[77]) Prime among the substances considered dangerous were cloth and clothing, which were mentioned in every set of instructions given to every guard in every town. Regardless of who was entering or from where, linens were closely inspected and often disallowed, as Pedro Gómez discovered in Madrid. Many stories about how plague often reached a given place mentioned the arrival of cloth, often carried by women, from elsewhere. Thus blame was attached and contagion was confirmed with an explanation that proved both hardy and mobile. Indeed, it was linens aboard the *"Rodamundo"* that had started it all. The illness was thereupon handed from one person to the next by way of something intimate and domestic, something essential to daily life that furthermore had once been the linchpin of Castilian commerce. It is worth pointing out that it was not just Spain that focused on cloth. A churchman in Cividale del Friuli, near Slovenia, attributed a 1598 plague there to Helena, a sick woman who had bought some cloth and whose house was not quarantined after an erroneous diagnosis from the apparently incompetent Dr. Spinelli.[78] The English town of Eyam, mythical site of self-sacrifice, first became infected in 1665 on account of a box of old clothing sent to the village tailor from London.[79] In Geneva in 1543, two servant girls who washed linens were arrested on suspicion that they were wilfully spreading disease.[80] In our epidemic, cloth-carrying meant apparel or bed linens (both *ropa*), be they linen or wool (silk was never mentioned). Raw wool was also a concern; wool-washers were expelled from Toledo and wool-washing was prohibited in Soria because sheep were thought to transmit the disease. The latter city made inquiries if it could conduct its wool-washing in the Sorian town of Vinuesa rather than in the capital itself and in June 1599 decreed ten

---

[77] Lasaosa Villanua, *El "Regimiento" municipal*, 348n90.

[78] Mario Brozzi, *Peste, Fede e Sanità in una Cronaca Cividalese del 1598* (Milan: Dott. A. Giuffrè, 1982), 30.

[79] Patrick Wallis, "A dreadful heritage: interpreting epidemic disease at Eyam, 1666–2000," *History Workshop Journal* 61 (Spring 2006), 31–56, p. 31.

[80] William G. Naphy, "Plague-spreading and a magisterially controlled fear," in *Fear in Early Modern Society*, William G. Naphy and Penny Roberts, eds. (Manchester: Manchester University Press, 1997), 28–43, p. 29. He writes, "The typical plague-spreader of 1545 was a woman, fairly poor, with no family connections, a hospital worker, a Genevan resident with no civic rights and a Savoyard." Sixteenth-century plagues in Geneva were notable for the number of arrests and executions of those who allegedly intentionally spread plague.

years' banishment for anyone caught washing wool there.[81] Constant *pregones*, the orders called out by town criers, warned town dwellers not to bring in cloth from pestilent places; at one point in Valladolid town criers announced that punishment for the crime would be death, hardly a practical solution under the circumstances.[82]

There is virtually no town or city with extant records that did not at some point believe that a certain piece or crate or shipment of clothing that crossed the barrier was or could be the start of a new chain. Thus the wall occupied a crucial place in the telling of the story, the spot, as if frozen, where it all began. We have seen several of these cases: Bilbao was worried to hear that a certain man who had been in San Sebastián when it was pestilent had sent several loads of clothing to Bilbao, prompting Bilbao to send a messenger to Guipúzcoa to track down the facts.[83] Burgos found out that in Oñate more than sixty people had died after clothing or linens had been brought from San Sebastián, and in Pasajes de San Juan, the local priest told authorities that the disease there had begun after bargain-seeking women had unwisely bought sheets, leading to the deaths of entire households.[84] The first deaths in Pamplona were the fault of a poor woman who exchanged legumes for two pieces of colored cloth and a curtain, setting off a chain of deaths in her neighborhood.[85] Those examples are all from the Basque Country, but similar cases can be found everywhere. The Valladolid city council entertained a complaint from Tudela de Duero about a man who had placed linens (or clothing) in Nuestra Señora de Duero (possibly today's Nuestra Señora de la Asunción) which had come from Santo Domingo de Silos, a town Tudela was guarding against, so the town asked the corregidor to order that the room where the linens now sat be locked and that no one be allowed to enter.[86] The corregidor of Segovia told Philip III that in the town of Vallamanta a widow had sent clothing to her daughters and daughters-in-law, and they all died.[87] After two women and a girl died in the village of Ciguñuela, Valladolid told the king that "the origin of the epidemic is well-known and is blamed on a headdress bought in

---

[81] Montemayor, "Una ciudad frente a la peste," 1120; Díez Sanz, *La Tierra de Soria*, 48–54, citing city council minutes.

[82] AMVA sig. 21-0, April 23, 1599.   [83] AFB libro 024, August 7, 1598.

[84] AMB-HI 3650, January 1598; José Ramón Cruz Mundet, *El mal que al presente corre: Gipuzkoa y la peste (1597–1600)* (San Sebastián: Kutxa Fundazioa, 2003), 31–2, citing Archivo General de Guipúzcoa, sec. 1, neg. 19, leg. 6.

[85] Baleztena, "Relación de la Peste," 187, 190, 199; the chronicle records all forty-seven dead in the epidemic's first burst.

[86] AMVA sig. 21-0, May 10, 1599.   [87] AGS-E leg. 183, doc. 253, May 30, 1599.

Valladolid despite all the prohibitions."[88] The corregidor of Burgos, Diego de Vargas Manrique, in yet another show of his nimble and sympathetic thinking, suggested to the people of the village of Los Ausines that they keep shepherds from Revilla out of their territory, but that if the shepherds should wander over anyway they be made to remove their clothes and leave them lying in the fields. The Revillans should be "provided with another set of clothing, and I will pay you for that right away."[89] When the city council of Burgos wrote to the marquis of Aguilar with news about one of the nobleman's towns in the Sedano Valley, it explained that it had received information that someone from the village had gone to Santander and brought back contagious clothing which had caused several deaths around two months earlier. The affected houses had been duly closed up, but now people working for second-hand clothes dealers had wrapped themselves in the infected linens, prompting Burgos to ask the marquis to immediately order that they be burned.[90]

Indeed, as the busy and benevolent Vargas, who unusually and regularly referred to himself in the first person in his letters to the beleaguered residents of outlying towns and villages, said in a letter to Melgar, "the peste hides and is contained not only in houses and in clothing but in even the smallest pleat of a tunic, from whence it can infect a kingdom." He wrote these words in February 1598 in response to Melgar's request to be declared pest-free, which the corregidor refused to do, despite how happy he was to hear of the town's improvement. He did not send this letter, but three days later wrote a shorter version of the same, again saying how pleased he was to hear that Melgar's health was better. "But as the peste has lasted so long," he added, "and being that in [Melgar's] 500 homes of *vecinos* 1,500 people have died [in the space of four months, according to the next letter], and as the town is encircled [by eight or nine pestilent towns, again according to the next letter]" he was regrettably forced to deny Melgar's request. Once again he used the same image: "In a corner, in the pleat of a tunic, corrupt air can be trapped that might infect all of Spain." This time he added a note after his signature: "There is no lack of people who say that in this phase of the moon more than thirty [more] people have died [in Melgar] and many have fallen ill, but I believe that much of this is due to some *vecinos*' envy [*envidia*], but let me know if there is any truth or substance to it." And the following day he returned yet again to the same idea, this time in correspondence with the Council of Castile. He told the council that he had sent

---

[88] Anastasio Rojo Vega, "La caridad, factor de mortalidad en la epidemia de peste de 1599 en Valladolid," *Medicina y Historia* 30 (1989), no source cited.
[89] AMB-HI 3651, December 1597.   [90] AMB-HI 3653, April 10 and 29, 1597.

investigators to Melgar with an out-of-town notary who reported back that the market town was suffering "extreme need." Even so, the corregidor stuck to his guns in refusing to declare the town open for business, "because with any misstep, the illness spreads from just one corner of a house, and the pleat of a tunic can enclose bad air that fills the entire kingdom with peste, and Melgar is the most pestilent town in all of Castile … it is another Torrejón de Velasco, in the Kingdom of Toledo, or Peñarranda de Bracamonte, in Castile," showing that Vargas was well acquainted with the plight of sick towns quite a distance away. He had enormous common sense, this man who was rightfully worried about cloth and meat and grains, though he was not quite ready to put aside the phases of the moon or pockets of bad air.[91]

The reasoning behind this universal interest in cloth deserves consideration and a slight detour. The degree to which peste was or was not contagious, and how, indicates which disease or diseases it actually was or was not. Historians over the past few decades have fiercely debated these points. Inconsistencies of seasonal timing, the speed with which the disease moved, symptoms, the impact of public health measures such as quarantine, and the absence of known hosts and vectors (bubonic plague as we know it today spreads from the rat to the flea to the human and is hardly ever contagious from one human to another) led critics, among them prominent scholars, to declare that the Second Pandemic, which includes the Castilian plague, was not bubonic plague and was not caused by the pathogen *Yersinia pestis*, and that historians had been led astray by retrospective diagnoses. Following those debates, a new wave of interdisciplinary plague research began thanks to startling advances in microbiology and paleomicrobiology, as a result of which the next generation of medical historians concluded that the undeniable inconsistencies between the two waves of plague must be embraced rather than be seen as evidence of two entirely different diseases. Archaeological work has produced evidence of *Yersinia pestis* in medieval plague victims in France and in England; thus the pathogen is constant, though the epidemiology is not. *Yersinia pestis* "can remain alive in a dormant form in soil for a period of several months or years," according to one recent scientific article, an assertion with enormous consequences for historians.[92] For our purposes, the most important point is that the array of vectors, hosts, and transmission agents of the plague might need to be expanded to account for discrepancies. Furthermore, there is

[91] AMB-HI 3650, February 2, 5, and 6, 1598.
[92] Didier Raoult, et al. "Plague: history and contemporary analysis," *Journal of Infection* 66 (2013), 18–26, p. 19.

evidence that *Yersinia pestis* left a reservoir population in Europe after the Black Death, the exact nature of which is unknown – though rats are not a good reservoir population because they quickly die of plague – which would explain the constant reappearances of the disease.[93] The fleas (and possibly lice[94]) and the mammals (probably not just rodents) were more complex creatures than thought, and the ecological settings in which they moved may have made an important difference. So possibly the cloth was, indeed, a danger. It was carried on pack animals, the wool came from sheep, and it might share space in carts with grain (and rodents). An article by Nükhet Varlik makes a strong case that "the various stages of handling wool and the process of manufacturing woolen broadcloth may have exposed the Jewish laborers in Salonica to an additional risk of contracting [plague]." Late-sixteenth-century Salonica was an urban textile center, she writes, as were Segovia, Toledo, Ávila, and others, though their decline was well under way by the end of the century, and many smaller towns throughout Castile also participated in the wool trade through the putting-out system or by washing and processing wool. Burgos had once been one of Europe's most important commercial centers for wool and, though its role was much diminished by the 1590s, wool still moved through it. According to Varlik, who cites scientific sources, "Investigations of the etiology and transmission of plague have shown that woolen cloth is a medium that hosts plague vectors … for extended periods of time." And, she goes on, "infected

---

[93] The bibliography is huge. Briefly, among the most prominent initial "plague deniers" were Samuel K. Cohn, especially his "The Black Death: end of a paradigm," *American Historical Review* 107:3 (June 2002), 703–38; and Robert E. Lerner, "Fleas: Some scratchy issues concerning the Black Death," *Journal of the Historical Society* 8:2 (June 2008), 205–28. A summary of "the new microbiological consensus" regarding the agency of *Yersinia pestis* can be found in Monica H. Greene's "Editor's introduction" to a special issue of *The Medieval Globe* 1:1 (2014), 27–62, along with articles in that issue by Ann G. Carmichael ("Plague persistence in Western Europe: a hypothesis") and Nükhet Varlik ("New science and old sources: why the Ottoman experience of plague matters"). The most recent review article is Guido Alfani and Tommy E. Murphy, "Plague and lethal epidemics in the pre-industrial world," *The Journal of Economic History* 77:1 (March 2017), 314–43. An earlier overview of the debate is Lester K. Little, "Plague historians in lab coats," *Past and Present* 213 (November 2011), 267–90. A summary of the inadequacies of the traditional transmission model is found in Hans Ditrich, "The transmission of the Black Death to Western Europe: a critical review of the existing evidence," *Mediterranean Historical Review* 32:1 (June 2017), 25–40.

[94] Raoult, et al., "Plague: history and contemporary analysis," 19, confirm lice as a vector, as do Katharine R. Dean, et al., "Human ectoparasites and the spread of plague in Europe during the second pandemic," *PNAS* [*Proceedings of the National Academy of Sciences*], February 2018, https://doi.org/10.1073/pnas.1715640115 (accessed January 2019); it is also referred to in Lilith K. Whittles and Xavier Didelot, "Epidemiological analysis of the Eyam plague outbreak of 1665–1666," *Proceedings of the Royal Society B* 283:20160618(2016), 2 (accessed January 2019).

fleas transported in woolen cloth could go for months without food in a state of hibernation and eventually transmit the disease to humans when they came into contact with a human host."[95] The surgeon José Estiche, working in Zaragoza in the 1650s, was ahead of the game when he wondered, assuming that cloth could be contagious, if it could remain that way for some time.[96] City and town officials throughout Castile, in other words, may have made the occasional gesture toward the moon, and perhaps they burned more aromatic herbs than strictly necessary, but their remedies to halt the epidemic and their insistence on the quarantine may have made considerable sense. Contagion was an empirical explanation for the disease and may in fact have existed in cases, though the epidemic nature of the disease can be explained only through vectors. So historians' occasionally condescending dismissals of the utility of quarantine in past centuries on the basis that the only vector of importance was the rat may have done Vargas and his colleagues a great disservice.

Melgar's insistent appeals prompted Vargas in April 1598 to once again convey the town's complaints to the Council of Castile. The townspeople had written to him saying they were running out of supplies, and they asked that each village council be empowered to appoint someone to go out and get wine and other foodstuffs and equipment and leave it at the shrines.[97] The townspeople's isolation "seems very harsh [cosa rigorosa], but considering it carefully, it is what piety and good government demand," he wrote, while at the same time asking the Council of Castile for permission to inspect the towns once again, a request he had made before but to which the Council of Castile had not replied. (The council must have consented this time, for this was when he dispatched Cristóbal de Morales to return to Melgar to interview inhabitants, as described in Chapter 2.) "Their complaints and demands are especially frequent regarding the harm that comes from prohibiting them from selling their wheat at a time when prices have risen so much," he said, "so we allowed them to take the wheat out to the shrines and to the countryside, where they can traffic with outsiders without direct contact." Storing wheat at the shrines had led to a new problem, however, which was that doctors believed "the illness can stick

---

[95] Nükhet Varlik, "Plague, conflict, and negotiation: the Jewish broadcloth weavers of Salonica and the Ottoman central administration in the late sixteenth century," *Jewish History* 28 (2014) 261–88, pp. 263, 273, and bibliography cited therein, esp. Kenneth L. Gage and Michael Y. Kosoy, "Natural history of plague: perspectives from more than a century of research," *Annual Review of Entomology* 50:1 (2005), 505–28, pp. 517–18.

[96] José Estiche, *Tratado de la peste de Çaragoça en el año 1652* (Pamplona: Diego de Zabala, 1655), 29r–v.

[97] AMB-HI 3651, early January 1598.

to wheat, especially when it is damp... Experience has shown this is true, as we have information from Boadilla de Villamar, where wheat was taken from pestilent villages to some shrines, and soon afterwards a *vecino* from the said place put his arm into the said wheat and felt pain in his arm, which led me to quickly put a stop to this and halt the commerce and communication they are asking me for."[98]

In this chapter and throughout the book, it should be clear that doors (or gates) were never really slammed shut or wide open, and even in the odd instance where they might appear that way, there was always room for maneuver.[99] The wall was a good place for observing who was who. A wide-open door meant to be interpreted as a sign of health might also be a sign of deceit. A closed door might reflect the confidence of health within or the fear of illness without. In any case, of course, quarantine was impossible to enforce. People were always going to sneak in and out, or successfully petition to cross unopposed. The challenge was to weigh the dangers of the disease against the dangers of one more day without the goods that were – even with pestilent pleats – their lifeblood. As Vargas wrote early on in the epidemic, referring to the quarantine, "We are harming ourselves with our own hands, we are killing ourselves as we close ourselves in."[100] Disease was never entirely certain, but there was no uncertainty about the fact that towns where people could not buy or sell or work in their fields or deliver their products were dying anyway. The open gate was worth the gamble.

---

[98] AMB-HI 3650, April 10, 1598.
[99] Daniel Jütte, *The Strait Gate: Thresholds and Power in Western History* (New Haven, CT: Yale University Press, 2015).
[100] AMB-HI 3653, August 14, 1597.

Site 4: Market

During quarantine, what did people do without? Food, for one thing. If they were not starving before the plague arrived, they probably were once it reached their town or reached the towns that normally supplied them. Virtually every plague report, whether from villages or major cities, mentioned that people were hungry, though many, of course, had been hungry before the plague arrived.[1] "Consider where we are, the disease hated above all others, and the number of poor people, and you will find hunger and need. And more are dying of that than of anything else, because the land here just yields stones," wrote a priest from Pasajes. "What little we got from the sea has ceased altogether, and thus those who used to care for the poor are unable today to take care of themselves."[2] The occasional open gate may have alleviated some towns'

---

[1] Here I will stipulate that being poor and hungry makes one susceptible to most diseases (especially typhus, which sometimes may have been mistaken for plague), and that plague and famine, fellow horsemen of the apocalypse, were also linked, if not causally or always in fact then in the popular (and historiographic) imagination. Previously we saw that the poor were sometimes expelled during the plague, but less because they were poor (and hungry) and therefore the "cause" of the epidemic, than because they were from elsewhere. On plague and famine in general see chapter 2 of Guido Alfani, *Calamities and the Economy in Renaissance Italy: The Grand Tour of the Horsemen of the Apocalypse*, trans. Christine Calvert (New York: Palgrave, 2013); Andrew B. Appleby, "The disappearance of plague: a continuing puzzle," *The Economic History Review* 33:2 (May 1980), 161–73; Appleby, "Disease or famine? Mortality in Cumberland and Westmorland 1580–1640," *The Economic History Review* 26:3 (1973), 403–32; and Appleby, "Epidemics and famine in the Little Ice Age," *Journal of Interdisciplinary History* 10:4, *History and Climate: Interdisciplinary Explorations* (Spring 1980), 643–63. On the Castilian case see Vicente Pérez Moreda, "The plague in Castile at the end of the sixteenth century and its consequences," in *The Castilian Crisis of the Seventeenth Century: New Perspectives on the Economic and Social History of Seventeenth-Century Spain*, I. A. A. Thompson and Bartolomé Yun Casalilla, eds. (Past and Present Publications, Cambridge University Press, 1994), 32–59, p. 39, where he states, "If famine was neither the principal factor nor the immediate cause of the crisis, it may certainly have increased both the rhythm and the intensity of mortality."

[2] Letter from Miguel de Villaviciosa, writing from Fuenterrabia about Pasajes de San Juan, in Luis Murugarren Zamora, "La peste en Guipuzcoa (1597–1599)," *Boletin de la Real Sociedad Bascongada de Amigos del Pais* 4:1–2 (1984), 247–69, p. 267.

needs for some products at certain times, but in general business was bleak. Meanwhile people were starving, "the most cruel of all deaths," as Don Quijote told Sancho.[3]

In the distant past, people might have thought that plague was somehow the outcome of unsavory commercial practices, a punishment for their excesses.[4] And later, in early-eighteenth-century Marseille, the site of what is usually considered Europe's last epidemic of bubonic plague, again the evils of commerce were conjured up. Only political and civic virtue, not corruption and craven material desire, would save the republic, it was said. At least rhetorically, Marseille turned away from commerce as it struggled to impose a new moral and sanitary order.[5] Nothing like that happened in Castile. The Iberian Peninsula was an eminently commercial place, and it was generally accepted by theorists, jurists, officials, and citizens that this brought not only prosperity and plenty but also that there was an inherent good in the give and take, the sociability, the provision of products and foodstuffs for the good of the republic – as long as the price remained just and the poor were attended to. By now readers should realize that Castilians at the turn of the seventeenth century believed it was the lack of commerce that was killing them.[6] Their hunger was the result of a failed economy. The establishment of Madrid as the capital, the decline of the cloth and wool industries, the subsequent severing of economic linkages between village and town, imbalances between rural and urban areas, inflation, and foreign competition all interacted as causes and effects.[7] Harvests were disappointing, taxes rose, towns and villages emptied out. Poor-relief efforts had halted, and the weather continued to be bad. There

[3] *Don Quijote* II chapter 59, said as Quijote was dying, though of sadness, not hunger.

[4] Mark Harrison, *Contagion: How Commerce Has Spread Disease* (New Haven, CT: Yale University Press 2012), 9.

[5] Junko Thérèse Takeda, *Between Crown and Commerce: Marseille and the Early Modern Mediterranean* (Baltimore, MD: Johns Hopkins University Press, 2011), 130, 133, 142. Messina and Tunis also suffered from that last wave.

[6] Though it is also true that passage of the disease through cloth was sometimes attributed to eagerness to make a sale or buy on the cheap. In this vein, Matías Escudero wrote in 1582 that an epidemic in 1564–1565 had made its way north from Africa because of greedy (*codiciosos*) French and Murcian merchants; Matías Escudero de Cobeña, *Relación de casos notables ocurridos en la Alcarria...*, Francisco Fernández Izquierdo, ed. (Guadalajara: Ayuntamiento de Almonacid de Zorita, 1982), 162.

[7] On cloth see Angel García Sanz, *Desarrollo y crisis del Antiguo Régimen en Castilla la Vieja: Economía y sociedad en tierras de Segovia de 1500 a 1814* (Madrid: Akal, 1986); and Angel García Sanz, "Castile 1580–1650: economic crisis and the policy of 'Reform'," in *The Castilian Crisis of the Seventeenth Century*, Thompson and Yun Casalilla, eds., 13–31; on wool see Carla Rahn Phillips and William D. Phillips, Jr., *Spain's Golden Fleece: Wool Production and the Wool Trade from the Middle Ages to the Nineteenth Century* (Baltimore, MD: Johns Hopkins University Press, 1997).

were important regional disparities, though, as some places took advantage of others' misfortunes; plague, like all disasters, provided economic opportunities, as we have seen, but the aggregate and the long term tend to be of little comfort to the afflicted.[8]

In 1597, the desperate town council of Castro Urdiales, where plague had attacked so quickly and so soon that no defense was possible, provisioned and armed several boats to set out and capture food from whatever other boats they could find. Six years later, some of the makeshift corsairs (one of them a boat captain, whose fellow defendants included his wife and a group of sailors) found themselves in court promising to repay the damages they had inflicted on a group of Galicians whose boat they had captured. The agreement between the parties states they were "sailing as corsairs, at war [*en corso y guerra*], procuring supplies during the peste that was in the said town at that time."[9]

Possibly other seaside towns acted similarly.[10] Interior townspeople, as we have seen, sneaked out to their fields or to other towns to collect supplies or glean what they could from fields and storage caves. Soldiers and sailors did not have that option unless they deserted. "If the plague doesn't kill them, hunger will," remarked the viceroy of Navarre, Don Juan de Cardona, to Philip III of his soldiers in Pamplona.[11] One of the most brilliant and acerbic of royal servants, Juan de Silva, was posted in Lisbon during these years, from where he wrote to Philip III while the latter was still in eastern Spain: "The soldiers waste away little by little from the disease, and most of them are affected, as hunger clears the way for illness." That same day Silva wrote to Andrés de Prada, a secretary of war to both Philip II and Philip III: "The progress of the *mal contagioso* is destroying these poor soldiers; three, four, or six of them fall ill every day, and never fewer than three … More would escape the disease if they could eat what they need and stay clean, but I suspect that what with the news from the fleet no one is paying any attention to this, as if we could eat news, and meanwhile more time is wasted in requests and

---

[8] On gains and losses as a result of plague and other disasters, see Alfani, *Calamities and the Economy in Renaissance Italy*, where he advocates (p. 8) a "holistic" approach that can account for the total context of economic and social data.

[9] Pedro Andrés Porras Arboledas, "La práctica mercantil marítima en el Cantábrico Oriental (siglos XV–XIX)," *Cuadernos de Historia del Derecho* 7 (2000), 13–127, p. 31, citing AHPC Prot. 1703, fols. 15–18.

[10] José Ramón Cruz Mundet, *"El mal que al presente corre": Gipuzkoa y la peste (1597-1600)* (San Sebastián: Kutxa Fundazioa, 2003), 65, reports that in April 1598 San Sebastián asked the king for permission to launch pirate ships against English and Dutch ships for similar reasons; the king said yes, but the city said it could not afford it.

[11] AGS-GyM leg. 548 doc. 3, Cardona to Philip III, October 29, 1599.

replies…"[12] Another of Philip II's envoys, Melchor de Teves, whom we saw earlier in Valladolid and before that in the military ports of Galicia, was of the opinion that it was not peste at all but rather hunger that was killing the poor, always the principal victims. Hunger caused *secas*, he told the king, and the obvious proof was that "men with black capes," or *letrados*, did not get sick, an opinion he would surely revise the following year once he arrived in Valladolid.[13]

Castile's overlaying networks of roads were particularly intense in the northern half of the peninsula. People lived off these roads. Valladolid and Burgos bought their meat in Extremadura, and cattle traveled from Galicia into Castile. Muleteers traveled from northern ports to Castilian cities, taking fish south and returning north with wine and grains. From further south, in La Mancha, they rode north with oil and soaps and took Castilian grains back with them, though grains seem to have traveled shorter distances than food, with most places producing at least some of their own bread.[14] Not all commerce was halted during quarantine. A city still had to take care of its people, it had to acquire the food, wine, wood, meat, medicines, and clothing from somewhere, and not necessarily from somewhere healthy. The sudden urgent demand meant prices would go up, of course, benefiting sellers and anyone else along the supply chain who could help get products moving down the roads and over the walls. As the Pasajes priest wrote, "All roads are closed to us, by land and by sea, so whatever used to cost us one, today costs us twenty."[15]

City council minutes throughout the region reflect the excruciating need for grain, mostly wheat, and bread even before the first person fell ill.[16] According to Paul Hiltpold's work on Burgos, this scarcity was not necessarily or entirely a supply problem but rather evidence that price ceilings were not being enforced or were enforced unevenly as a result of subterfuge or royal privileges, making price controls useless. As a result,

---

[12] BN mss. 6.198, fol. 108, Torre de Caparica, March 13, 1599. The reference to the fleet may concern last-gasp adventures by Spanish fleets against the English. The always quotable Silva two months later wrote to his friend and colleague Cristóbal de Moura about the plague in Lisbon: "The world is falling apart here while people think only of their own problems and pleasures"; BN ms 6.198, fol. 114.

[13] AGS-GyM leg. 515, doc. 177, June 13, 1598.

[14] José Ubaldo Bernardos Sanz, *Trigo castellano y abasto madrileño: Los arrieros y comerciantes segovianos en la Edad Moderna* (Valladolid: Junta de Castilla y León, 2003), 32. The words "bread" (*pan*) and "grain" or "wheat" (*trigo*) were often interchangeable.

[15] Murugarren Zamora, "La peste en Guipuzcoa, 267.

[16] One small but relevant example: Isabel Testón Núñez, et al., "Los problemas del abastecimiento del pan en Extremadura: La ciudad de Trujillo (1550–1610)," *Studia Historica. Historia Moderna* 5 (1987), 159–75.

grain moved to better markets, a shift made possible by, precisely the region's complex and far-reaching roads. That said, it is also true that towns had to buy high during the waning years of the century, having exhausted their stocks, and then sell low to their own townspeople.[17] Most towns and cities had municipal granaries (*pósitos* or *alhóndigas*), used to store grains during plentiful years and thus control supply and prices, but local measures could be undermined by market disturbances elsewhere. In theory, and sometimes in fact, *pósitos* were what saved people. But they also were frequently in the hands of unscrupulous local figures who might use them for their own benefit, both political and financial, or the buying and selling by town officials might turn out to be unprofitable.[18] Bilbao, for example, suffered from the plague starting in 1598, and this once and future hub of northern shipping and nascent industry was starving. "Given the great need and hunger that people and *vecinos* of this city are suffering, and that many are obviously dying of hunger, the city agreed to send Dr. Villarreal, priest of this town's church, to find out which people are suffering from need and, at the city's expense, give them decent help [*honesto sustento*] so they do not suffer so much hunger," the city council minutes read. A few days later bread was distributed at the city's expense, and later that month the minutes report that the bishop of Álava had sent his condolences and had offered to *sell* Bilbao 2,000 *fanegas* of wheat. Bilbao accepted the offer and sent someone to Álava to negotiate a "good price" with the idea of distributing bread among the poor.[19]

Bread was the currency of disaster. If the granary still had grain, as was the case at first with Burgos, the king might give permission for the city to simply distribute it among the poor, bypassing the usual price and supply rules.[20] But some towns were obliged to buy grain from other places,

---

[17] Paul Hiltpold, "The price, production, and transportation of grain in early modern Castile," *Agricultural History* 63:1 (Winter 1989), 73–91.

[18] For one example of how a *pósito* functioned, with the added appeal that the *sobras* of the *alcabala* were involved, see Linda Martz, *Poverty and Welfare in Habsburg Spain: The Example of Toledo* (Cambridge University Press, 1983), 138–9. Philip II reformed the *pósito* system in 1584: see María del Carmen Fernández Hidalgo and Mariano García Ruipérez, *Los pósitos municipales y su documentación* (Madrid: Abad, 1989), 83–8.

[19] AFB libro 023, September 12, 16, and 26, 1598. A *fanega* is a dry measure equivalent to around 1.5 bushels of wheat.

[20] AMB-HI 2376, "*Provisión facultando a la ciudad para que pueda repartir por una vez entre los pobres enfermos de peste hasta 500 fanegas de trigo del pósito,*" April 30, 1599. Francis Brumont, "Le coup de grace: la peste de 1599," in *La Ciudad de Burgos: Actas del Congreso de Historia de Burgos* (Valladolid: Junta de Castilla y León, 1985), 335–42, p. 338, refers to nearly ten times that amount being distributed in Burgos over the summer; see also his "Le pain et la peste: Épidémie et subsistances en Vieille-Castille a la fin du XVIe siècle," *Annales de Démographie Historique* (Paris: EHESS, 1989), 207–20,

which meant paying transportation costs, subject to controls, and borrowing money by mortgaging their own municipal properties, an operation that required the king's permission. The resultant guarantees, or collateral, over time became something like credit default swaps that could be handed off to new investors. One of Bilbao's neighbors, Lequeitio, left a record of a deed of deposit stating which town properties had been handed over to Nicolás de Olaeta and his wife, María Pérez de Insaurraga, who for some reason then transferred the properties to their neighbor, Nicolás de Jauregui, after which the deposit was renewed at the request of a *vecino* of Aulestia named Sancho Martínez de Iturrioz, one of Lequeitio's creditors, all "for a shipment of grain delivered as a result of the plague epidemic."[21] The usual operation was for a town to request permission to raise revenue through a *censo*, a sort of annuity or mortgage loan, the most widespread credit instrument in early modern Castile. City councilors and well-off people often placed their money in these bonds and annuities, thus making themselves beneficiaries of the very taxes they levied. At the height of the plague, in August 1599, Segovia requested permission to take out a *censo* worth 40,000 ducats on its granary, a huge amount; the city, like others, was resorting to the expedient of selling *censos* to investors in order to maintain its granary, a slippery slope that often ended badly.[22] A much smaller town, Mañeru (Navarre) left behind the careful testimony it gathered in order to justify its request to float a *censo* worth 1,000 ducats "to help the poor in the said town and buy wheat and fix the dam at the mill." Mañeru is near Estella and Puente la Reina, among the Navarrese towns worst hit by plague. Both the wheat and grape harvests had been very poor, its own workers were being turned away elsewhere out of fear of infection, and, on top of that, guarding the town was an expensive proposition. So the poor were starving, and the little wheat the town had that normally would be sold was staying within its walls, partly because no one would buy it and partly to feed its own. The town needed 1,500 or even 2,000 ducats (both are mentioned) but was asking for permission to mortgage just 1,000. Six *vecinos* provided almost identical testimony regarding the situation, which was received by the Navarrese Royal Council. The first of the

pp. 214–15, which contains detailed information about Burgos's wheat purchases during 1598.

[21] AFB Notarial Lequeitio, escr. Amezqueta 15.

[22] AMS Actas leg. 1016, August 13, 1599; I do not know if the request was successful. Toledo took similar steps, with its *pósito* eventually going bankrupt in 1608; see Martz, *Poverty and Welfare*, 145. For examples of 1630s regidores investing in their cities' own *censos*, see Ruth MacKay, *The Limits of Royal Authority: Resistance and Obedience in Seventeenth-Century Castile* (Cambridge University Press, 1999), 71–2.

witnesses – they all were men, all except the priest sixty years old or older – Martín de Beriain, said he knew the town had 130 or 140 ducats worth of municipal properties (*propios*) and rents, plus whatever the mill took in, which this year was hardly anything. The town's debts reached 250 ducats, borrowed from *vecinos*, mostly to feed the poor so they would not die of hunger or wander off in search of food. "Because of the peste and because we are so close to Puente de la Reina, no one will come here to buy wine or livestock and people here cannot find buyers and thus they have no money with which to hire laborers and other people to work in their fields, and thus everyone is in great need..." Town leaders and the vicar, Martín Martínez, had scoured the region at great expense looking for bread, which they said they had bought only at a very high price.[23]

With granaries empty or being trafficked by town governments, and with roads increasingly off-limits to vendors whose products anyway would not be allowed through, it was essential that villages that had the grain with which to produce their own bread be allowed to do so. As usual, Burgos and its towns offer examples of ingenuity and both good and bad behavior. After the town of Cogollos became pestilent, it leased a mill from the nearby town of Hontoría de la Cantera so that, as Corregidor Diego Vargas Manrique wrote, "The *vecinos* would not go lacking and would be able to support themselves." But now, the corregidor wrote, Hontoría had decided to kick the people from Cogollos out, saying they were not following the rules. This was not right, he said, it was not just. He ordered Hontoría to immediately let those from Cogollos return so they could grind their grain. In turn, he instructed the latter that they indeed had to follow the rules: they could not wander off from the direct road, and they must appoint just one or two people to be in charge of carrying and grinding the grain.[24] Similarly, Tobar had blocked people from Susinos from using a mill that might actually have belonged to Susinos though it was within Tobar's limits. Tobar said those from Susinos were pestilent, which they were, but the corregidor pointed out that depriving them of bread was most harmful to them. Therefore, he decided that Tobar should send someone to the shrine between the two towns to pick up the grain that Susinos would leave there to be milled; Tobar should grind it and return it to the shrine. Furthermore, Toribio Ortega, a resident of another nearby town (probably present-day Pedrosa

[23] AGN TR Procesos 017710. The quote is from fol. 2r.
[24] AMB-HI 3651, fols. 38r–9r, September 1597. This was the same month that Vargas sent shoes to Cogollos.

del Páramo), was hired to supply Susinos with any supplies they might need in this regard.[25]

Fish was the most common food product being transported from the north, and it was a ubiquitous item on most people's plates, which was only logical given the number of church-mandated feasts. But immediately there were problems. Once news reached Burgos that Santander was infected, Corregidor Gerónimo de Montalvo and his plague commissioners prohibited all fish from northern ports from entering.[26] Ávila in December 1597 prohibited *besugo* from Santander and its towns, instead recommending fish from Asturias and Galicia; possibly the Galician route would have worked, but the Asturian route (via León) seems an unlikely solution. Serafín de Tapia writes that gradually "fresh" fish in the interior was actually salted and soaked or in escabeche (brined or marinated), which might have been safer but might also have disguised bad fish, or at least raised fears in that direction.[27] Indeed, escabeche caused problems in Valladolid, and possibly elsewhere; at around the same time as Ávila halted sea bream, Valladolid's city council was dealing with a shipment of brined fish sitting outside the Río Mayor gate, a matter of sufficient importance for a full council meeting to be called on October 29, 1597 to discuss the entry of fresh and salted fish. It was not simply the matter of consumer safety but, naturally, of money; fishmongers and tax farmers who had successfully bid to collect the *renta del pescado* were very keen on having the fish be admitted and had made their wishes known. The majority of the council ended up approving what seems to have been a compromise: the council agreed that no fish could enter the city unless it was bought in the same port where the fish had died and furthermore that it be accompanied by notarized testimony to that effect. The brined fish that had inspired the meeting and which had not been allowed to pass through the city gate had been purchased on the outskirts of Medina de Rioseco, most certainly not a port (though it was one of the region's most important fair towns), and was said to have come from "suspicious parts." The majority council vote was followed by the presentation of a petition by tax farmers asking that the city appoint someone to go with fish buyers to the markets

---

[25] AMB-HI 3650, October 9, 1598.
[26] AMB-HI 3653, January 4 and February 6, 1597.
[27] Serafín de Tapia, "Los factores de la evolución demográfica de Ávila en el Siglo XVI," *Cuadernos Abulenses*, no. 5 (January–June 1986), 113–200, p. 169. Bacalao, dried-salted cod, was present along the coasts, with Bilbao as its main entry point. But it had not yet started being widely consumed in the interior, though Regine Grafe points out that Don Quijote sampled some; *Distant Tyranny: Markets, Power, and Backwardness in Spain, 1650–1800* (Princeton, NJ: Princeton University Press, 2012), 58.

(though it is unclear at which markets they bought their fish) and watch them make their purchases and examine the certificates accompanying the fish. They protested that they would lose income as a result of the city's precautions and said they would insist in this regard to the Chancillería.[28]

Just a few weeks later in Burgos the health commission entertained petitions from fish vendors and asked them to propose safe routes over which fish could travel from the coast to the city.[29] That may have been because the Council of Castile around that time got involved in figuring out how to safely move fish from the infected north coast all the way down to Madrid, and for some reason the corregidor of Burgos was coordinating the effort, leading to extraordinarily detailed correspond-ence in which each party essentially repeated what the other had said. The men who carried fish from the Cuatro Villas down to Madrid generally hailed from Suances and Comillas, while delivery men from San Vicente (itself one of the Cuatro Villas) more often went to Valladolid and its countryside to pick up bread (or grain) and wine, the corregidor told the council. The other ports of the Cuatro Villas were all infected. The challenge was to prevent fish from a sick town being transported to a healthy one. So, he proposed, those from Suances, Comillas, and perhaps San Vicente should each pass through a series of towns where they must obtain signatures from local officials, all of whom he named in his correspondence not only to all the towns of origin but also to the Council of Castile; one town did not have a notary (a remarkable occurrence, it must be said), so muleteers should meet there with aides to the Duke of the Infantado who would verify the operation. Muleteers from the healthy Vizcayan towns of Bermeo, Mun-daca, Motrico, Placencia (in present-day Guipuzcoa), and Portugalete also had routes laid out for them which all led straight to Pancorbo. As mule trains would have to make their way down through that beautiful, narrow town nestled in a steep gorge, he instructed the *alcalde mayor* there, Lic. Garay Martinez, to carefully examine everyone's papers, and the corregidor naturally sent copies of all these instructions to the Council of Castile. Once the travel papers passed muster in Pancorbo, another of the corregidor's aides would once again certify everything, checking the notar-ies' seals against a list of seals he had been given to ensure that the "sea bream and other fresh fish" would be allowed to enter the capital city.[30]

---

[28] AMVA sigs. 21-0 and 22-0, covering the same period, October 15–19, 1597.
[29] AMB-HI 3653, November 20, 1597.
[30] The Council's involvement in fish transport: AMB-HI 3650 fol. 9v–10v, January 1598; AMB-HI 3651, fol. 181v–2r, December 1597; and probably nearby entries.

Seafood was just one of a long list of foods whose journey inland was being interrupted or rerouted by the plague. At least in theory, meat was possible to raise oneself, and it was favored over vegetables. (Even today, vegetables are not high on Spaniards' list of favorite foods.) Lamb was generally preferred to beef, pork, or goat. During the plague, unless it could absolutely be proven that meat or cattle had not passed through suspicious parts, it probably was being halted, and townspeople had no choice but to be self-sufficient. Stews thinned out. One indication that meat had vanished from Burgos markets is that by late 1600 the city council prohibited anyone from taking tallow outside the city, "given its scarcity for making candles, owing to the lack of cattle as a result of the 1599 peste." (In one of Vargas Manrique's earlier, periodic reminders to Cogollos on proper plague precautions, he said he had been informed that there were not enough candles with which to light the holy sacrament, "so I am sending you wax that costs 400 maravedies."[31]) Whether the cattle had died or had been slaughtered, or none had been able to enter the area, or both, is not clear. But we know that meat of all sorts was recommended for people who had to live, work, or travel in pestilent areas; employees in the Alcalá de Henares hospital, we saw earlier, ate "good meat, very good wine, and good bread."[32] Luis Mercado recommended poultry of all sorts, lamb, veal, and stews with aromatic herbs and a shot of lemon, and he said fruits and vegetables should be avoided.[33] Half a century later, the Zaragoza surgeon José Estiche, who worked with plague patients, wrote that appropriate meals included "lamb, chickens, hens, capons, sour grapes, oranges, lemons, sour apples and other foods that are easy to digest, feeding each patient according to the seriousness of the illness, strength, age, and custom. The illness itself demands little food, but it must be good, administered on a schedule according to the orders of a prudent doctor. Usually patients were fed twice a day, and those who needed it were fed three or four times a day." They drank water, not wine, as the latter attracts heat and enables toxins to communicate with the heart.[34]

---

[31] AMB-LA 131, October 7, 1600; AMB-HI 3651, fol. 39r. Different words are used: *sebo* is tallow, *cera* is wax.

[32] RAH Jesuitas 9-3662/182. Carolyn A. Nadeau, *Food Matters: Alonso Quijano's Diet and the Discourse of Food in Early Modern Spain* (Toronto: University of Toronto Press, 2016), 45–6, notes that food was considered a remedy for mental illness.

[33] Luis Mercado, *El libro de la peste del Dr. Luis Mercado con un estudio preliminar acerca del autor y sus obras por el Dr. Nicasio Mariscal*. [1598] [Biblioteca Clásica de la Medicina Española, vol. 1] (Madrid: Imp. de Cosano, 1921), 251.

[34] José Estiche, *Tratado de la peste de Caragoça en el año 1652* (Pamplona: Diego de Zabala, 1655), 53r–v.

What little food there was, was often taxed. So on top of being sick and frightened, caring for relatives, and eating less, now people would pay more. We have seen that the most frequent fiscal mechanism for offsetting the cost of fixing walls, outfitting guards, paying medical salaries, and building and supplying hospitals was to levy a *sisa*, an excise tax placed on foodstuffs. *Sisas* required royal permission, which was generally granted though sometimes with modifications on the amount and length of time they were levied. *Sisas* could be used as collateral for municipal bonds and therefore often might benefit city council members and tax farmers. They were most frequently placed on wine and meat, though also on oil and vinegar; some foods, such as bread and wheat, were generally exempt. The burden of *sisas* was local; they were self-imposed. There was virtually no town that did not resort to them, not only for plague expenses but for any unexpected financial burden. Alcalá de Henares told Philip II in August 1598 that it needed to increase its guard force, including men on foot and on horseback who were circling the town to make sure no one entered, to which end it requested permission to place *sisas* on up to 300 ducats worth of unspecified food; the king and the Council of Castile responded with permission for 100 ducats, excluding bread, instructing that everyone must pay and that the *sisa* not be extended once the specified amount was collected.[35] The provision that no one be excepted is a reminder that all municipal tax arrangements were an opportunity to take advantage of one's neighbors; in Madrid later in the seventeenth century, when very strict anti-plague measures were in place, Philip IV's Council of Castile told the king it had received word that though the ongoing *sisa* of two maravedies on every *azumbre* of wine to pay for plague guards was supposed to be applied universally, wine suppliers to both houses of the palace (probably meaning the queen and the king) were not paying. Such inequity was not only unfair, the council pointed out, it was potentially dangerous being that religious establishments and ambassadors, who also had their own wine suppliers, would soon be doing the same, and the resulting holes in the city's security would hurt everyone.[36]

The wine country today known as La Rioja suffered massively during the late sixteenth-century plague; it had done so before and would do so again. It sits between Burgos, Bilbao, and Pamplona, so really there was

---

[35] AMAH leg. 569/001. The warning: "mandamos paguen y contribuyan todos y qualesquier personas de qualquier calidad y condición que sean." A 1581 *sisa* in Segovia related to plague precautions referred to "exempt and non-exempt" people, the former not liable for ordinary taxes; AMS leg. 23/8, July 6, 1581.

[36] AHN CS leg. 7236 (Archivo Antiguo del Consejo de Castilla), June 22, 1637. An *azumbre* was a liquid measure of around two liters.

not much hope. In 1600 the town of Badarán, on the route between Burgos and the Rioja capital city of Logroño, asked Philip III if it could levy a *sisa*.[37] Its spokesman was one Domingo Ochoa Alaiza, who began typically by outlining all the terrible burdens the town had suffered. Over the past year the town, whose 150 *vecinos* worked in the fields, had spent more than 1,000 ducats on doctors, druggists, surgeons, barbers, and gravediggers, he said, and the town was close to collapse. The town suggested two remedies: first, that the crown grant permission for the town to sell thirty *fanegas* of common lands (*dehesas*), which it said it had done in the past when faced with similarly dire financial emergencies (what the common people who used these common lands thought about this we do not know); and, second, the town wanted to levy a *sisa* for at least four years and for up to 2,000 ducats, also "according to custom and to what has been done in the past." The king's reply, as is often the case, reflects information contained in the town's missing original: the town had borrowed and/or mortgaged 3,000 ducats as a result of the plague, of which the city council had assumed up to 300 ducats, but the remaining amount, the town had said, would have to be covered by *sisas* on wine, sugar, meat, and fish.[38]

The king ordered Badarán's townspeople to gather in an open meeting to discuss the matter, "as is your use and custom," and to vote and collect information on "the nature of the contagious disease in the town and how long it lasted and how many people died and if indeed in order to remedy and cure the sick and pay the doctor … you sought loans and mortgages for the said three thousand ducats, or how much it was," and what the collatoral was. An open meeting was held on April 17, but the *alcalde mayor*, Diego de Boas del Bosco, said not enough people had come, so a larger meeting was held on April 27. There, a priest, Andrés de Arenzana, who was around sixty-three years old, led off the testimony by saying that more than 180 people had died of peste during nine months of 1599, which he knew because he had administered last rites.

---

[37] The entire Badarán discussion comes from AHN CS 30.168, exp. 12. Logroño itself received permission to levy a *sisa* for 1,000 ducats but was unable to implement it because by then the well-off had all left, leaving the city council no recourse but to mortgage off town properties; Fernando Pons Ibáñez, "Epidemia de peste en Logroño (Año 1599)," *Berceo* 73 (1964), 387–406, p. 395, citing city council minutes for July 12, 1599.

[38] Santo Domingo de la Calzada, a more important town just to the northwest of Badarán that appears frequently in Burgos documentation, obtained permission to pay for a doctor by placing *sisas* on lamb, beef, salted and cured fish, cooking and whale oil, candles, wine, and fresh fish; Diego Téllez Alarcia, "La peste Atlántica en Santo Domingo de la Calzada (1599)," *Berceo* 162 (2012), 85–119, p. 99, citing city council minutes for August 2, 1599.

He also knew that in order to pay the medical expenses the town had borrowed 100 ducats from Juan López, a *vecino*, and also that the towns of Nájera and Anguiano had given (pending payment) cooking oil and whale oil and shoes (or perhaps shoemakers) and many other things worth more than 200 ducats, and that "the said city" (probably Logroño) had given medicines worth more than 39,000 maravedies. The apothecary, doctor, and surgeon were all owed back salaries; the former barber-surgeon Pedro de Montenegro, was one of the first to die "in the fury of the said disease," meaning a new one had had to be hired. The priest also knew that four gravediggers had been hired from the town of Zacastro, four leagues away, because no one in the town dared do the job, and the four men were owed 250 ducats in salary and meals. Everyone remaining in the town, the priest concluded, was very poor indeed, their clothing and linens and furniture had all been burned, and therefore he knew it to be true that the fiscal requests would not harm any *vecino*. Arenzana was followed by a long line of witnesses who said essentially the same thing; among them, seventy-year-old Juan Muñoz reiterated all the town's debts and said that just ninety *vecinos* were left of the 200 who used to live there. The *alcalde mayor*, taking every precaution to ensure that the testimony would be acceptable to the crown, now decided that people from other towns should also offer information.[39] So the following day's meeting featured men from the nearby village of Cordovín. One, Juan de la Bastida, confirmed that Badarán had been isolated for more than nine months, that he had heard that 180 people had died there, and that it was deeply in debt. Another, Pedro de Cerinula, said the people of Badarán "are so poor and needy because of the said illness that if [the crown] does not give them the said license they will all leave the town, leaving behind their houses and children." A neighbor added that wives would also be abandoned. All the witnesses from Cordovín agreed that the *dehesas* being proposed for sale were highly appropriate. Around a month later the *alcalde mayor* asked the town council to draw up a list of all town properties, presumably following a request from the crown, and a few days later the town had its answer. The crown had determined that Badarán had spent 1,160 ducats on the plague, half of which it could raise by levying a *sisa*, but the other half would have to be divided up among the *vecinos*. There would be no selling-off of *dehesas*. The town appealed, but it is highly unlikely it succeeded. Its patron saint, San Roque, would have to suffice.

---

[39] At the end of Chapter 1 we saw Ávila towns seeking reductions of the *alcabala* similarly asking neighboring towns to provide corroborating testimony.

Towns and villages levied new taxes during plague years because they needed to pay for emergency health services, but also to offset losses owing to the drastic diminishment of other taxes as a result of the disappearance of commerce. The reduction of those taxes meant that tax farmers, many of them members of the municipal elites and town councils, were taking in far less. Devices we have seen such as sales taxes, sale of common lands and grain, and the mortgaging of public properties were generally decided upon by town and city councils whose members were far from neutral. They were economic agents, especially during times of crisis. Tolls (*el portazgo*), for example, whether of travelers into a city or the merchandise they carried, were obviously decreasing, and the town council of Pancorbo in 1600, through which just about all travelers from the north had to pass, complained to Burgos that the meager commerce from Vitoria and Bilbao during the plague had had serious implications for their tolls.[40] In an earlier episode, the *sisa* farmer in the seaside town of Guetaria (Guipúzcoa) sued his own city council asking that the terms of his lease be renegotiated to make up for his losses during the plague or that he be compensated for goods that were not allowed to enter the town, thus depriving him of income.[41] The man who leased the job of collecting revenue on cooking oil in Pamplona also sued, unsuccessfully, pointing out that he had been unable to find muleteers willing to travel with loads of oil in 1599, and even if he had, the towns of Aragon would not have let them in, instead greeting them at the gate with arquebuses and other weaponry. So he himself had to put together carts and mule trains and ended up losing money, or so he said.[42] One of his neighbors, Gaspar de Montalvo, who held the lease for fresh fish sales, also sued to be compensated for his alleged losses; he won a partial victory. In that case, Pamplona argued that though the lease contract did specify a discount in the case of warfare or plague as long as fewer than six regidores remained in the city, in fact the epidemic had been "so benign" that nobody in office had left, a blatant lie.[43] Another tax that suffered was the *renta del peso*, paid on all incoming products weighing over a certain amount.[44] There was a scale for assessing this tax

[40] AMB-LA 131, fol. 224r, July 3, 1600; the Burgos city council agreed to consider the matter, which does not seem to reappear in the minutes.
[41] ARCV Registro de Ejecutorias, caja 1242,6, suit filed by Juan Ortiz de Leizate dated 1572, but it is unclear when the plague visited Guetaria.
[42] AGN TR Procesos 296565.   [43] AGN TR Procesos 329929.
[44] José María Monsalvo Anton, "Poder municipal y mercado urbano precapitalista: Una introducción a las ordenanzas de la renta del peso mayor del concejo de Salamanca," *Salamanca: Revista Provincial de Estudios* 8 (April–June 1983), 63–76; the article includes the city's ordinances for the *renta del peso* from the early sixteenth century.

in a public and visible place where villagers from outside could also go, knowing they would pay an officially set price for their purchases. The tax farmers in charge of inspecting the weights (*pesos*) and collecting the amounts leased their post or were appointed; in the city of Salamanca they earned 5 percent of the value of all products bought and sold, though that amount was not necessarily charged elsewhere.[45] In Palencia in the wake of the plague, the tax became the focal point of a lawsuit. In April 1599 the corregidor there had told the king that the city and the surrounding six leagues were "entirely healthy," which may have been true at that moment, though probably not for long, given that the city is midway between Burgos and Valladolid. (The city's population in 1591 has been estimated to have been 10,218 inhabitants; by 1599 it had plunged to 5,143, though it gradually recovered.)[46] Its alleged and relatively good health may have been the result of especially stringent efforts to halt incoming merchandise, but those same efforts reduced revenue for the lessees of the *peso*, who sued the city demanding that the monetary value at which the *peso* had been set now be lowered to account for the fall-off in business. The lead plaintiff was Diego de Céspedes Lobera, who lost his initial case and appealed to the Chancillería in late 1599. One of his attorneys argued that "after my clients won the bid for the *renta del peso*, nearly all business and commerce of merchandise to be weighed ceased owing to the *enfermedad de peste* in this city of Valladolid [they were speaking in the Chancillería] and in the cities of Burgos, León, and Seville and in Villalar, Cisneros, and others..." When they had bid for the *renta del peso*, according to the brief, the only sick towns were far away on the north coast, meaning the guard did not much affect their revenue. But the guard in Palencia quickly became so intense that not only were people from nearby sick towns not allowed to enter, those from healthy towns were not allowed in either, as the lawyers demonstrated in their depositions, and as a result the lessees' revenue had gone down by three-quarters. Céspedes won the case. The city countered by saying any lessee had to run the risk of "fortuitious cases of peste and similar things," which was not part of the contract and anyway had been true

---

[45] Monsalvo Anton, "Poder municipal y mercado urbano precapitalista," p. 64.

[46] AGS-E leg. 183, doc. 300. The city did not suffer from the economic collapse to the same degree as the rest of Castile, according to Guillermo Herrero Martínez de Azcoitia, "La población palentina en los siglos XVI y XVII," *Publicaciones de la Institución Tello Téllez de Meneses* 15 (1956), 5–30. Population figures are from the same author, in "La población palentina en la Edad Moderna," in *Historia de Palencia, vol. II: Edades Moderna y Contemporánea* (Exma. Diputación Provincial de Palencia, 1984), 62–82, p. 68. Similar figures can be found in Annie Molinié-Bertrand, *Au siècle d'or l'Espagne et ses Hommes. La Population du Royaume de Castille au XVI siècle* (Paris: Economica, 1985), 156.

since time immemorial. And, the city added in its January 24, 1601 brief, "in the said city there was absolutely no peste," which actually did not contradict claims by the plaintiffs, who were talking about excessive prevention, not illness. If the plaintiffs had lost a great deal the previous year, the city said, that just meant they had made a lot of money in the years before that. But the appeals court held to its decision, ruling that Céspedes and his co-plaintiffs should get a reduction of 200,000 maravedies.[47]

As if the quarantine and the subsequent drop in commerce and tax revenue were not enough, there were also the instances, to which we have referred earlier, in which a town was said to be pestilent when it was not, making bad things considerably worse. Two towns with similar products and similar markets might easily be tempted to whisper here and there that it was said, one had heard, that just maybe the town down the road had had some unexpected deaths. We're not sure but, really, one can't be too careful. Such apparent libel seems to have descended upon the town of San Martín de Valdeiglesias, under the jurisdiction of Toledo (today it is part of the region of Madrid). Toledo had heard the bad news but wanted to make sure, and so it sent one Fernando Ruiz de los Arcos to find out. Rather than go straight to the target, the wily Ruiz de los Arcos circled. In his report, he said people in the villages of Almonte and Pelayos told him they weren't bothering to guard against San Martín being that they had heard that the news was due to differences between San Martín and Cebreros over wine sales. Cebreros wanted to sell more, so it had said San Martín was pestilent. (Though, in the previous chapter we saw that someone from Cebreros was sick in July 1599.) After hearing that, Ruiz de los Arcos decided to visit a nearby monastery, where the abbot assured him San Martín was fine, though he conceded that around twenty people had died in the past three weeks, including three or four men with *carbuncos* because they had not sought aid and had worked too hard in the sun-baked fields. On Thursday morning Ruiz de los Arcos entered San Martín itself and spent the whole day wandering around dissimulating, confirming, he said, that the town's health "has not been

---

[47] ARCV Pleitos Civiles Pérez Alonso (F) 1357-2. In a similar case in Pamplona, *peso* leaseholder Sancho de Berrio sued his city and won, as the Navarrese Royal Court ordered the city to discount forty ducats to offset his losses in 1599 (he had asked for seventy); AGN TR Procesos 013108. Disputes as a result of tax losses owing to the plague raises the interesting question of insurance, in this case financial protection against acts of God. I have found no reference to such coverage, though late medieval and early modern theologians and economists were debating its permissibility; see Giovanni Ceccarelli, "Risky business: Theological and canonical thought on insurance from the thirteenth to the seventeenth century," *Journal of Medieval and Early Modern Studies* 31:3 (Fall 2001), 607–58.

this good in years." He visited an apothecary (he bought sugar, to throw the man off) and learned that of around 7,000 inhabitants there, only twenty had died recently (the same number mentioned by the abbot), and indeed he wandered through the plaza and saw lots of happy people who were apparently unaware of what was being said about their town. Toward evening he loitered by the church to see if by chance there was a burial or if a priest might suddenly dash out to deliver last rites, but he came up empty. Finally, he visited the town of Cadagalso, which belonged to the marquis of Villena, and the estate guards told him they were not guarding against San Martín. What was good enough for the marquis was good enough for Ruiz de los Arcos, and he assured Toledo that San Martín de Valdeiglesias was not suffering from plague. Restoring its lost reputation, however, was a steep climb, and it would be nice to know by how much Cebreros's wine sales rose in 1598–1599.[48]

Cities and towns all either had regular markets or their inhabitants attended markets nearby, though the decline in the wool and cloth industries, along with reduced demand from the colonies, meant there were fewer such exchanges toward the end of the century.[49] During the plague, when muleteers and other vendors were halted at city gates with their cloth or fish or wool, they probably were aiming to get into the city for its weekly or biweekly market, diminished though it may have been. Burgos, as we saw when looking at the distribution of supplies at shrines, had markets at least twice a week; they were noisy, crowded, stinking, highly entertaining traffic jams.[50] Ávila had Friday markets in the Mercado Chico, as well as a yearly grand fair in September. Tudela's was every Thursday. The Palencian town of Carrión de los Condes, west of Burgos along the road to Santiago, had a Thursday market as well, but the usual system changed once plague threatened, which drove the town into a court of law. It would seem that originally the market was held inside the town walls but the council had moved it outside to the San Juan parish to protect the town from plague. The plaintiffs, residents of San Juan, on August 1, 1598 asked the town council to shut down the

[48] AMT Libro de Salud 176, unfoliated, sometime in 1598. Toledo sent several other men, councilmen and physicians among them, to inspect the surrounding towns; see Julián Montemayor, "Una ciudad frente a la peste: Toledo a fines del XVI," in *La ciudad hispánica durante los siglos XIII al XVI: actas del coloquio celebrado en La Rábida y Sevilla del 14 al 19 septiembre de 1981*, Emilio Sáez, et al., eds., 3 vols. (Madrid: Universidad Complutense, 1985), 1113–31.

[49] Michael R. Weisser, *The Peasants of the Montes: The Roots of Rural Rebellion in Spain* (Chicago, IL: University of Chicago Press, 1976), 12–13.

[50] Paul Jacob Hiltpold, "Burgos in the reign of Philip II: the Ayuntamiento, economic crisis, and social control, 1550–1600," PhD diss., University of Texas at Austin, 1981, 66–7.

transplanted market because it was attracting people from pestilent towns who apparently encountered no obstacles to entering not only the marketplace but also local houses. Closure would be "for the common good of the said town, and because of the urgency and the royal order [probably a routine plague warning from the king] the town should order the market closed, as everyone is of one same body and the same as all the rest."[51] In other words, San Juan residents should not be burdened with dangers not shared by the rest of the town. But the town council insisted the market should remain where it was and that there were sufficient guards in place to prevent contagion. The neighbors presented a second petition, and then a third, to the royal appeals court, insisting the market should be held where it had been since time imme-morial, that the city council should spend its funds on protecting the extramuros *vecinos* – for example by paying for guards to let them in and out of the town gates, which had been closed – and that they were "*vecinos* of the said town of Carrión and contribute just like the rest and therefore should benefit from the same privileges as the intramuros vecinos." They won their appeal, and the town council did not even bother appearing before the Chancillería.

In addition to its regular markets, Old Castile was famous for its regional fairs, often held on saint's days, and these, too, were altered. A contemporary *relación* praised Medina del Campo's fairs, among the most prominent in Europe in the late Middle Ages, because they "enriched the kingdom and supplied everything necessary for human life and good government," a nice summation of the virtues of commerce, though with the requisite caveat that bad habits and greed must be avoided at all cost.[52] Two other important, albeit much smaller, fairs in northern Castile were in Melgar de Fernamental, which we have seen was severely affected by plague, and Villalón de Campos, which used shrines as supply depots during these years, a sign that it also was suffering.[53] Towns were self-sufficient in certain products but relied on markets for others. As David Vassberg wrote: "It is difficult to make generalizations that stand up, because of the widely varying conditions between years, between regions, and even between villages in the same

---

[51] ARCV Registro de Ejecutorias, caja 1896, 87; "por ser todos ellos un cuerpo y un mismo con los demas."

[52] "Relación de la antigüedad y sitio de Medina del Campo y sus ferias y de la contratación de ellas, y del estado que tienen hasta hoy 18 de octubre de 1606," in CODOIN, vol. 17, 541–74, p. 543.

[53] Elena Maza Zorilla, "Villalón de Campos y la peste de 1599," *Cuadernos de investigación histórica* 2 (1978), 363–86.

region. But it is clear that Castilian villagers often had surpluses to market, and sometimes these surpluses were quite substantial."[54]

These fairs were social occasions as well as commercial ones, and as such they were immediately banned once an area had been declared pestilent, depriving people of both sustenance and distraction. The cancelation of a fair was perhaps the most obvious moment when officials weighed commerce and health against one another. In 1599 the king prohibited anyone from entering Valladolid to attend the San Miguel fair, which the city council protested, though earlier we saw that a town crier in Valladolid was owed money (from the city, no less) for announcing two markets before the San Miguel fair that anyone violating that order would suffer death.[55] The 100-ducat *sisa* that Alcalá de Henares was permitted to levy to pay for guards was of particular interest, the king remarked, given the upcoming San Bartolomé fair there on August 25, so that fair apparently was allowed.[56] But when Diego de Vargas Manrique quit his post as corregidor of Burgos in January 1598 because lower-level judges had violated his orders, one of his many complaints was that a certain *alcalde mayor* had allowed the San Martín and Santa Catalina fairs (it is unclear where) to proceed when he had explicitly prohibited them.[57] In May 1599, after the king told Segovia it would have to cancel its San Juan fair in late June 1599, the city council debated the matter, recognizing the "damage that might be done to His Majesty's royal patrimony" if the pestilence raging through the surrounding region and villages were to enter the city and put an end to the cloth trade. So the city council resolved in mid-May to go along with the king's order, but that was followed by a petition from outlying villages whose people depended upon the fair just as much, if not more, as the city did. Their spokesman, Juan de Vergara, explained that Segovia had not properly communicated to the king the opposition of some of its own city council members and of the villages, who argued that cancellation would be "very prejudicial and pernicious both to [the royal] service and the common good of the entire kingdom and the said city and its district." Vergara's petition was examined by the Council of Castile and, remarkably, the crown appears to have reversed itself. Despite the prior decision by the Segovia city council, the crown now ordered that the fair should be held as usual, though guards must be in place to ensure that no one from an infected

---

[54] David Vassberg, *The Village and the Outside World in Golden Age Castile: Mobility and Migration in Everyday Rural Life* (Cambridge University Press, 1996), 26, and in general chapter 2. See also chapter 1 of Bernardos Sanz, *Trigo castellano y abasto madrileño*, on the overlapping food networks that supplied Madrid.

[55] AMVA sig. 22-0, September 1, 1599; AMV-CH 130 a-4 (ant. leg. 321), fol. 56.

[56] AMAH leg. 569/001.   [57] AMB-HI 3651, fol. 196.

town enter the city.[58] So there were many interests in play: the host town, the outlying towns, the merchants, the innkeepers, people who wished to buy food and clothing and livestock, people who wished to sell, and authorities who needed to issue reasonable orders that stood a reasonable chance of being obeyed.

Documentation in the Burgos municipal archive offers one an especially rich and detailed account of the fair of San Lucas, in the beautifully preserved town of Villadiego, which though small, accounted for reams of correspondence. The town, part of the estate of the powerful Constable of Castile (it remained in the hands of that aristocratic clan until the nineteenth century), had 212 taxpayers (*pecheros*) in 1528 and 246 in 1591, so it was fairly stable at around 1,000 inhabitants, around half the present-day population.[59] Its spacious, lively, and irregularly shaped central square, entirely surrounded by a double stone and wood colonnade offering deep shade and shelter, depending on the time of year, is evidence of the town's prestige and importance.

In late September 1597, Vargas Manrique wrote to Villadiego saying he had learned the town held fairs on the feast days of San Lucas and San Andrés that were attended "by people from the mountains of the Kingdom of Toledo, Castile, Andalusia, and Vizcaya, and many people come to buy and sell all sorts of merchandise and livestock, and as the town is wide open and also surrounded by pestilent villages there is great danger of the peste or *mal contagioso* entering the town and then spreading throughout the kingdoms." He told the town that he would be in touch with the king (still Philip II) and the Council of Castile, and in the meantime he ordered Villadiego to meet and discuss the matter.[60] On September 30, the town wrote back, saying the majority of *vecinos* had met and had considered the drawbacks of both holding and canceling the fair. People from far and wide "have their hopes placed on the benefit of the said fairs, some because they buy food, others because they sell their animals." Therefore the *vecinos* "were unanimous in their agreement and desire that the said fairs not be canceled and that they go forward as is the custom and as was done in the cities, towns, and villages of Valladolid, Burgos, [and] Nájera, areas near this town that suffered from this danger which Our Lord has seen fit to bring upon them." They proposed a series of safety measures and promised to abide by them: town council

---

[58] AMS leg. 1016, May–June 1599.
[59] Molinié-Bertrand, *Au siècle d'or l'Espagne*, 148. The Palacio de los Velasco, the condestables' family name, stands just off the main square on a smaller square called Plaza de los Cerdos, perhaps because livestock was sold there.
[60] AMB-HI 3651, fols. 66–7, probably September 29, 1597.

members and other officials would guard the town; guards on foot and on horseback would be placed on all the little paths leading to pestilent villages in addition to on the roads; the corregidor and his law enforcement agents could inspect during the fair to ensure no one from a sick town was there; and innkeepers (whose livelihood naturally was threatened every time a fair was canceled) would receive the usual admonitions about pesty guests.[61]

The corregidor was torn, he explained to the Council of Castile. It was dangerous to hold the San Lucas fair, scheduled for October 18, but the towns needed it so badly.[62] In fact, the day before he wrote to the council he had gone to Villadiego himself to inspect. He met there with the town council and the *vecinos* and visited the site of the livestock fair and the areas just outside the town and confirmed that it would not be difficult to guard the entrances. He agreed that the town was well protected and that all the gates were closed except two, which had guards, and that they led onto the main square where the food market would be held. And yet, upon finishing this inspection, Don Diego told the townspeople he still had doubts. He was worried about needy buyers and sellers coming south from San Sebastián and Laredo, and also from Melgar de Fernamental and other pestilent towns in the area. We can assume that these doubts led him to deny permission, because Pedro de San Martín de la Portilla, the town's *procurador general*, presented a petition objecting to the ruling.[63] Edicts and orders were issued and copied and sent from Burgos to Villadiego and to Madrid, the upshot being that the fair would not be allowed.

The documents then jump to just after the day of San Lucas. Though the fair officially had not been held, people appeared to have gone anyway, ignoring the *pregones*. That was bad enough, but in addition authorities in the town of Briviesca (quite a distance away) had taken it upon themselves to punish its townspeople who had attended the fair that wasn't, and if there was one thing Vargas could not abide it was lower-level judicial officials taking matters into their own hands. He instructed them to immediately cease their policing on this point. Officials in Pancorbo, however, for some reason were allowed to prosecute their townspeople who had gone to the fair. Vargas had "personal orders from His Majesty that the Villadiego fair not be held," he told the Pancorbo *alcalde mayor*, despite which people there had allegedly gone to the fair, and so he ordered Pancorbo to find out who they were and punish them.[64] At the same time, he deputized two officials, Francisco López

[61] AMB-HI 3651, fol. 81, September 30, 1597.   [62] AMB-HI 3651, October 3, 1597.
[63] AMB-HI 3651, fols. 93v–5v.   [64] AMB-HI 3651, fols. 111r–12r, October 20, 1597.

and Diego de Frías Salazar, as constables and sent them out to find out what they could about the distressing fact that "many people had gone to the fair and bought and sold many products."[65] But the situation in Pancorbo turned oddly complicated as Vargas slowly became aware that in fact the Villadiego fair had not been held, neither legally nor illegally, and that therefore Pancorbo (and Briviesca, it turned out) for some reason were punishing people who had done no wrong. "Great rigor was used against the poor, because really there was no fair," Vargas told Pancorbo and Briviesca in his order to officials there to immediately drop the phony cases and stop stalling and send him the documentation he had requested.[66]

Villadiego's second fair, that of San Andrés, was next on the calendar, November 30, and by then Vargas was a bit overwhelmed by all the festivities. "From one hour to the next one learns of fairs about which one knew nothing before," he complained to the Council of Castile. In Santibañez, just three leagues away from the city, for example, there was yet another San Andrés fair, and meanwhile the peste was spreading rapidly, though mercifully it had not yet slipped through the Burgos city walls.[67] After hearing back from the Council of Castile that the San Andrés fair could not be held, he delivered the bad news to Villadiego, but, as before, the town pushed back. The fair would not increase the likelihood of the spread of disease, the town's leaders assured the corregidor, "because the lack of business affects poor people as much as the plague itself," the very same point the corregidor himself had made to the Council of Castile. Again, Vargas appears to have seen reason in the town's insistence, and he told the Council of Castile that the pestilent towns and villages, especially Melgar and Cogollos, in fact were improving and would continue doing so with the cold weather. "People's inability to go out to their crops means they are in need, and this is the reason why wheat is not being sold," he wrote, adding that he had heard that townspeople, in their desperation, were going to pestilent places and buying wheat there. But if shepherds from healthy places took healthy livestock to market there would be no danger, "because the benevolence of God is such that the illness is not contagious through the air," he argued, quite correctly, once again illustrating how determination of the epidemic's mechanisms, no matter how tentative, was crucial in the weighing of economic and commercial strategies.[68]

It seems unlikely that the San Andrés fair was held that year. Vargas surely was dismayed to see San Lucas back on his desk the following

[65] AMB-HI 3651, 112v–13r.   [66] AMB-HI 3651, fol. 133.
[67] AMB-HI 3651, fol. 138.   [68] ANB-HI 3651, fol. 142.

October (1598), when Villadiego naturally once again assured him that the town was perfectly healthy. Vargas sent one of his men to investigate and seems to have decided this time that the fair could be held but that no one from diseased towns was to attend. An order to that effect was cried out in all the relevant towns, villages, and along the roads, but it was probably impossible to faithfully enforce.[69]

So business was never entirely halted, but blockades (be they bureaucratic, physical, or fiscal) were set up everywhere, getting in the way of products, people, and money. Underlying it all was the question of trust. The fact that assurances of good health were generally met with a small invasion of messengers and spies whose job it was to determine the true state of affairs indicates that most towns distrusted the claims of others, probably because they knew that, were the situation reversed, they too would lie, saying they were healthy when they were not. Reputation was at stake, and there were few more important concepts in Castile. Later I will address the more theoretical aspects of truth and falsehood in the exercise of good government; here we will look just at commerce, at the crucial need to keep the goods moving and to be able to count on other people to trust one's claims. As Mark Harrison wrote, commerce during times of plague is "a game of chess with many players, each of which attempts to second-guess the actions of the others."[70] Lies, or simply breezy assurances of health, obviously work only if they are credible; but if everyone is doing it, then credibility is strained. Liars, in other words, have good reason to distrust others. On the other hand, the more good news floating around, the less the potential risk of lost reputation. Lies thus reflected a way of doing business within a network of political relations. Officials everywhere who reported early calamities assured the palace that great care had been taken to keep the matter quiet, to avoid *ruidos*, to alarm no one. Such subterfuge is typical of any disaster with potential social manifestations, not just plague; Richard Cobb, for example, writing about hunger in eighteenth-century France, said that "public authorities ... had to move carefully as soon as dearth, and its more dangerous outriders, rumour and credulity, were announced once again in a province. It would be unwise to take large-scale action immediately, for this might indicate alarm on the part of those who knew the true state of affairs and would confirm the people in their worst fears; a panic would ensue, and would make matters much worse."[71] Likewise, in plague-infested Venice in 1575, people did everything they could so as

---

[69] AMB-HI 3650, fols. 108–14.   [70] Harrison, *Contagion*, xvi.
[71] Richard Cobb, *The Police and the People: French Popular Protest, 1789–1820* (Oxford: Clarendon Press, 1970), 216.

not to alert the Republic's trading partners, who might otherwise declare Venice off-limits. Its ambassadors simply denied the epidemic had crossed the waters and invaded the crowded city.[72]

If this was a game, albeit in difficult conditions, there were no more important players than the commercial cities of Burgos and Bilbao, which critically needed each other and needed to be believed by the other. Both had brokers, agents, and traders stationed throughout the Iberian Peninsula and Europe. The Catholic Monarchs in the late fifteenth century had licensed the Consulate of Burgos to, among other things, make decisions regarding fleets and merchant insurance for goods arriving in the port of Bilbao, which did not please the latter city, and Queen Juana later gave Bilbao its own trade guild in 1511. Throughout the sixteenth century the two interdependent cities, while continuing to squabble, together "represented one of the most important pillars of the Spanish economy, one of its great poles of growth."[73] By the time of our plague, Bilbao still had a substantial foreign commercial community, and in fact in August 1599 the city ordered Flemish, French, and Portuguese merchants living there to immediately contribute to the anti-plague effort with a set amount of money, under pain of prison and confiscation of goods.[74] Shipowners in Bilbao had close commercial and family links to merchants in Burgos, from whence most northern coastal production was distributed throughout the peninsula and which also channeled peninsular products north to the ports. Bilbao was a center for fishing, timber, shipbuilding, and iron. It also served as a stopping-off port for products that would later be shipped around the peninsula to Andalucía. It was an inexpensive port to operate out of, a storage depot, and a market in itself, and by the end of the sixteenth century, it had emerged as the leading Cantabrian port; in 1568 when Laredo (anyway in a less favorable location) fell to epidemic, ships from the Low Countries had shifted their cargo to Bilbao, so everyone knew the lesson.[75] Bilbao,

---

[72] Paolo Preto, *Peste e società a Venezia nel 1576* (Vicenza: Neri Pozza Editore, 1978), 31–4.

[73] Jean-Philippe Priotti, *Bilbao et ses marchands au XVI siecle: Genese d'une croissance* (Villeneuve d'Ascq: Presses Universitaires du Septentrion, 2004), 31; on the consulates see Hiltpold, "Burgos in the Reign of Philip II," p. 44.

[74] AFB Consulado 0051/013. Twenty-eight names are listed, each one paying between 100 and 400 reales, to be collected by Rui de Aguirre, a *vecino*.

[75] The Laredo item in Priotti, *Bilbao et ses marchands au XVI siecle*, 116, citing Simón Ruiz correspondence; see also William D. Phillips, Jr. "Spain's northern shipping industry in the sixteenth century," *The Journal of European Economic History* 17:2 (Fall 1988), 267–301; and Phillips and Phillips, *Spain's Golden Fleece*, 218, which notes that relations between the two cities became strained as Bilbao merchants began acting on their own account. I do not know if European nations stayed away from Bilbao's port during this plague, but I have to assume that they did, meaning that the game of mutual deceit among Spanish cities was reproduced more widely; on this subject in general see

despite having been infected earlier by the plague than inland cities, which put it at an immediate disadvantage, was on the rise, while Burgos was most certainly past its prime.[76] But the great Castilian city, which had the honor of being addressed above all other cities as "the very noble and very most loyal city of Burgos, *cabeza de Castilla*," was not quite yet out of the picture, if for no other reason than geography.[77] Eventually, though, the long wars with the Low Countries, along with incessant attacks by English ships, hurt Burgos more than any other city, spelling the end of the wool trade. Much of its business, including its role as Spain's leading insurance broker, would end up being picked up by Madrid.

A letter from Vargas Manrique to the Council of Castile in early 1598, the year during which Burgos and Bilbao played their deadly game of deceit and false hope, shows he understood perfectly the pitfalls of relying on other people's word. "In Burgos," he wrote, "it is said, and it has been written, that Vitoria has peste, with five or six houses closed up. Many times I have determined that similar news turns out to be false, the result of various sorts of enmities and jealousies, which I would like to put a stop to with punishments." But, he told the council, public health was of such urgent importance that he had to proceed as if the news were true, given that Vitoria – midway between Bilbao and Burgos – "has so much business and commerce, as it is the place where all the merchandise and supplies coming from the Vizcayan ports and much of the Cuatro Villas pass through."[78] Vargas also wrote to Vitoria, stressing the need to "put the common good before the particular good." Judging from the Burgos end of the correspondence, Vitoria had complained that Bilbao was lying about Vitoria's state of health; Vargas seems to have heard that Bilbao was halting all messengers from Vitoria and refusing all contact with anyone coming from that city. "I do not know if this is the result of jealousy or greed or anything else," Vargas wrote, "but if it were discovered that there had been false testimony and the person or persons

Harrison, *Contagion*, chapter 2; and, concerning a later plague, Cindy Ermus, "The Spanish plague that never was: crisis and exploitation in Cádiz during the *Peste* of Provence," *Eighteenth-Century Studies* 49:2 (Winter 2016), 167–93.

[76] Paul Hiltpold, "Política paternalista y orden social en la Castilla del Renacimiento," *Cuadernos de Investigación Histórica BROCAR* 13 (1987), 135–6, citing his own dissertation, p. 51, says Burgos's population dropped from 4,000 *vecinos* in 1550 to 1,500 by 1600.

[77] BL Eg. 356, vol. 1, fol. 32, "Los títulos que Su Magestad pone a las ciudades y villas de estos reynos de Castilla de boto en Cortes quando las escribe." Burgos is *"la muy noble y muy mas leal ciudad de Burgos cabeza de Castilla nuestra camara"* while the rest are just *"noble," "muy noble," "muy noble y leal,"* or *"muy noble y muy leal."*

[78] AMB-HI 3651, fol. 196, January 1598.

who were guilty were from my district, they would be punished such that you would be very satisfied, because such testimony can be very costly and harmful." Similar falsehoods born of enmity had been uttered in his jurisdiction and had been punished, he said. In any case, he assured Vitoria, his city had "never given credence to the news nor denied communication with anyone from Vitoria nor put the city's name on the list of sick places.[79]

The year 1598 was, indeed, the year when Vizcaya was badly infected. (The neighboring Basque province of Guipúzcoa suffered, as we saw in Chapter 1, already in 1597, indicating the disease probably had arrived by sea, not by roads, given that Vizcaya actually sits closer to Santander.) In April 1598, Burgos officials took safety measures after hearing that Laredo and other nearby ports were still pestilent. The city decided that only goods coming from Bilbao, a "healthy port," would be allowed to enter, which one has to imagine gave rise to a flood of false certificates.[80] But a few months later word reached Burgos that maybe Bilbao was not so healthy after all. "This city has received information about [Bilbao] regarding the *mal contagioso de la montaña*," Burgos wrote. "We have been told that coastal towns are guarding against [Bilbao]... In order that business and commerce with [Bilbao] not stop, given the great harm that would ensue, we have not wished to put it on the list until hearing back from you," Burgos told Bilbao, adding ominously at the end: "A spark can set off a great fire, and we pray to Our Lord that that not happen."[81]

Four months later, Bilbao was still cheerfully telling Burgos, and presumably other places, that things were fine, and Burgos appears to have been willing to go along, though there must have been information to the contrary by then. "We will let other cities that had gloomy news [*información siniestra*] know," Burgos reassured Bilbao.[82] Bilbao was grateful for the courtesy, its city council wrote on August 31, and returned the favor with the wise tactical move of finally admitting that in fact there was a little illness there after all but everything was under control. In the Ascao neighborhood, "populated by many artisans and people with few possibilities, given the general dearth this year ... in the

---

[79] AMB-HI 3650, January 23, 1598. *Enciclopedia General Ilustrada del País Vasco*, vol. 53 (San Sebastián: Editorial Auñamendi, 2001), 195, says (with no source) that Vitoria suffered greatly, with the first plague case inside the city being recorded in May 1599. A contemporary said 2,000 people died in the city and its villages (Vitoria then had barely 4,000 inhabitants).

[80] AMB-HI 3653, April 14, 1598.

[81] AMB-HI 3653, August 9, 1598; "*una centella prende un gran fuego que plega a nuestro señor no sea.*"

[82] AMB-HI 3653, August 20, 1598.

past twenty days some *vecinos* have fallen ill," Bilbao conceded. Security measures were being enforced; women and *vecinos* had been moved out, "more out of precaution and because of their weakness than out of necessity," the city hastened to add, which it was telling Burgos only "because a case like this calls for telling the truth in a straightforward manner." All the sick people were workers and/or poor people, who were receiving money, medicine, and medical care. Some twenty people had been moved into a house outside the city that had been turned into a hospital, and around thirty had died altogether during the distressing event (*sobresalto*). "Given the large number of people living in this city, that is not excessive," especially given that August and September were generally sickly months, "and at present thanks to the glory of God and His infinite goodness there is general health everywhere." Were anything to change, Burgos could rest assured Bilbao would let them know.[83]

In early September 1598 Burgos sent an emissary to Bilbao in the person of Francisco López, a city notary (probably the same López whom we saw earlier investigating illicit town fairs). He carried a letter from Burgos full of gracious sympathy and offers to help, meaning that by then the epidemic was assumed to have entered, but he also had instructions to ferret out the truth. The corregidor of Burgos was being cautious about actually putting Bilbao on the list of pestilent cities. A great deal was at stake. Burgos had heard, Vargas told his counterpart in Bilbao, Juan Pardo, that Bilbao was sick, that houses were shut, streets blocked, people were leaving, and many other towns would not allow communication with Bilbao. His information came from witnesses and correspondence, he said. Nonetheless, and having sifted through the information he had, "with the esteem I have for that city [Bilbao] and my desire to preserve good relations and be a good neighbor, I have not permitted that Bilbao be added to the list, though it is true, as you know, that the slightest carelessness can allow the illness to enter."[84]

A few days later, the Bilbao city council, which by now was meeting in Portugalete (where López had arrived), quite obviously an indication that the city itself was pestilent, wrote again to Burgos. "Some merchants and neighbors" had moved to Portugalete, Bilbao explained, to better ensure that merchandise be safely unloaded from the ships and moved to Burgos and the rest of Castile. Now that Burgos knew of the "great health" reigning in the north thanks to the quarantine, Bilbao hoped Burgos would allow mule trains to enter from there, continuing the age-old

[83] BL Eg. 356 vol. 2, fols. 354r–v, August 31, 1598, six signatures: "La villa de Bilbao por su orden su alcalde regidores diputados y secretario."
[84] AMB-HI 3650, September 4, 1598.

custom of mutual recognition and respect of the two great cities. "In my land and jurisdiction thanks to God there is total health and so much security that I am shut off from all people from Bilbao and from all other suspicious parts, and thus Your Lordship may with all satisfaction and security admit and conduct business with me..."[85]

The next day, September 11, Bilbao wrote again to say it had seen López's letter and thus knew of Burgos's willingness to help however it could. The city explained again that it had moved to Portugalete merely to better oversee the transfer of merchandise from the port to elsewhere in Spain. Cargo had been moved along the river to other towns, where it was being securely watched. As an example, a shipload of cod had just arrived on a boat from Newfoundland, and the fish was being unloaded safely, "and the same will be done with all the other cargo that arrives from there and from elsewhere, and many are expected both from there and from Flanders and Ireland and Andalucía and France and elsewhere. We beg Your Lordship, who has always supported us, that you do everything you can to ensure that merchandise from here be moved and admitted, with authenticated testimony, so that commerce and business not leave this coast, as those from San Juan de Luz and Bayonne [in France] and elsewhere wish it to, places that are spreading bad stories about Bilbao, with which for the moment, and until God says otherwise, they are not dealing, dealing rather only with this town [i.e. Portugalete] on which God in His mercy has bestowed great health..."[86]

But the same day that Bilbao wrote this letter, Burgos decided not to take any chances, and Bilbao was declared off limits. Two days later, Corregidor Vargas issued his formal order to that effect, and Bilbao was added to the Burgos list.[87]

After that, the correspondence took on a more business-like tone. If Bilbao and the other Vizcayan towns wanted to continue doing business with Castile, they would have to abide by Burgos's conditions. First, given that Bilbao was so close to Portugalete, and given the large number of Bilbao *vecinos* who had moved to Portugalete, Burgos was severing ties with the latter town as well: "Communication is cut off, as well as with the people there, so that neither directly nor indirectly shall they do business or speak or receive any clothing or paper or anything else from the said town." Furthermore, given that Bilbao was such an important business center and a depot for so many goods and that "owners will

---

[85] BL Eg. 356 vol. 2, fols. 353r–v, September 10, 1598, nine signatures. Bilbao addressed Burgos as *Su Señorio*.
[86] BL Eg. 356 vol. 2, fols. 352r–v, September 11, 1598, five signatures.
[87] AMB-HI 3653, September 11, 1598; AMB-HI 3650, September 13, 1598, auto.

want to remove [those] goods so as to be able to use them, and they have done so secretly and placed objects in houses outside the said city, you [the Bilbao city council] must order that under severe penalties no one must ship any items out of the city, either to Portugalete or to anywhere else, and that the things that have already been moved out must stay where they are and be guarded, and it does not matter if no one has gotten sick or died in these storage places because one cannot know if the workers who carried them there were sick, which would be the total perdition of this Kingdom." Bilbao must keep perfect track of all goods, separating those already there from those yet to arrive at the docks. Someone must be appointed to oversee the packing of outgoing goods, which must all bear a certificate and must travel straight to Burgos. Burgos would send one of its own to Portugalete to oversee this work. That same day Burgos sent Francisco López to Vitoria. The capital of Álava, Vargas suggested, had spoken too highly of its own health; essentially, he said, he did not trust Vitoria anymore, a wise course of action.[88]

Sure enough, two days later (September 18) the corregidor of Bilbao had to admit that people were now dying in Portugalete, prompting the exasperated Vargas to write to the Council of Castile: "The avarice of those in Bilbao who wanted to protect their goods in Portugalete has led the illness to spread." He had wanted to protect the fish and other goods coming from Newfoundland, but it was too late, and Portugalete had now joined Bilbao on the list, he said.[89] From Portugalete, matters shifted to Baracaldo, the next supposedly clean town the Vizcayan authorities chose as their headquarters. (It actually is closer to Bilbao than Portugalete, so the decision is hard to figure out.) Burgos now sent one Mateo Enríquez north to supervise the movement of merchandise from there at a daily salary of 500 maravedies, to be paid by the sick towns. He carried a letter from Burgos to Baracaldo, asking that the latter town "take great care that no merchandise that has been in Bilbao or in Portugalete directly or indirectly be allowed to enter, nor any merchandise that has been in contact with the said towns, and that sailors and masters from the ships there not be allowed to wander around and that they have no contact with people from those towns, nor should they go there."[90]

In mid-January Enríquez was still in Baracaldo, presumably still earning his 500 maravedies per day, an arrangement that frankly puzzled

---

[88] AMB-HI 3653, September 16, 1598.
[89] AMB-HI 3650, September 18, 1598; AMB-HI 3650, Vargas to council, September 1598.
[90] AMB-HI 3653, October 1598.

Burgos: "We do not know why those who are paying your salary are keeping you there so long, but if they are paying you, we are very pleased, and let us know if anything changes." Bilbao's health seemed to be improving already in December (though Portugalete was still sick), and Enríquez and Burgos both expressed concern that residents of Bilbao were returning too quickly to their city.[91] But Enríquez's long and lucrative tenure as Burgos's eyes and ears came to an end on January 19, when it emerged that he was at the center of a fraudulent ring. One Caspar Duarte was immediately dispatched northward to bring the culprit back, along with the city's stamps and stamped paper, which he appeared to have been using freely and illicitly. Duarte received the usual instructions to avoid pestilent places at all costs. Once he located Enríquez he was to hand the city's letter to him, and if Enríquez refused to accompany him Duarte was authorized to call for the police.[92] While he was there, he was also supposed to carry out renewed investigations into the true state of health in Bilbao, which once again was assuring everyone that it was just fine. By February it appears Burgos was coming around to believing that Bilbao really was healthy once again.[93] Burgos – which itself would be ravaged in the coming months – may have taken Bilbao off its list, but Bilbao and its towns experienced the return of the disease (as did many other places) in the following months. Like most places, they were anxious to save on guard money and desperate to go back to business.

It would be Burgos's turn during the spring, summer, and fall of 1599, by which time Vargas was dead. The first plague deaths to be acknowledged in the city council minutes occurred in March, though the new corregidor, Francisco Valencia, had admitted to the king that there were deaths earlier in the San Esteban neighborhood.[94] The city, which had been devastated by plague in 1565, continued in apparent denial, insisting to the crown, at the urging of its doctors, that the disease was not really peste. The city council's indignation when Valladolid refused to allow the Burgos notary through the gate in April, an incident we saw

---

[91] AMB-HI 3653, December 13, 1598 and January 9, 1599.
[92] AMB-HI 3653, January 19, 1599 (minutes and a letter).
[93] AMB-HI 3653, February 7 and 9, 1599.
[94] AGS-E leg. 183, doc. 267, as seen in chapter 3. The January deaths appear in a report by the Burgos regidor Andrés de Cañas, in BL Eg. 356, vol. 2, fols. 329–37; published by Francis Brumont originally in *Boletín de la Institución Fernán González* 26 (1984–1985), 167–82, and which appeared subsequently as "La peste de 1599: una relación del regidor Andrés de Cañas," *BROCAR: Cuadernos de Investigación Histórica* 13 (1987), 155–66. A man named Lerma, his wife, and two children died on January 4 or 5; some said the fault lay with a ragpicker who had stayed with them, while others said Lerma had brought infected blankets from a town near Villadiego.

in Chapter 3, and its insistence that refusals to allow *burgaleses* to pass through gates were the result of personal enmity, coincided with the hospitalization of hundreds of people there; by May 15, the regidor Andrés de Cañas estimated that more than 400 had died.[95] But no matter how strained the city's credibility, it seemed safer to risk not being believed than to risk being put on the list.

When Fernando Ruiz de los Arcos was stealthily inspecting towns in Toledo to verify if San Martín de Valdieglesias was or was not sick, he went to the town square and saw lots of people, a sure sign that things were just fine. Marketplaces were a way of measuring social welfare, and not just during epidemics. Commerce was health, it was civility; indeed, the Spanish word "plaza" is a synonym for market. But as people left, supplies disappeared, and those who remained preferred the safety of their homes – or they followed physician Luis Mercado's advice and sent the servants to do the shopping – plazas became lonely places.[96] The landscape had shifted.

[95] Brumont, "La peste de 1599," 157–8; on p. 162 Cañas discusses the bad relations between Burgos and the *alcalde mayor* living in Lerma, who the city held responsible for spreading the news that Burgos was sick; on p. 165 Brumont publishes a draft of a letter from the city to the king, also today in BL Eg. 356 vol. 2, scoffing at towns' insistence that Burgos was sick; if it were sick, the city reasons, then it would have told the king. Actually, the corregidor had the opportunity to do just that, in the letters contained in AGS-E leg. 183, but instead maintained the city was healthy.

[96] Mercado, *El libro de la peste del Dr. Luis Mercado*, 247.

Site 5: Street

As stalls in the marketplaces thinned and fewer products were allowed to enter, the dwindling inhabitants of towns and cities – at least the healthy ones – might have to leave their homes every day to see which meager foodstuffs had found their way through the gates. Except for them and the ever-present *pregonero* shouting aloud the city council's most recent edicts, the streets were mostly empty. People must have been desolate and afraid as news, true and false, drifted in along with travelers lucky or able enough to squeeze past the guards. "A healthy, upright woman arrived here yesterday at eight in the morning, apparently from Valladolid," wrote a correspondent from Salamanca, "and by eleven o'clock she had been buried."[1] Better to stay inside than to deal with that. Most artisans, whose workshops were usually in the interior of their homes or in the back but who sold out in front, adding noise and color to streets, were gone. There were no bills of mortality, but no lists were needed for people to know that neighbors had left, died, or had been moved to the hospital. As Defoe's fictional protagonist remarked of London, "It was a most surprising thing, to see those Streets, which were usually so thronged, now grown desolate, and so few People to be seen in them."[2]

Luego, lejos, largo was the rule in Spain as everywhere else: leave quickly, go far, return late. When town leaders in Alcorcón (today a large Madrid suburb) gathered to respond to Philip II's request for information on his Castilian dominions, they would remember that around eighty years before that their ancestors had been felled by pestilence that was passed from one person to the next, though they could not say which sort it was, "and so it was necessary for many *vecinos* of the said place to leave the town, and a little bit away they built cabins where they lived until the fury of the said illness had

---

[1] RBP II-2163-107, García Sarmiento de Acuña to Diego Sarmiento de Acuña, July 20, 1599.
[2] Daniel Defoe, *A Journal of the Plague Year* (New York: Meridian Classic, 1960), 25.

passed."[3] In some places city councils and church chapters vanished as
well, and even doctors joined the flow, though other town officials,
churchmen, and medical personnel stayed through it all. Miquel Parets
wrote in his 1651 journal that two-thirds of Barcelona's inhabitants had
fled, but the editor of the diary, James Amelang, adds that governments
had the obligation to leave during plague.[4] Undoubtedly there were
those who packed a bag and abandoned their flock or their citizens with
no notice and no effort to make up for the loss, but one gets the
impression that these were the exceptions, and that if officials left, as
in the case of Barcelona, it was because that made more sense for the
community and that furthermore there were laws and customs backing
them up. As with the Valladolid Chancillería, officials moved elsewhere
en masse and sometimes had to move again as the plague chased them.
Bilbao's city council moved to Portugalete (and its corregidor may have
moved to Durango[5]), Portugalete appears to have moved to Baracaldo,
Laredo went to Ampuero, the viceroy of Navarre went from Pamplona
to Olite (and the Navarrese Royal Council went to Tafalla, leaving
Pamplona without a criminal court, prompting the city to deputize
new officials), Logroño went to a variety of extramuros villages.[6]

Not suprisingly, the wealthy left almost immediately. The Duke of
Medina Sidonia wrote to the royal secretary Martín de Idiaquez from
Segovia in May 1599 to say he and his family were leaving that very
afternoon.[7] When the future Count of Gondomar was corregidor of
Toro, his friends in Valladolid kept him up to date on who was going
where. The apparently very well-informed Francisco de Villapadierna,
for example, wrote that his wife was going to a village five or six leagues
away, Don Antonio Cabeza de Vaca and Don Juan Quijada y Pliego and
their wives had all left on Thursday for Castrillo, on Wednesday Doña
Inés de Negrón and her children went to Salamanca, Hernando Muñoz
and his wife and sister went to Ávila, the chief postman along with his

---

[3] Carmelo Viñas y Mey and Ramón Paz, eds. *Relaciones de los pueblos de España ordenadas
por Felipe II* [Provincia de Madrid y Reino de Toledo], 4 vols. in 3 (Madrid: Instituto
Balmes de Sociologia [CSIC], 1949), vol. 1, p. 42. James S. Amelang, ed. and trans.,
A Journal of the Plague Year: The Diary of the Barcelona Tanner Miquel Parets, 1651 (New
York: Oxford University Press, 1991), 63–6, also describes huts built outside Barcelona
during the 1651 plague that housed those unable to go far away.
[4] Amelang, *A Journal of the Plague Year*, 44 and 133n95.
[5] AMB-HI 3650, September 18, 1598.
[6] Olite: AGS GyM leg. 548; Logroño: Fernando Pons Ibáñez, "Epidemia de peste en
Logroño (Año 1599)," *Berceo* 73 (1964), 387–406, p. 394; Tafalla: Ignacio Baleztena,
ed., "Relación de la peste desta ciudad de Pamplona del año 1599," *Príncipe de Viana* 23
(1946), p. 392.
[7] AGS-E leg. 184, doc. 77, May 26, 1599.

wife and his brother-in-law and another couple moved to Simancas, Doña Catalina González and her children were in Torre de Lobatón, the Countess of Buendía had left that same afternoon for Cabezón and from there would move on to Dueñas and Palencia, and Catalina del Rio and her brother and her children were leaving the next day for Portillo, though her husband was staying in Valladolid.[8] Recalling the exodus from Florence a few centuries earlier, the Marquis of los Vélez, on his estate in southern Spain, wrote to Gondomar that he had heard that all the best sort had indeed left Valladolid for Toro, which had become a sort of satellite court, "and you must be very content with all your friends there … I have heard such sad stories, that all of Castile must have lost people, they say many have died and that *secas* are everywhere…"[9] An indication of the logical resentment toward those who left and came back once it was all over can be seen in the city council minutes of Soria, where Councilman Antonio Beltrán was punished with a 50,000-maravedi donation to the hospital. Antonio de Neya, who had been asked several times to return but stayed wherever he was, was assessed the same, and Pedro de Barnuevo, whom the city had sent out to buy wheat and who then simply vanished, was fined 20,000, as was his colleague Josep Heras de Sarabia. In addition, four noblemen were told they would have to pay 30,000 maravedies if they wished to reoccupy their houses in the city.[10]

Churchmen acted similarly. When plague struck Galicia in August 1569, the cathedral chapter of Santiago de Compostela voted to allow honorary canons to leave town as long as some among them remained to conduct services. In October, possibly having moved to the town of Padrón, it organized shifts ("whether by lot or by some other method"), and after that it seems that most of the canons left, leaving behind just nine men, three of them, according to the contemporary source, cardinals. By February 1570 everyone was back in Santiago.[11] A later plague in Málaga during the reign of Philip IV offers a less exemplary case. In May 1637 the Council of Castile told the king that people in Málaga and nearby towns were dying of a disease that "by all signs is the plague" that may have been triggered by the arrival of an English ship,

[8] RBP II-2163, doc. 87, Villapadierna to Gondomar, July (?) 24, 1599.
[9] RBP II-2184, Vélez to Gondomar, October 7, 1599.
[10] Enrique Díez Sanz, *La Tierra de Soria: Un universo campesino en la Castilla oriental del siglo XVI* (Madrid: Siglo Veintiuno, 1995), 48–54, citing minutes from November 15, 1599.
[11] López Ferreiro, *Historia de la Santa A. M. Iglesia de Santiago de Compostela*, vol. 8 (Santiago: Seminario Conciliar Central, 1905), 233–4, citing "Tumbo E," a volume of privileges and other documents. He says 8,000 people died in Santiago during that epidemic.

which the council knew because the corregidor of Antequera had written. No word was forthcoming from Málaga, however, a much more important city, prompting the king to note, "It is very odd that there are no letters from authorities in Málaga." Silence can be as informative as news. By July what was left of the city council was asking for permission to impose *sisas* to help the sick and the poor, who were one and the same being that the rich and well-off, in addition to the church, had all abandoned the city. "[Your Majesty's] duty to help Málaga, both spiritually and temporally, is absolute [*inescusable*]," the Council of Castile advised the king, especially as the regidores had left and the corregidor had not obeyed orders to summon them back. Not only that, but the bishop had moved to the city's fortress, the Alcazaba ("he might as well have left Málaga" the council remarked), the canons had left, and the convents and monasteries had closed themselves off.[12] Departure of church personnel might lead to arguments with the city, which frequently relied upon priests and other religious authorities to provide care and information; in general, the city needed the church. In Santo Domingo de la Calzada, in present-day La Rioja, the town council fought furiously – and fruitlessly – to prevent the church chapter and the bishop from closing up shop and leaving during the pestilent summer of 1599.[13] In Burgos, the cathedral chapter in April 1599 asked the city council to allow churchmen who wished to leave to do so; some had already tried but had been halted at the city gates by vigilant guards. Civic leaders there may still have been trying to hide the fact that plague was about, but churchmen were not so reticent: "Although the doctors are not saying it is peste, it is known and notorious that it is contagious, as one can see the dying, and how the disease sticks, and as it is so notorious they begged the city to allow people to leave if they so wished." The city council, regretfully, gave them permission.[14] The archbishop himself, however, stayed, and was reported to be a model of charity and sacrifice, tirelessly and bravely visiting the sick and spending his money on them.[15] The council in Bilbao also faced religious reluctance; in September 1599 it heard complaints that parish priests were not administering last rites, so people were dying "with no spiritual comfort, causing *escándalo y murmuración*." A city official was

---

[12] AHN CS leg. 7236 (Archivo Antiguo del Consejo de Castilla), docs. 2–6.
[13] Diego Téllez Alarcia, "La peste Atlántica en Santo Domingo de la Calzada (1599)," *Berceo* 162 (2012), 85–119, pp. 104–6.
[14] AMB LA-130, April 27, 1599.
[15] Francis Brumont, "La peste de 1599: una relación del regidor Andrés de Cañas," *BROCAR: Cuadernos de Investigación Histórica*, 13 (1987), 155–66, p. 161.

given the task of speaking to the priests, reminding them of their duties and promising punishments in the future.[16]

The royal physician and treatise writer Luis Mercado demurred on whether it was permissible to leave, saying it was up to the theologians to decide, though he suggested he was not in favor.[17] Martín González de Cellorigo also was among those who weighed the moral and practical implications of leaving, saying the latter was certainly the "most efficient remedy," though he admitted it could be compared to desertion from one's militia unit and abandonment of duty. On the one hand, leaving was *buena política*, defended by jurists and physicians, because that way fewer people would get sick and once people returned their towns could "recover their grandeur." But there were negative consequences as well. One truly had to leave quickly, go far, and return late, otherwise one just made things worse. Inhabitants of Valladolid, Cellorigo said, had foolishly gone to the countryside and gotten sick just the same, trading the "clarity and love" of their city's nobility for "rustic, ignorant, timid, and unschooled" villagers who could and would do nothing for them. Many of those who left Valladolid had violated all sense of *buena política*, both in substance and in form, he wrote, leaving families unprotected, spreading the disease themselves instead of staying at home where they could be attended to, and returning too early, repentant for having left, and thus infecting even more people.[18] Jesuits generally left affected towns, balancing their duties to the sick with their duties to their students, and they seem to have gradually opted for the latter as the Company shifted its emphasis to education.[19] Though not directly relevant to this case, Luther in 1527 published a pamphlet entitled "Whether One May Flee From a Deadly Plague," the answer being that one should stay and tend to neighbors while taking precautions oneself. Calvin and his followers were less keen and also frankly divided; during the plague of 1542–1544, church leaders drew lots to decide who would stay and who would go,

---

[16] AFB libro 024, also in Bartolomé Bennassar, *Recherches sur les grandes épidémies dans le nord de l'Espagne a la fin du XVIe siècle. Problèmes de documentation et de méthode* (Paris: SEVPEN, 1969), 87.

[17] Luis Mercado, *El libro de la peste del Dr. Luis Mercado con un estudio preliminar acerca del autor y sus obras por el Dr. Nicasio Mariscal* [1598] [Biblioteca Clásica de la Medicina Española, vol. 1] (Madrid: Imp. de Cosano, 1921), 247–8.

[18] Martín González de Cellorigo, *Memorial de la política necesaria y útil restauración a la república de España* (Madrid: Instituto de Cooperación Iberamericana, 1991), 24–8.

[19] Lynn Martin, *Plague? Jesuit Accounts of Epidemic Disease in the 16th Century* (Kirksville, MO: Sixteenth Century Journal Publishers, 1996), 115–22; Bernard Vincent, "Les épidémies dans l'Espagne des années 1555–1570," in *Le corps dans la société espagnole des XVI et XVIIeme siècles*, ed. Agustin Redondo (Paris: Publications de la Sorbonne, 1990), 141–52, p. 151.

with the losers refusing to abide by the result, about which Scott Mantetsch has remarked that this "was hardly the Company of Pastors' finest hour." One of Calvin's most outstanding heirs, Theodore Beza (or Bèze), wrote in a 1579 treatise that flight was not incompatible with Christian duty and piety. "When the choice was not clear," Mantetsch wrote, "Beza suggested that those Christians were less culpable who remained behind when they might have fled, than those who fled when they should have remained behind."[20] The choice, in fact, was usually not clear at all.

If people were leaving, they obviously were going somewhere, but that somewhere could not be the home of friends or family members in communities guarding against the peste. Though the apostle Luke had said that one must love one's neighbor as oneself, and the book of Matthew, quoting Jesus, says "I was hungry and you gave me food, I was thirsty and you gave me drink, I was a stranger and you welcomed me," such hospitality – mentioned even in the Partidas as an obligation of the clergy toward the poor – had no place in the world of quarantine.[21] Later in this chapter, Andrés Alonso will pay dearly for allowing travelers from Santander into his home just outside Burgos. Another Burgos man, Pedro Giménez, and his family also were punished, "for having taken into their home a woman named María, married to Pedro, a rich shepherd and a *vecino* of Revilla del Campo," one of the towns we saw earlier that shared access to shrines; the corregidor told an official to go to the village of Salguero with his staff raised high and order the local *alcalde* to arrest Giménez and within twenty-four hours send him and everyone in his house into two years of banishment.[22] Innkeepers were subject to banishment for the same crime, as we saw earlier, and so were families of

---

[20] Scott M. Manetsch, *Calvin's Company of Pastors: Pastoral Care and the Emerging Reformed Church, 1536–1609* (New York: Oxford University Press, 2013), 284–9. The English version (1580) of Beza's treatise is *"A LEARNED TREATISE OF THE PLAGUE: WHEREIN, The two Questions: Whether the PLAGUE be Infectious, or no: And Whether, and how farr it may be shunned of Christians, by going aside? are resolved."* To the best of my knowledge, no comparable treatise was produced in Spain. For a similar discussion in the Muslim world see Justin K. Stearns, "Public Health, the State, and Religious Scholarship: Sovereignty in Idris al-Bidlisi's Arguments for Fleeing the Plague," in *The Scaffolding of Sovereignty: Global and Aesthetic Perspectives on the History of a Concept*, Zvi Ben-Dor Benite, et al., ed. (New York: Columbia University Press, 2017), 163–85, esp. 177–8; additionally, Nükhet Varlik, in "Plague, conflict, and negotiation: the Jewish broadcloth weavers of Salonica and the Ottoman central administration in the late sixteenth century," *Jewish History* 28 (2014), 261–88, pp. 287–8, says Ottoman plague treatises weighed the pros and cons of flight (by everyone, not just officials) and generally permitted it, leading to opinions that later entered the legal canon.

[21] Luke 10:17; Matthew 25:35; Partida I tit. V law 40; also Partida I, VI, 34.

[22] AMB-HI 3651, October 22, 1597.

students in Burgos who took in their children when they returned from boarding school. After neighbors and officials in the Navarrese village of Irujo in 1599 noticed that a woman (a wet nurse, it turned out) and a two-year-old had suddenly appeared in the home of Juan de Irujo, a merchant who was away at the time, they immediately set about investigating the newcomers. Irujo's wife and children, one of whom was an abbot, were there but refused to cooperate, making the officials certain that even more suspicious people were being hidden. All residents were told to stay put and not to leave "on their feet nor on anyone else's," and meanwhile reports were filed with the Navarrese Royal Council. Reason prevailed eventually, as the court lifted the quarantine, sent the nurse and child back to Estella, and told the Irujo family to stop receiving guests.[23]

It was the same throughout the country. As towns expelled the non-native poor or single women and as other people chose on their own to leave, these new refugees could not go back home until it was all over, nor could they find lodging with friends or family. But, clearly, they did, probably in points further south as they moved just ahead of the plague, being pushed from one place to the next. In fact, northern towns may have been freer with the expulsion orders, figuring that people could always move south, managing to slip into the next town down the road with lenient guards where they had a relative with an extra mattress. Two guards in the Bilbao neighborhood of Ispaster named Juan Pérez de Esuneta and Juan de Chumategui, a father- and son-in-law appointed to inspect houses, turned out themselves to be harboring nuns from the very diseased town of Lequeitio who had fled, one of whom was now dead. More nuns from Lequeitio showed up in a complaint filed against one Pedro de Arrupe, a vecino of another Bilbao neighborhood (Ereño), who was denounced by Juan de Gueztarean Bidarrueta, the virulent local treasurer, who said creditable (but unnamed) sources had told him that Arrupe had walked hand-in-hand with a nun, one of whose sister nuns had recently died of plague. "And the said Pedro de Arrupe talked with the said nun and took her hand and walked with her and asked her things," the complaint read, all of which was "in great disservice of God our Lord and showing little respect for His Majesty's royal service, and thus he should be shut up in his house for eighty days."[24] In Lequeitio's pathetic appeal to Philip II that fall, the town implicitly

---

[23] AGN TR Procesos 040251.

[24] AFB Notarial Merindad de Busturia, escr. Aurrecoechea 23, docs. 23/0094 and 95, December 1 and 8, 1597. I believe this is the only instance I have seen of people being enclosed in their homes as a punishment, and I do not know if the punishment was carried out. The two guards were fined. These papers state that testimony was not recorded because there were no notaries left.

pointed to hospitality and charity as among the victims of the plague: "The illness of peste that because of our sins has spread throughout the maritime regions has entered the town of Lequeitio, one of the largest towns of the *señorío* [Vizcaya] where many people go to sea every year to serve Your Majesty ... most of them are dying of hunger and the other towns of the *señorío* are in such need that everyone can barely take care of themselves without being able to help others."[25] To not be able to help one's family – the nuns surely were sisters or daughters of the men – was the most cruel thing. (Though there also were relatives who chose their own health over their kin's; in Barcelona, Miquel Parets in 1651 recorded that when his wife was sick and then died of bubonic plague, neither of her sisters in the city came to see her: "Although the sick woman sent for them because she wanted to talk with them and see them before she died, there was no way to convince them to come, as everyone fled from the plague. And there were many cases of this sort."[26]) Fray Domingo de Soto, the author of the famous treatise on poverty mentioned earlier, considered freedom of movement and of refuge to be natural rights whose benefit to the poor was most obvious in times of dearth or disease; indeed, Charles V's 1544 Poor Laws had drawn objections from him and others precisely because they attempted to curtail these rights. When mendicant orders at Ypres protested against begging reforms (part of the same package of laws) they turned to Virgil: "What land so barbarous is this that we are barred the hospitality [*hospitium*] of the shore?"[27]

Occasionally, though, records reveal moments of defiance against this new way of treating neighbors and relatives, versions of the open gate when towns opted to bend the rules in the name of common sense or benevolence. We saw earlier how Burgos Corregidor Diego Vargas Manrique, showing ingenuity along with compassion, stepped into the middle of a dispute when one town would not allow a neighboring, infected town to use its mill, which in the past had always been shared. He essentially reminded people of their duty to one another at a time when neighborliness was too easily abandoned. A more inspiring case was recorded by Dr. Valentín de Andosilla, who for a time treated plague patients in Navarrete (La Rioja), a town of 700 *vecinos* with no funds or properties left. "The *vecinos*," he wrote, "tired of these endless and intolerable burdens, unanimously agreed that all those who died, would,

---

[25] AGS-GyM leg. 490 doc. 114, October 6, 1597.

[26] Amelang, *A Journal of the Plague Year*, 59.

[27] Annabel S. Brett, *Changes of State: Nature and the Limits of the City in Early Modern Natural Law* (Princeton, NJ: Princeton University Press, 2011): on Soto, p. 29; on Ypres, p. 19, citing *The Aeneid*, I: 539–40.

according to their abilities and devotional duty and after paying for their burial, leave something for the poor and for matters relating to the said illness, and this act of charity did so much good that though there were 150 *pobres* or many more, they never lacked medicine, meals, attendants, or care … This is what happened to our town when it seemed our republic would be annihilated and consumed, our forts toppled … and the devoted and noble mother of our district [*comarca*], the city of Logroño … came and sent everything it had for us in our fight against this frightful monster of a disease."[28]

In times of pestilence, those who remained were the sick, the poor, the ghosts, the orphans, a few shopkeepers, craftsmen, and vendors; the doctors and officials and churchmen who stayed behind to do their duty; the survivors, the abandoned, the men who had sent wives and children elsewhere, the inhabitants secretly harboring relatives. They waited, and they prayed. "To those of us who waited for it to strike it seemed as if it carried a registry of our names, of those who would live and those who must die," Cellorigo wrote.[29] An average household probably had two parents, maybe three children, perhaps a servant, perhaps grandparents. If the man of the house was an artisan, there might be an apprentice or two. One estimate for Madrid in 1597 gives seven people per house, though the number was higher in the more crowded parishes and Madrid houses were smaller than those in towns and villages.[30] Those who stayed probably were lonely and had less to do than in normal times; if they were making or selling things, their customer base had pretty much vanished. If they worked in the fields, their movements had been checked. If they were children who had lost their parents, then they were living in someone else's house, with relatives or neighbors.[31] If they were parents who lost their children – like those in Aranda, where sick children "nearly all died if they were younger than ten, as their blood is weaker and curing

[28] Valentin de Andosilla Salazar, *Libro en que se prueba con claridad el mal que corre por España ser nuevo y nunca visto: su naturaleza, causas, pronósticos, curacion, y la prouidencia que se deue tener con él …* (Pamplona: Mathias Mares, 1601), 134v–5v.

[29] González de Cellorigo, *Memorial de la política necesaria*, 23.

[30] Alfredo Alvar Ezquerra, "Espacios sociales del Madrid de los Austrias," in *El Madrid de Velázquez y Calderón: Villa y Corte en el siglo XVII*, Miguel Morán and Bernardo J. García, eds., vol. 1 (Madrid: Ayuntamiento de Madrid, 2000), 151–68, p. 155, citing AGS-EH leg. 121.

[31] In Pasajes, Villaviciosa said, there were 130 orphans, along with 80 children who had lost their mother to the epidemic while their father was at sea. Many had no close relatives, he said. Letter from Miguel de Villaviciosa, writing from Fuenterrabia about Pasajes de San Juan, in Luis Murugarren Zamora, "La peste en Guipuzcoa (1597–1599)" *Boletin de la Real Sociedad Bascongada de Amigos del Pais* 40:1–2 (1984), 247–69, p. 267. Portions of the letter also appear in José Ramón Cruz Mundet, *"El mal que al presente corre": Gipuzkoa y la peste (1597–1600)* (San Sebastián: Kutxa Fundazioa, 2003).

them is more difficult, given their tender age" – then somehow they kept going, taking care of the children who remained.[32] They might even have taken in other people's children, as in Burgos, where there were so many orphans that foster parents were needed, requiring city funds.[33] If they were men who liked to drink a few glasses with their neighbors, the local tavern may well have been closed down. But cooking, cleaning, laundry, tending to animals, maybe foraging, all continued.

Indoors, if someone in the household was sick, of course the duty of the others was to report the case, but many people remained quiet, hiding the ailing (and the dead, who would have died without last rites), giving rise to incessant inspections. If outsiders were discovered concealed inside homes, they might be expelled or might be cared for; probably the former as time went on. The most frequent solution seems to have been not to shut people up but rather to remove everyone and only then shut the house. Once the plague had clearly moved on these houses were reopened, though occasionally they were demolished, with cleaning crews in charge of moving through them one by one, checking them off their list.[34] Far less often, judging from the documents, were people isolated inside their own homes, sometimes with their healthy (for the time being) relatives. Thus in Burgos, sick people in the Villatoro neighborhood remained inside their homes with the rest of their family while everyone else in the neighborhood was prohibited from having contact with them.[35] In Pamplona, however, the sick person was lowered to the street in his or her bed, followed by everyone else who lived in the house, "even if there were many of them," and the whole group was housed outside the city walls, after which their house was scrubbed.[36] But the most common recourse seems to have been to quickly isolate the sick, if possible in a hospital, or otherwise alone in their homes. The discovery of three sick people in Logroño led to their enclosure together, with a servant assigned to feed them and the keys to the house placed strictly in the hands of the city doctor.[37] Likewise, in the Segovian village of

[32] AGS-E leg. 183, doc. 315, May 11, 1599. In the town of Santo Tomé del Puerto (Segovia), 205 people died from February to the end of May 1599, of whom 150 were children under the age of 16; AGS-E leg. 183, doc. 295.
[33] AMB-LA 131, 54r–5r, March 16, 1600.
[34] For example, in Burgos, AMB-HI 3653, April 8, 1600. Doctors in Madrid, including Mercado, in their suggestions to the king in April 1599, also said houses should be cleared of sick people and then either boarded up or knocked down; AGS-E leg. 183, doc. 279.
[35] AMB-LA 130, April 6, 1599.
[36] Baleztena, ed., "Relación de la peste desta ciudad de Pamplona,"191–2.
[37] Pons Ibáñez, "Epidemia de peste en Logroño," 387–406, 400–1, citing Logroño city council minutes, August 23, 1599.

Fitençuela, after a woman who had buried her husband and her two sons soon developed a *seca* herself, village authorities shut her up in a house (not necessarily hers), passing food to her through a slot or a window; she recovered.[38] Not much imagination is required to see that shutting people up might also be punishment or revenge, an unexpected opportunity. Juan de Gueztarean Bidaurreta, who had denounced his neighbor for talking to nuns in Lequeitio and demanded that the neighbor be shut up for eighty days, might well be such an example.

But not everyone was behind closed doors enclosed, sick, or waiting. Those who could were working. Corregidor Vargas and his colleagues throughout Castile were not on their own. They had messengers, guards, law enforcement, cleaners, and a reserve army of people to carry out the necessary and unpleasant tasks aimed at ensuring, first, that the disease remain at bay and then, once it entered, that it kill as few people as possible.

If contradictory news and faulty science made it difficult to truly discern what was going on, townspeople in addition may literally have been blinded, for once they set foot in the street, the smoke in the air might have made it impossible for them to see their few remaining neighbors. With prohibitions against cloth a fixture in instructions for guards, the need to burn all contaminated cloth, especially bed linens of the dead, was an essential component of towns' anti-plague arsenals. As soon as cities learned the plague was on its way, they immediately put up guards, separated the sick from the well, sealed up sick houses, and burned the clothes, in that order. Bonfires of pestilent objects took place outside the town, and often fires were in contained spaces so as not to spread the harmful bits, but the smoke must have wafted back, and in any case within the town there were ongoing bonfires of aromatic materials deemed to be good for one's health. This was true even in times of no plague, as it was widely thought that bad, putrid air could cause a variety of diseases. As in the *Aeneid*, plague could strike "out of some foul polluted quarter of the skies," so it was best to keep pollution to a minimum at all times.[39] Once the plague had receded and houses were reopened and aired out, they were washed down with bucketfuls of vinegar and perfumed with juniper and rosemary, which could ensure that the last of the harmful vapors would be vanquished.

The model public health effort in Alcalá de Henares described in Chapter 1 included clothes-burning as soon as the Council of Castile's envoy arrived there. There, as elsewhere, this was an employment

[38] The village may not exist anymore; AGS-E leg. 184, doc. 182, June 14, 1599.
[39] Virgil, *The Aeneid*, 3:168.

opportunity. At a "moderate salary" the envoy hired three men dressed
de bocacín (a rough cloth like burlap; hospital workers and gravediggers in
Alcalá de Henares and other places were also dressed *de bocacín*) to pull
diseased clothing out of houses, load it onto carts, and take it to the burn
site, a brick oven a quarter-league away from the town by the banks of the
Henares River. There, "another honorable man" helped them pitch the
clothes in. ("They say the three men have gone to Guadalajara to work
because it went so well for them here," the official wrote.) Town criers
told inhabitants to report all dead and sick people so their clothing and
linens could be picked up, and doctors and religious personnel worked as
inspectors to that end. There were days when ten cartloads were collected.[40] Burgos hired thirteen laborers and shiftless people (*ganapanes y
pícaros*) to burn clothes after removing them from houses all along the
Calle de la Alberdería, an early focal point for plague. The clothesburners were housed for nine days in the shrine of Rebolleda, where
the Burgos plague hospital was first established, and the city council
agreed on March 8, 1599 that nine of them would be dismissed within
three days. Each would get twelve reales and their clothing would be
washed for them. The other four would remain, however, and were to
receive a suit of clothing made of rough linen (*vestidos de anjeo*).[41] Nearly
a year later the city had run out of firewood, and instead of burning
the final bedclothes being removed from the now empty hospital, it
was burying them.[42] In the Basque fortress town of Fuenterrabia, two
military surgeons were in charge of fires, assisted by town officials and
the notary, who wrote everything down in his sixteen-page notebook.
Along with them went an ox driver leading the cart, and two women,
whose job it was to enter closed-up, pestilent houses and haul everything
out while the notary made an inventory of all the items. The women
carried the mattresses on their heads, though if the goods were very heavy
the ox driver helped out. Weapons, including arquebuses, were held
above the flames in the street to be disinfected. Money, jewels, and
valuable objects were deposited somewhere. Pots and dishes, papers,

---

[40] RAH Jesuitas 9-3662/182. The not entirely reliable Antonio de León Pinelo reported
that gravediggers in 1599 had stolen infected clothing and sold them in Alcalá, which he
said was the cause of the epidemic there; *Anales de Madrid (desde el año 447 al de 1658)*,
Pedro Fernández Martín, ed. (Madrid: Instituto de Estudios Madrileños, 1971), 173.

[41] Burgos discussion is from AMB-HI 3653, March 8–19, 1599. The inhabitants of
Alberdería were removed even if they had had no contact with the dead, and when
they demanded to be allowed to return, doctors were dispatched to check on their health.
The *pícaros* in Burgos were supposedly being supervised by a policeman but were such
uncontrollable scoundrels that they would steal any clothing that seemed usable and
then sell it; Brumont, "La peste de 1599," 160.

[42] AMB-HI 3653, February 9 and 16, 1600.

unopened linens, and good furniture were disinfected. Townspeople were instructed not to throw their clothes into the sea.[43]

The incessant burning meant that some people were losing their only set of clothes or their only set of sheets, and municipal accounts often included line items to reimburse the loss, though one has to wonder what the poor in these situations would do with cash, or where they might buy replacements. One of the most dramatic recognitions of this plight came in Ávila, whose city council appears to have been somewhat dysfunctional, with members absent or talking out of turn and a corregidor, Pedro Ortiz Ponce de León, who seems to have gone missing for at least part of the time.[44] His irregular correspondence with Philip III in spring, summer, and fall of 1599 admitted to very few plague-related deaths in Ávila, and he spun positively about those he recounted, though he apparently simultaneously painted a dire picture to the city's cathedral canons, who suspected him of exaggerating the disease in order to squeeze more taxes out of them.[45] For some reason, clothes-burning either did not take place at all during the months the plague was in the city or the bonfires were insufficient. In January 1600, a very cold month in Ávila (in the late twentieth century the average temperature was 3°C; temperatures obviously have warmed since the late sixteenth century, and the 1590s anyway was an exceptionally cold decade), the city seems to have realized that there was still pestilent clothing stuffed away in houses, along with sick people, and that something needed to be done about this. Their realization coincided with orders from Madrid's Junta de la Salud, an arm of the Council of Castile, to burn clothing. City health officers summoned medical personnel to testify on January 12 regarding how many sick people remained in the city, after which the local junta decided to take action and then did nothing for two weeks

---

[43] Cruz Mundet, "El mal que al presente corre," 76–7, no source cited, but probably Guipuzcoan local records. Cortes records from April 1598 state that the people of Castro Urdiales had thrown clothing and household decorations into the sea (ACC vol. 15, p. 579), and earlier we saw that the people of Pasajes did the same with their beds.

[44] Ponce de León was on the job in 1598–1603. On September 10, 1600, he warned regidores that if they kept interrupting each other they would each be fined 500 ducats. The following discussion is based on AHMA Libro de Actas 25, covering 1600, roughly fols. 26r–93r; and AGS-E leg. 183, scattered documents on Ávila, some of which are reproduced in Bennassar, Recherches sur les grandes épidémies, 114–29.

[45] Andrés Sánchez Sánchez, La beneficiencia en Ávila: Actividad hospitalaria del cabildo catedralicio (Siglos XVI–XIX) (Ávila: Diputación Provincial, Institución Gran Duque de Ávila, 2000), 71, citing cathedral documents. On the corregidor's unwarranted optimism, not to say dishonesty, see Serafín de Tapia, "Los factores de la evolución demográfica de Ávila en el Siglo XVI," Cuadernos Abulenses 5 (January–June 1986), 113–200, pp. 170–3.

except hold useless meetings (this according to one of its members). The junta's commissioner, Luis Pacheco, then took it upon himself to organize the collection of infected clothing from the hospital, during which the hospital's wooden beds and crockery were also smashed, burned, and buried.[46] But the junta appears to have been as inoperative as the city council, with meetings canceled for lack of attendance. Members were ordered to appear on January 23 with a notary to draw up a list of houses where there were still sick people (though apparently not all of them suffered from plague) and infected clothes. Regidor and junta member Vela Núñez pointed out that burning clothes was a measure that mostly affected the very poor, who would be left with nothing, and he asked the city to obtain blankets and sheets and wool for mattress stuffing which could be paid for by loans from townspeople. (It appears the church did not contribute, though this is not certain.[47]) On January 27 there was another expedition to collect clothes, starting with the Calle de San Francisco, and there indeed officials found that people were so poor that upon turning over their clothes and linens they had nothing left: "Giving up the clothing they wore when they got sick, they must go to bed naked, and others don't even have a bed, and the weather is so cold that many are dying." So the city, with the king's permission, decided to disburse 66,840 maravedies left over from the granary and proceed with the clothes-burning.[48] In February the city requested permission to levy a new *sisa* to pay for blankets and clothing. Still in April 1600 there was another round of fires, and the following month Philip III announced he was coming to Ávila, a visit that would end up costing the city at least 11,000 ducats, which the city asked to pay for with a variety of new *sisas*.[49] One has to wonder how much of the sheets-and-blankets fund was raided for this purpose.

Poor people might be tempted to hide their clothing or grab items off the carts as they went rumbling by on their way to the bonfires, and plenty of town councils warned their police to be on the alert for just that. The corregidor of Toledo on August 27, 1599 told the king that 244 people, mostly women and children, had died in the city since August 1, and many more had died in the city's smaller towns and villages. "The clothing and linens of the sick are regularly collected and burned, not just

---

[46] AHMA Libro de Actas 25, fol. 28v.
[47] Sánchez Sánchez, *La beneficiencia en Ávila*, 72–4.
[48] Tapia, "Los factores de la evolución demográfica," 180, says Calle de San Francisco, the road to Valladolid and Arévalo, was the likeliest place for plague to have entered Ávila. In Valladolid, too, the city found that the remaining convalescents in the hospital could not be sent home because they had no clothes: AMVA sig. 22-0, November 22, 1599.
[49] AHMA Libro de Actas 25, fols. 190r, 264r.

in the city but also in the villages so that there is no opportunity for the illness to return, because clothing is where it sticks the most, and some people try to steal clothing and hide it, and when they are caught I have given them exemplary punishment, quite rigorous, because I believe it is appropriate," he wrote.[50] Some people may have taken (or kept) items of clothing and waited until the epidemic moved on before putting them on the market. That seems to be what happened in Valladolid, where in November 1599, when the city was at last tolerably healthy, the city council asked the corregidor to put a stop to ongoing public auctions or sales of bed linens, mattresses, and clothing because, according to one regidor, "everything they sell, or most of it, comes from poor people who died of *mal de secas*." Another council member disagreed, pointing out that if the open sales were prohibited, they would simply continue illegally, and that the poor needed to acquire bed clothes from somewhere. The corregidor agreed with the majority, saying that anyway he had issued such an order previously and would now reiterate it.[51] Segovia may have avoided these problems, judging from an accounts ledger, by paying people to wash pestilent clothing rather than burn it.[52]

The notary in Fuenterrabia was there to write everything down because sooner or later, once the smoke cleared, an accounting would have to be made. If desperate people would steal dirty clothes, equally desperate but possibly more sophisticated people would claim that things had gone up in flames when they had not. Thus the notary. A 175-folio ledger in Valladolid covering 1598–1599 includes many cases of reimbursement after fires: Lucía Ruiz, married to Francisco de la Vega, received twenty-two reales for a doublet, a tablecloth, a new blouse, and two trunks of something, all of which had been burned. Diego Bravo and his wife Mariana de Tejada were compensated for five men's and women's shirts and a handkerchief and a collar. Francisco Pérez had lost two new shirts and another old one, three collars, four pieces of linen, and three pairs of cuffs. The fire that took place the day Dr. Santa Cruz discovered the man he thought was the city's first plague victim also led to reimbursement. It turned out that the city had seized all the clothing in the possession of laundress María Sainez and burned everything in order to get at the dead man's clothing. She was compensated (though there is no indication if the clothing's owners also were.) So too was the *alguacil* in charge of that fire, Antonio de Medina, who received twenty-three

---

[50] AGS-E leg. 183, doc. 310, August 27, 1599.
[51] AMVA sig. 22-0, November 15 and 19, 1599.
[52] AMS leg. 394, fol. 46v. The clothing was taken from the sick, washed, and then kept under lock and key.

reales to cover his expenses, including vinegar which he had had to buy and the wages for his helpers, plus an additional eight reales for his own time.[53] The collars, cuffs, shirts, and handkerchiefs probably were taken because someone in the house had gotten ill or died, though it is hard to explain why everything else was not taken as well. Maybe, as in the María Sainez case, items had somehow erroneously been mixed in with some-one else's dirty linens, which is likely in these cases as none mention bedsheets, which would certainly indicate illness or death.

Pedro de Mendoza, owner of a house in the Begoña district (*anteigle-sia*) of Bilbao, lost his entire house to fire, the fate that the Basque fishing town of Pasajes had barely avoided. Mendoza testified in the corregidor's first-instance court that he had pleaded with the burners not to do it, and now he was demanding that they compensate him with 200 ducats to cover his losses and the rent he had to pay in his new lodgings. The defendants – Juan Martínez de Salcedo, Bartolomé de Goiti, and Juan de Zurbarán – responded that Mendoza's claims were unjust and baseless because the so-called house that had gone up in flames was actually just a hut where cattle would find shelter. They said it was the plaintiff's fault that plague had entered the *anteiglesia* to begin with, in a house called Aguirreleta, because he had sheltered sick people there. Those people included his wife, his daughter, and two sons, who all died. Two other sons survived, and with them he went to the dwelling that eventually burned, called Mendiaga, where one of the remaining sons also died. The defendants, two of whom were town officials (*fieles*), said they spoke with Mendoza and the surviving son and that then Mendoza himself lit the hut on fire for reasons not entirely clear, though it is logical to assume that by then he was broken with grief. But even had it been they who burned it, that would have been perfectly acceptable, they testified, "because in such times where everyone's life is at stake (and if God in His mercy does not free this town [of the disease] we may lose most of the kingdom) not only could we burn the said hut but we could do anything to prevent such danger. But, as I say," continued one of the plaintiffs, "neither I nor the *fieles* did anything of the sort, and it is truly audacious for [Mendoza] to say there was neither cause nor pestilence because it is quite notorious that he brought the disease to the said *anteiglesia* and five people died and that is why they are not buried in the church [*fuera de sagrado*]."[54]

Along with the pestilent clothing, the sick and the dead also were transported along city streets, taken away by men who called out to one

---

[53] AMVA-CH 130 a-4 (ant. leg. 321), fols. 45 and 72.
[54] AFB Corregidor 3969/002. The case took place in the latter half of 1598.

another and to the inhabitants to bring out their dead, pushing and pulling carts that groaned and creaked all day long. The sick were borne on the carts themselves or on cots or stretchers, taken to hospitals outside the city walls or, if they arrived too late, to common graves well outside the city limits. Instead of being buried with their friends, whether inside or outside the church, they would lie forever outside their town; that was the fate of Pedro de Mendoza's kin. In Madrid in 1597 people were being buried in deep pits sprinkled with lime at the shrine of Santa Barbara, near the present-day plaza of the same name, which then was just outside the northernmost gate.[55] Some people, such as inhabitants of towns outside Ávila who went up to the mountains, fled and left their dead behind with no one to bury them.[56] Someone had to find the bodies, though, and towns everywhere found men willing to do the job, though not always right at hand and certainly not at the price towns would have wished to pay. This, again, was a seller's market, with time on the sellers' side. The town of Bandarán (La Rioja) reported it had had to hire gravediggers from elsewhere because no one in the town wanted the job.[57] Valencia at a later date solved the problem of gravediggers' high wages by using slaves, which the city bought, and prisoners, to whom the city offered a reduced sentence or freedom.[58] Juan de Olaiz, a vecino of Puente la Reina (Navarre), went off to Pamplona to dig graves and returned to find his furniture gone.[59] In Pasajes, Padre Villaviciosa told provincial authorities that of the eight gravediggers, who were locals and did the job "just to serve God," two had died, four quit (or left), "and the remaining two persevere in their good works."[60] In July 1599, at the height of the Castilian plague, Segovia found Alonso Manzano and Juan Bernaldo, who were to "dig graves and bury everyone who has died, regardless of what time it is and whenever we are called to do so, be it day or night, wherever we are sent, from today until St Michael's day of this year," when they were to be paid thirty ducats. They could draw advances if they needed to, with the money coming out of

[55] RAH Salazar leg. 23, carp. 4, no. 11, fol. 390r–v, yet another indication the capital was hit earlier than recognized.
[56] AGS-E leg. 183, doc. 243, June 30, 1599.   [57] AHN Consejos leg. 30.168 exp. 12.
[58] Fray Francisco Gavaldá, *Memoria de los sucesos particulares de Valencia y su provincia en … tiempo de peste* (Valencia, 1651), part 4. This plague took place in 1647.
[59] AGN TR Procesos 120945. He blamed a neighboring couple, who said the town had requisitioned and then burned all his beds. He seems to have won the case, though he got less than he asked.
[60] Letter from Miguel de Villaviciosa, writing from Fuenterrabia about Pasajes de San Juan, in Murugarren Zamora, "La peste en Guipuzcoa," 266.

Segovia's *propios*.[61] A ledger of expenses incurred in 1598–1599 in Segovia itemizes payments to men for carrying beds to the hospital, delivering firewood to Santa Catalina hospital so clothes could be burned, transporting the poor, cleaning the street, carrying the clothes, burning the clothes, carrying a woman "in my arms to Santa Catalina," supplying barley and wheat and straw, pulling or pushing carts, and carrying stretchers with patients on them. Someone made two litters or stretchers of walnut wood and four poles to carry them on. Men picked up dead bodies on the street, outside the bakery, in the *casilla de* Doña Isabel de Savedra.[62]

Putting aside the plague for a moment, it appears that by the late sixteenth century people were clamoring to be buried inside their churches or in convents and monasteries. Religious authorities frowned upon this "invasion of the churches," both for sanitary and for space reasons, and popes issued repeated injunctions that appear to have been ignored.[63] People wanted to be inside, preferably with a good vantage point, where their spirits could hear the prayers being said for them, where they would be protected from the devil and accompanied by their friends. Cathedral canons told the Seville city council in April 1581 during an epidemic that "the dead do not fit anymore."[64] Carlos Eire refers to old churches in Madrid such as San Ginés as "cities of the dead," constantly being torn up to accommodate new bodies, and he also says few outdoor graveyards were being used by the late sixteenth

---

[61] Manuela Villalpando Martinez, "Tres noticias de la Segovia antigua: Un brote de peste en la Segovia de 1653," *Estudios Segovianos* 95 (1997), 17–26. In Denmark, poor men were paid in beer to bury plague victims, a custom that governments tried to halt because of the entirely predictable results; Peter Christensen, "'In These Perilous Times': plague and plague policies in early modern Denmark," *Medical History* 47 (2003), 413–50, p. 436.

[62] AMS leg. 388/7, unfoliated. In her study of the confraternities of Zamora, Maureen Flynn wrote that "during years of pestilence, cofrades were particularly active, coming out two by two into the streets with wooden planks and coffins to recover plague victims and bury them in cemeteries." I have not found evidence of confraternities helping out in this way, though that does not mean it did not happen; *Sacred Charity: Confraternities and Social Welfare in Spain, 1400–1700* (Ithaca, NY: Cornell University Press, 1989), 65, citing AMZ leg. 1097, no. 1, the parish archive of San Lázaro no. 1, and the parish archive of San Juan de la Puerta Nueva, libro 12. Nor have I found anything similar to the fascinating role played by older women as described by Richelle Munkhoff in "Searchers of the dead: Authority, marginality, and the interpretation of plague in England, 1574–1665," *Gender and History* 11:1 (April 1999), 1–29.

[63] Fernando Martínez Gil, *Muerte y sociedad en la España de los Austrias* (Madrid: Siglo Veintiuno Editores, 1993), 434–5. On p. 444 he says it was only in the seventeenth century that church authorities used health as a reason to prohibit burial inside.

[64] Alexandra Parma Cook and Noble David Cook, *The Plague Files: Crisis Management in Sixteenth-Century Seville* (Baton Rouge, LA: Louisiana State University Press, 2009), 87.

century.[65] If true, this would mark a change from what had gone on before. Ordinary people – which is most people – certainly were buried in cemeteries, sometimes next to hospitals. The 1611 dictionary by Sebastián de Covarrubias states clearly that a cemetery is "the place right next to the church where the bodies of the faithful are buried." Late sixteenth-century synodal documents cited by Martínez Gil indicate cemeteries were being used for markets, games, dances, and even gambling, all of which naturally was deemed improper.[66] More broadly, an eighteenth-century treatise on burials and funerals reported that in the sixteenth century and long before, Spaniards generally were buried in cemeteries next to their church; indeed, the Partidas instructed that cemeteries should measure forty steps around the church.[67] There was no shame in being buried outside, and it did not suggest excommunication or ostracism; on the contrary, the treatise says that "people of distinction" wanted that honor, and plenty of nobles and royals lay outdoors just as the ancient Christians had done, and people who demanded to be indoors simply misunderstood ancient rites. Outdoor graves could be and were places of respect, though possibly as the plague progressed in the late 1590s they became less so. Thomas Laqueur offers a beautifully evocative image of burials in late medieval England which is worth quoting, allowing for the disparate time and place: "An orderly, that is, properly aligned burial mattered in the old regime. Even in the crisis of the first great plague epidemic of 1348–1349, when the dead in their thousands were placed in the mass graves of emergency burial grounds, they were put there with care. They were not dumped. They were not scrunched up. Small coins and other signs of caring were often placed on them. They would face east when the resurrection came. Their bodies are carefully aligned. By contrast, the mass grave of soldiers after the Battle of Towton (1461) in the War of the Roses is a jumble, bodies stripped and mutilated. So were many early modern military graves. To be disordered is to be dirt."[68]

---

[65] Carlos M. N. Eire, *From Madrid to Purgatory: The Art and Craft of Dying in Sixteenth-Century Spain* (Cambridge University Press, 1995), 91–4. James Casey's brief study of death in Granada suggests people were buried inside the church and five years later were removed to a common ossuary: James Casey, "'Queriendo poner mi ánima en carrera de salvación': la muerte en Granada (siglos xvii–xviii)," *Cuadernos de Historia Moderna Anejos* (2001), 17–43, p. 34.

[66] Martínez Gil, *Muerte y sociedad*, 446–50. See also Leonor Gómez Nieto, *Ritos funerarios en el Madrid medieval* (Madrid: Ak-Mudayna, 1991), 60–6.

[67] Fr. Miguel de Azero y Aldovera, *Tratado de los funerales y de las sepulturas, que presenta al excelentísimo señor Conde de Floridablanca* (Madrid: Imprenta Real, 1736), 69–75; Partidas I tit. XIII law 4.

[68] Thomas W. Laqueur, *The Work of the Dead: A Cultural History of Mortal Remains* (Princeton, NJ: Princeton University Press, 2015), 126. An article in *The Times* of London about a graveyard dating from that city's seventeenth-century Great Plague

People in pestilent Castilian towns in the late 1590s indeed faced the prospect not only of not being buried inside the church but, far worse, of being buried in a disorderly fashion, in a mass grave far away. One could not know if gravediggers would be as careful as their colleagues in England. So, unwilling that their loved ones' bodies be picked up in carts and taken outside the city walls, some inhabitants of Bilbao were organizing their own funerals late at night with the surreptitious cooperation of the clergy. "After night falls," the city council instructed on July 30, 1599, "there shall be no gravedigging nor shall any cadaver be carried to the church nor shall the nuns of the churches open their doors, and if they do they will be severely punished." There was talk (*nota y murmuración*) in the city about these night vigils when bodies were being buried, the council worried. "Outsiders [*forasteros*] are scandalized to see [such things] at such an hour, late at night, without priests and only laypeople," according to the minutes, "and on another day priests went to the homes of the said deceased, and the neighbors gathered, and they held a vigil, and it was inferred that there were two bodies in one house…" These bodies were carried to the church for interment, fairly remarkable at this late date, but the practice did not survive long, with or without priests. A month later, the city council, worried that plague victims' bodies buried in churches and monasteries might harm inhabitants, ordered that a large pit be dug near the infirmary and that the dead be placed there and covered with lime. Like most cities, Bilbao had divided itself up into districts for the purpose of collecting bodies and detecting illness, and it was the neighborhood bosses who should ensure that improper burials cease.[69]

Gravedigging was not a high-prestige job at the best of times, but there are indications that people believed that contact with bodies of plague victims might make one infectious, making the job even worse than usual. The very fact that bodies were buried in lime, away from the town, makes this clear. In Chapter 3 we saw that Ávila expelled a father who buried his son. Similarly, Nicolás Suárez, the envoy who inspected the Tagus River valley in 1582, made inquiries in Aranjuez as to the death of Esteban de Valencia, who had arrived at mid-day on Saturday and died Monday night. The constable Juan de Soto told him that Valencia seemed to be ill when he arrived and that once he died the governor (*gobernador*) had ordered that the body be taken to the town of Ontígola,

shows that then, too, plague victims were "buried with care and reverence"; Ben MacIntyre, "Blitz spirit dates back to the Black Death" [an historically incorrect headline], December 23, 2017.
[69] AFB libro 024, July 30 and September 6, 1599.

a half-league away, where he was buried, and all the clothing and the bed were burned. The house where he died was sealed, and both the owner of the house and the gravedigger were banished.[70] On the other hand, one person who did not seem worried about possibly pestilent bodies was María Ortiz, a *vecina* of Puente la Reina, who three years after the demise of her husband decided to go out to the vineyard where he was buried, dig him up, and rebury him properly in the church of Santiago, which she said had been his wish. She claimed there was nothing left but bones, as lime had been dumped there three or four times, and that the bishop had assented to the translation. But after some town council members blocked her attempts, she and her daughter-in-law not only sued, they tried to disinter him. Witnesses claimed the body emitted a strong smell and that the head still boasted a beard. They also said that when the two women had picked out some bones, the witnesses promptly grabbed them (the bones) and put them back into the grave. Ortiz and her daughter-in-law were jailed and later released, and the deceased, Juan de Elordi, remained where he was.[71] Dr. Valentin de Andosilla was of the school that believed dead bodies were contagious. Classical experts had said the opposite, he conceded, but in the case of this epidemic – which he believed constituted an entirely new disease, caused not by the air but by the "poison of death" – bodies were highly dangerous: "I witnessed a dog eating a body that had been dead for eight days, which the dog had uncovered in a shrine, and the owner of the dog was advised to kill the dog, which he did not do, and that same day as the dog was being petted he infected five people and they all died," he wrote. "And that same week I heard of another dog who had eaten poorly buried cadavers in the same shrine. (This was because a woman had tied her husband to her foot with a rope and was dragging him along the ground and she left him somewhere badly buried.) In short, that dog infected three people in its house and they died, and I have seen many cases like these."[72] Andosilla mentions dogs and goats as infectious agents; throughout Castile town councils ordered that cats, dogs, pigs, and sheep be removed or killed (as they were in Defoe's London), and, as we saw in the discussion of commerce and markets, fish from the north was also highly suspect.[73]

[70] AGS-CR leg. 115 no. 4, fol. 25r.   [71] AGN TR Procesos 013202.

[72] Andosilla, *Libro en que se prueba con claridad el mal que corre*, chapter 4, fols. 18v–19v.

[73] Defoe, *A Journal of the Plague Year*, 123. As mentioned in a long footnote to chapter 3, medical historians, epidemiologists, and microbiologists are broadening the list of possible vectors and hosts of plague. Cats are on the list, as are many other mammals (camels, goats, most rodents) and even birds. I am grateful for recent (2017) communication on the MEDMED-L listserv concerning scientific advances in this area.

The noise, the smoke, the emptiness, and the collecting of the sick and the dead were described in compelling detail by a Dominican friar who stands a bit outside our framework: he worked in Valencia, which avoided the great Castilian plague but was severely affected during 1647. The Dominican, Francisco Gavaldá, ran one of the plague hospitals, where "on Tuesday, October 29, 1647, at four in the afternoon, we entered," the "we" being six religious fathers and four laypeople. Two of the ten would die. "I will say what I saw," Gavaldá announces. The previous weeks had been terrible, with so many bodies that the gravediggers could not bury them all, which is why Valencia had hired slaves and prisoners. Many inhabitants fled, leaving houses and belongings. Carts maneuvered their way through streets bearing bodies wrapped in sheets or naked, some of them passed down to the gravediggers from windows above. Regardless of their social class or if they were religious or lay, bodies went onto the carts. Mothers might try to bribe officers in order to stay with their children, he said, but the city stood firm. "At first the living looked at the carts with horror and desperation because they were like ordinary wagons, with nothing covering up the deceased. Some were wearing ordinary clothes, others were wrapped in a sheet, others with a blanket, and others with just a shirt. Who could not feel horror and outrage at such a spectacle? Later things got better because the carts were covered with cane canopies over which a black cloth with a painted cross was draped. Two men worked on each cart, helping each other to load the bodies, and because they were there by force, because some were slaves and the rest had been taken out of jail to purge their sins, in burying the dead they did not exhibit the charity of Tobias. Maybe because they did not want to make a second round on one street, they tried loading the living as if they were dead, which happened. Others ... did not want to pull the dead out of the houses, like the time there were five dead in one house and one of them dared to demand six pounds [*libras*] to bury one cadaver. This disorder and indecency created confusion, and so did the fact that in Valencia no paper or manuscript notice could be found to shed light for those of us walking through such darkness."[74]

When city councils at last began dismissing gravediggers and the legions of opportunistic laborers shuttling the sick and the dead, it was

[74] This long quote is from Gavaldá, *Memoria de los sucesos particulares de Valencia*, part 14. Tobias in the Old Testament performs acts of mercy to the dead. The apparent lack of documentation to which he refers would be astonishing if true; I will return to the matter of institutional memory in Chapter 6. Our Gavaldá must not be confused with another Francisco Gavaldá, a Hieronymite who became Bishop of Segorbe.

because this darkness finally was beginning to fade. Burgos on September 15, 1599 decided that the two *picaros* whose job it was to carry litters could be let go. People peering out their doors from their refuge would no longer hear their comings and goings all day long. On October 8 it was time for the four remaining gravediggers to be laid off.[75] It was over.

However, town criers would continue their plague-related work for a bit longer, calling out the last of the city council's measures and decisions. In small towns *pregoneros* probably would limit themselves to the main square, church steps, and a few other important gathering places, but in larger cities they were ubiquitous, and they walked defined routes; in Madrid on June 12, 1602, *pregones* warning residents about all the towns in the south suffering from plague were cried aloud at as many as thirty-four sites.[76] The sound of the town crier's voice must have been an accepted, if annoying, part of daily life in early modern Spain (and probably elsewhere). Several times a day one might hear them calling out guild regulations, price ceilings for bread and other foodstuffs, tax-farming agreements, punishments for a variety of offenses, sumptuary laws prohibiting any number of frills and styles, upcoming *autos-da-fé* or celebrations, the names of those appointed by the city council to do one thing or another, or the opportunity to bid on city jobs. During plague years, as we have seen, they read (and reread) the lists of pestilent towns, warned innkeepers to reject travelers without proper identification, ordered people to report their dead and hand over their linens, threatened punishments for tearing down portions of walls, and summoned the poor to gather at a certain location for sorting and expulsion after distribution of some alms. They were, naturally, accompanied by notaries, not only to make sure the correct information was being read aloud, but also to have a witness to testify that the act had, indeed, occurred. When several muleteers were prohibited from entering Burgos, an instance mentioned in Chapter 2, very few people in the city would have missed the news: "In the city of Burgos on the said day month and year, before me, the public notary, in the plaza of this city, Francisco de la Cruz, the city's public *pregonero*, read in a loud and intelligible voice what had been ordered and agreed upon by the above-noted gentlemen ... and I, the said notary [declare] that there were many people in the plaza of this city ... and it was *pregonado* again ... before many *vecinos* and people in the arrabal of San Esteban and in the little plaza of San Esteban and in

---

[75] AMB-HI 3653.
[76] AV Secretaría 1-138-4. Thirty-four streets are listed, but some are repeated, meaning either that they were to visit twice or possibly the notary made a mistake.

many other places ... where such *pregones* usually are by custom read aloud, and there were many people present..."[77]

To some extent this never-ending voice cemented notions of public order in people's heads and confirmed or reaffirmed memories of similar instances, of having heard the same orders and carried out the same practices. There was a cyclical, persistent aspect to epidemics. When plague arrived, communities stepped outside their usual rhythms for a while, albeit in familiar ways, and then returned, having regained their footing, though it would never be the same. Novelties, *novedades*, were frowned upon by Aristotle and contemporary political theorists; according to Castillo de Bovadilla, a corregidor "must try to conserve the state of the city and neither invent nor devise *novedades* but rather follow the path of the ancients, the path taken by his predecessors, because *novedades* generally cause harm rather than good in the Republic."[78] One should do what one had done in the past, walk the same paths, and hearing something might make remembering those experiences that much easier. Orality reminded people of the rules, but it may also have helped them reenact past practices, especially as they were all hearing the same thing. J. G. A. Pocock wrote many years ago: "Awareness of a past, then, is a social awareness and can exist only as part of a generalised awareness of the structure and behaviour of a society. Almost any society preserves statements of some kind concerning events which occurred in a past time; its awareness of these events is its awareness of its past; and this awareness plays some part in its life in the present. Since all societies are organised consciously or unconsciously to ensure their own continuity, we may suppose that the preservation of statements about the past has in various ways the function of ensuring continuity, and that awareness of the past is in fact society's awareness of its continuity."[79] Such a lofty and significant mission seems a bit beyond the capacities of the average town crier, but it was not the men themselves but rather their voices, their scripts, their authority that awakened townspeople's awareness of the past.

Town criers were public employees, and every town or city had one or more, but because of the increased workload and the likelihood that some had left town to escape the plague or died, more were added.

---

[77] AMB-HI 3653, January 18, 1597.

[78] Jerónimo Castillo de Bovadilla, *Política para corregidores y señores de vasallos* (Madrid: Instituto de Estudios de Administración Local, 1978), 2 vols. (facs. of Antwerp: Juan Bautista Verdussen, 1704). [1597], vol. 1, p. 63. Similarly, Giovanni Botero's *The Reason of State*, translated into Spanish in 1593 by chronicler Antonio de Herrera, has a section called "The avoidance of novelty."

[79] J. G. A. Pocock, "The origins of study of the past: a comparative approach," *Comparative Studies in Society and History* 4:2 (1962), 209–46, p. 211.

(Lazarillo de Tormes, one of Spain's most famous *pícaros*, after many tribulations was named *pregonero* in Toledo, the culmination of his rocky professional journey.) Given the legal formalities involved in reading aloud edicts and public announcements, most temporary criers seem also to have been notaries; unlike with manual laborers, cities could not hire just anyone. Because they were not salaried, these extra *pregoneros* submitted invoices. For example, Valladolid's city treasurer dealt with one Juan García de Juria, a royal notary (perhaps employed by the Chancillería, where his hours undoubtedly had been cut back), who said the city had ordered him, among other things, to cry aloud prohibitions against guests and products from pestilent places, instructions to innkeepers that patrons and merchandise carry documents with the seal of the city, and warnings against punching holes in walls.[80] Another notary in Valladolid, Juan de Auría, who appears to have been somewhat of a tattle-tale, delivered *pregones* in tanneries and announced on two successive market days that no one was to attend the San Miguel fair and that if they did they would be punished with death.[81]

The *pregonero* carried with him the *vara de justicia*, the staff that showed he embodied royal authority. If the king sent edicts to a city that later were to be sent on to smaller towns, it was the crier who carried those orders and read them aloud, and his physical person represented the crown. But an unlucky *pregonero* who worked for Burgos Corregidor Diego Vargas Manrique found he was unprotected, and Vargas found himself ensnared in a typical jurisdictional contest. When in January 1598 Vargas – who was officially referred to in government correspondence as a member of the Order of Alcántara, Corregidor of Burgos by the king our lord, and appointed judge for matters concerning the guard and defense of the twelve leagues around the city – issued orders prohibiting the towns of San Martín and Santa Catalina from holding fairs, this was not to the liking of Lic. Arriola, the *alcalde mayor* of the *adelantamiento* de

---

[80] AMVA-CH 9-7 (ant. leg. 287) fols. 10–11, November 1597. García de Juria also listed many "notifications" he had carried out which probably were not cried aloud, such as telling people in the marketplace not to sell fish from Santander, telling millers not to accept guests, telling his fellow notaries to keep track of all the trials and fines concerning peste, reporting on guardsmen who had not shown up for duty, instructing friars at the Nuestra Señora de Prado monastery to tie up their boats, and "many other things" for which he had not been paid. The city authorized payment of sixty reales.

[81] AMVA-CH 130 a-4 (ant. leg. 321) fol. 56. Like García de Juria, Auría also conducted inquiries for the city. He looked into the death of a man near the Tudela gate, investigated guards who did not properly demand safe conducts from travelers, reported on innkeepers and *vecinos* who were taking in people from Galicia, searched for a man in the Santa Clara neighborhood who was said to have been in Bilbao, informed on servants of a man named Medina who were said to have broken down a wall, and undertook "many other" tasks.

Burgos, an administrative and judicial entity dating from the Middle Ages whose jurisdictions (essentially unincorporated areas) inevitably overlapped on others'.[82] So Arriola neatly imprisoned Vargas's councilmen, envoys, and *pregonero*, ripped up the corregidor's papers, and ordered that the *pregonero* be whipped. He also apparently ordered the fairs to go on, according to what Vargas later gleaned from the town of Belorado. Vargas's complaint to the Council of Castile suggests that Arriola was offended at the judicial interference implicit in Vargas' orders: "He considered my orders to be a slight to his office, as if in courts and the Chancillería there were no procedures against negligence or to supplant ordinary judges," he wrote, adding that Arriola "says he has the same commission as I do from the Chancillería of Valladolid." And now the corregidor of Reynosa was following Arriola's regrettable example. Vargas requested that the Council send him (Vargas) a statement from the Chancillería stating how much work he had done for his endangered province, which thus far had been spared, credit for which must also go (he added) to God's mercy. A week later, the Chancillería apparently had not given him the backing he had requested, so Vargas simply quit. "Although I could take personal offense at this, I am thinking only about the lack of respect for the Council and the public good, for which reason I beg you to honor my request... I cannot continue in this post if I do not receive the favors I beg of you. The Council will lose a faithful and diligent servant, but I will be freed from much work and no small amount of danger."[83] Two weeks later the king stepped in, seemingly at the Council's suggestion, ordering Arriola's replacement, Lic. Mosquera de Figueroa, (it is unclear when the substitution took place) to free the prisoners from Burgos and explain himself. The corregidor of Reynosa was similarly reprimanded. Neither was to "interfere or get involved with what our Corregidor of the said city of Burgos decides regarding our letter and commission" empowering him in plague matters. Vargas withdrew his resignation.

Corregidores like Vargas stood at the intersection of many jurisdictions. Prime among their responsibilities was to ensure that cities kept the money flowing to the crown and to prevent the city's Cortes representatives or local nobility from challenging the monarchy. They or their lieutenants chaired city council meetings and could break tied votes. They rotated in and out for approximately two years, with their salary being paid by municipalities, and generally they were on their way up the

---

[82] On *adelantamientos*, see José Luis de las Heras Santos, *La justicia penal de los Austrias en la Corona de Castilla* (Salamanca: Universidad de Salamanca, 1991) 57–60.

[83] AMB-HI 3651, January 20 and 27, 1598.

administrative and judicial ladders; many leading political figures of the sixteenth and seventeenth centuries, both noble and commoner, had been corregidores. It was not an easy job, as they had to balance not only competing jurisdictions within Castile's vast and tangled judicial network, as Vargas found in this case, but also competing economic needs and demands. *Sisas*, for example, which paid for public health measures, were financed not by the crown but by townspeople who asked the king (with the corregidor as mediator) for permission to tax themselves. The crown was continually asking the kingdom for ordinary and extraordinary "donations," and the corregidor's job entailed strong-arming city councils to get what the king wanted even when city coffers were empty and people were going hungry. But there are also instances where one can clearly see the corregidor stuck in the middle, trying to defend the interests of both parties; squeezing municipal treasuries of all their funds and assets was neither financially feasible nor politically advisable. They had to be pragmatic, the keyword of Hapsburg rule in Spain. In the oft-quoted words of Castillo de Bovadilla, "Truly, there is no task among the courts and government like bullfighting with city councils."[84]

Because they were judges, corregidores imposed punishments. They made good on the incessant threats being cried aloud on town streets. We have seen plenty of examples of stiff fines and banishment decrees for violations of plague rules, but there also were more public penalties, visible to everyone. The Partidas spelled out the twin objectives of punishment in general: to penalize the wrongdoer, obviously, but also to deter others, "so that everyone who hears and sees the punishment take it as an example and a warning to ensure that, out of fear of punishment, they will not err."[85] Judging from the documents, during this plague epidemic there were surprisingly few crimes other than quarantine violations, of which there were an infinite number. There were no social disturbances that I can find. Apparently there were hardly any criminal cases against people who entered locked homes, marking a stark contrast with Italy (and Marseille, where, in the 1720s, according to Junko Takeda, "The commonest crime throughout the [plague]

---

[84] Castillo de Bovadilla cited by Benjamin González Alonso, *El corregidor castellano 1348–1808* (Madrid: Instituto de Estudios Administrativos, 1970), 212. On corregidores see also Heras Santos, *La justicia penal*, 60–5; on Castillo de Bovadilla see Ronald W. Truman, *Spanish Treatises on Government, Society and Religion in the Time of Philip II: The "de regimine principum" and Associated Traditions* (Leiden: Brill, 1999), 164–82 and bibliography cited therein. Chapter 1 included an account of how military authorities considered the corregidor of Guipúzcoa to be too close to local interests, to the detriment of the crown; he had "the difficult task of balancing the suspicions of some against the urgent needs of others": Cruz Mundet, *"El mal que al presente corre,"* 147.

[85] Partida VII, tit. 31, law 1.

outbreak was burgling abandoned buildings, for which the standard punishment was imprisonment for life in the galleys"). Gavaldá said that when Valencians who fled returned they found their houses empty, and the Burgos city council during the dreadful 1565 plague placed guards in the city to hinder robberies "which in similar occasions tend to occur." Pamplona also had foot patrols to impede robberies of empty houses, and there is a later reference to "certain thefts in suspicious [i.e. diseased] houses."[86] Miquel Parets's diary during the 1651 plague in Barcelona says "the death penalty was decreed for anyone entering these [closed-up] houses to rob or even to touch anything in them before they were well cleaned and fumigated."[87] But these examples do not demonstrate that robberies were frequent or actually even took place. It may be that in Castile lower-instance case files for this period were destroyed, but it is notable that no city council minutes include references to theft as a problem during these years. The royal tribunal of Navarre has a few cases that might be construed as theft, but in every one the defendant, sometimes a town council member, has a logical explanation; for example Puente la Reina responded to allegations of missing wine by saying that when the well-off residents left town, it was only natural that the poor ate their food and drank their wine.[88]

Nor were there criminal cases in Castile associated with the allegedly deliberate spreading of the disease. According to Paolo Preto, stories of deliberate infection were a topos ever since Thucydides described the plague of Athens. They resurfaced in Italy in 1576, he writes, when doctors wrote about evil people, the *untori*, who spread peste on saddles and reins, and again in 1629 when two men disguised as friars were arrested for trying to infect Milan. Philip IV of Spain wrote to the Spanish governor of Milan at that time to warn him about four Frenchmen who had fled Madrid after allegedly trying to spread "poisonous and pestilent ointment" in Spain's capital. The news from Milan explains the one

---

[86] Junko Thérèse Takeda, *Between Crown and Commerce: Marseille and the Early Modern Mediterranean* (Baltimore, MD: Johns Hopkins University Press, 2011), 144; Gavaldá, *Memoria de los sucesos particulares de Valencia*, part 13; Gonzalo Diez de la Lastra y Diez de Güemes, "Datos curiosos para la historia de la ciudad, sacados de los Libros de Actas del Excmo. Ayuntamiento de la M. N. y M. M. L. Ciudad de Burgos, Cabeza de Castilla y Cámara de S. M.: Peste bubónica en Burgos en el año 1565," *Boletin de Estadística e Información del Excmo. Ayuntamiento de Burgos* 263 (1944), 51; Baleztena, "Relación de la Peste desta Ciudad de Pamplona," 392.

[87] Amelang, *A Journal of the Plague Year*, 57. In contrast see Giulia Calvi, *Histories of a Plague Year: The Social and the Imaginary in Baroque Florence*, trans. Dario Biocca and Bryant T. Ragan, Jr. (Berkeley, CA: University of California Press, 1989), based on an enviable 300 criminal trials for breaking and entering.

[88] AGN TR Procesos 089003. And the wine probably wasn't very good, the town added.

reference I have found to the phenomenon in Spain, which came in 1630. On September 28 of that year, the king ordered *pregoneros* to call out an order (*bando*) promising rewards to anyone denouncing the presence of foreigners who had entered Spain with pestilent powders (*polvos*) (Figure 5.1). [89]

But Castilians' apparent reluctance to burglarize empty homes does not mean the judges and constables were not kept busy. We just saw that a notary in Valladolid, Juan de Auria, hyperbolically announced the death penalty for those illicitly attending a market. The death penalty was also cried out there for all people who had "gardens, chicken coops and houses outside the barrier of this city." Anyone who sheltered any person, item of clothing, or product from outside likewise was "under penalty of their life and the loss of all their property," a punishment so dire as to make it doubtful indeed. [90] But in Burgos, Vargas in December 1597 ordered that new gallows be raised near the city gates and in all its jurisdictional towns where there were fairs and markets, and he specifically targeted anyone committing violent acts or robberies or "stirring the waters." Clearly he was getting alarmed, though the problem seems to have been people wandering about rather than engaging in acts of violence. A few weeks later he thanked one of his commissioners, Cristóbal de Morales, for the attention the latter had given to punishments, though in the same letter he cautioned that Morales must tell local authorities not to prosecute villagers for debts, at least for the time being. Still, all towns within six days must "raise new gallows in the most public place within their town limits." To the town of Padilla de Arriba he wrote separately, like a disappointed father: "There is such disorderliness, with the pestilent communicating with the healthy and carrying goods from one to the other, and seeing that our orders and exortations have not sufficed, for the common good of all I am obliged to place guards and issue orders [*pregones*] and raise gallows, as you have seen." He only wanted to help them, he insisted. [91] A few months later he dispatched a Jesuit, Father Diego de Angulo, to Melgar de Fernamental, Villasandino and the rest to hand out alms, tally up those in need of medical help, and

---

[89] Paolo Preto, *Epidemia, paura e politica nell'Italia moderna* (Rome: Editori Laterza, 1987), 11, 43; The *bando*, available on the Biblioteca Digital de la Comunidad de Madrid without a call number, is called *Pregón y vando ...*" and was issued in 1630. The cataloger, probably in the mid-twentieth century, classified it under "Chemical warfare" (*guerra química*). The 1630 plague in Milan was enormous; its best-known account is Alessandro Manzoni's novel, *The Betrothed*, which includes famed descriptions of the *untori*.

[90] AMVA sig. 21-0, April 23, 1599.

[91] AMB-HI 3651, fols. 169–70, 180. December 1597.

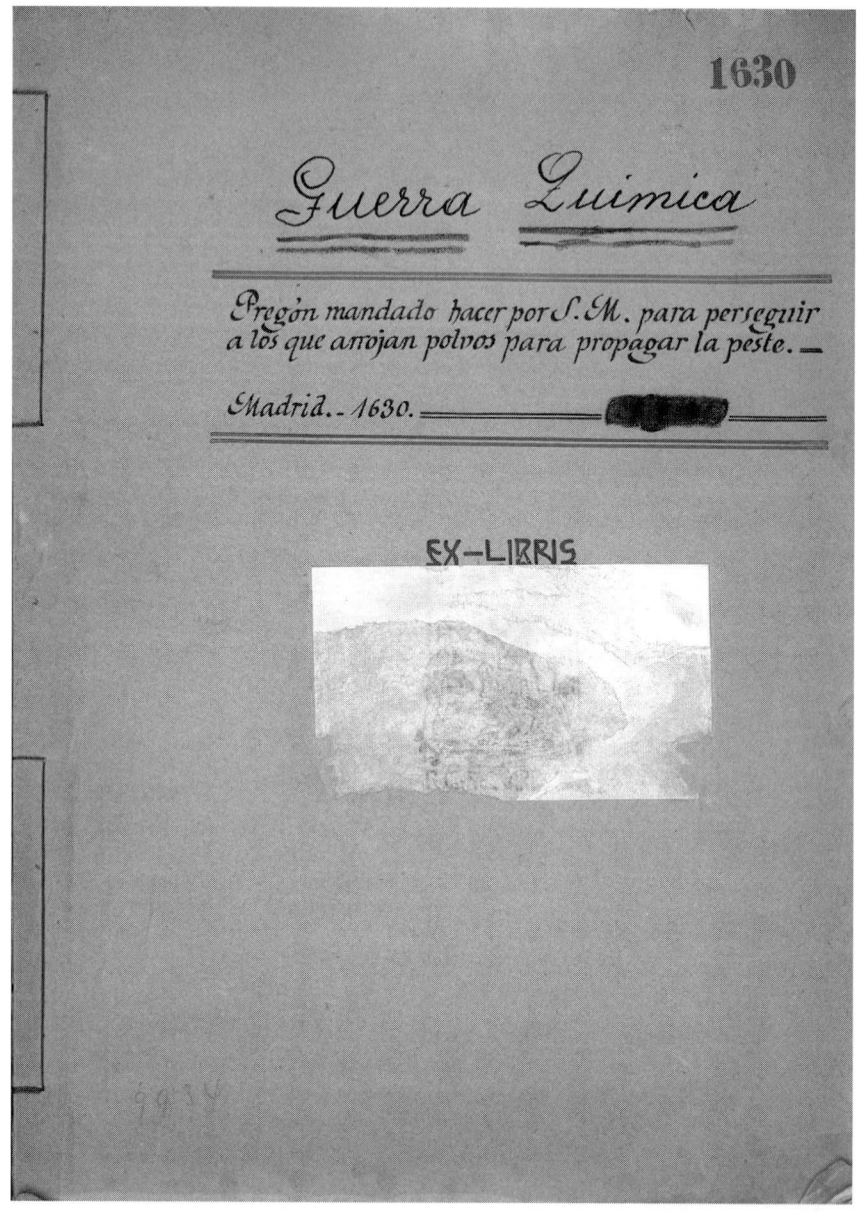

Figure 5.1 An edict by Philip IV against spreading pestilent powders in Madrid and the rest of Spain originating from the 1630 plague in Milan. It offers rewards for denouncing those who bring in powder and prohibits foreigners from entering Madrid without first spending two months in the kingdom.
Source: Biblioteca Regional de Madrid, A-Caj. 186/9

PREGON Y
VANDO, QVE POR MAN.
dado de su Magestad se ha publicado en
su Corte, para que se guarde en ella, y en
las demas Ciudades, Villas, y Lugares
destos Reinos, conforme a lo acor
dado por el Consejo.

CON LICENCIA.
EN MADRID, POR LA VIVDA DE ALONSO
Martin. Año 1630.

Vendese en casa de Martin Gil de Cordoua.

Figure 5.1 (*cont.*)

178   Life in a Time of Pestilence

conduct the usual survey of villagers ("with people who Your Reverence
believes will tell the truth, and in this respect distinterested widows are
no less appropriate.") He was also to conduct a sort of internal performance review by asking all town authorities "if they had been harmed in
any way by the corregidor of Burgos or by commissioners and guards
placed there by the corregidor for the defense and protection of the town
or village, and if so they must declare what the offense was and how it
transpired." A week later, Vargas was feeling less Christian about
matters. There had been a nasty case in Arenillas where the executioner
(*verdugo*) had "gotten him in the throat," meaning either a bad hanging
or a bad garrote, and the man took five or six days to die. So that did not
help. "No one wants justice in their own house," he complained sadly to
Father Angulo, adding that if people had grievances it was probably
because they had behaved badly. He had installed the gallows there only
because his rules were being violated, Vargas insisted, adding that punishments had been moderate. But, even so, if his commissioners had
committed some crime, he wanted to know about it, and people should
not be afraid to testify: "My desire is that justice be done."[92]

At the same time as Vargas ordered new gallows to be built, he also said
that anyone caught entering the city with counterfeit papers would suffer
public shaming (*verguenza pública*), by definition a punishment that took
place before the eyes of the already traumatized community. As with the
hangings – and, as we saw earlier, with banishment – there is no indication
how often these punishments actually were carried out. Crimes for which
public shaming, generally including lashes, was deemed the proper sentence included resisting authority (which can mean anything), vagrancy,
prison escapes, perjury, bigamy, prostitution, and theft. But there was
enormous discretion, and sentences frequently were reduced or altered
upon appeal. A study of 191 criminal cases in sixteenth-century Galicia
shows that just thirteen defendants were sentenced to public shaming;
a subsequent group of 775 cases in the seventeenth century yielded
forty-six.[93]

Possibly under the rubric of resisting authority, one unfortunate man
was picked up for violating the quarantine and sentenced to public

[92] AMB-HI 3650, April 12, April 20, 1598.
[93] Pedro Ortego Gil, "La pena de vergüenza pública (siglos XVI–XVIII): Teoría legal
castellana y práctica judicial gallega," *Anuario de derecho penal y ciencias penales* 51:1–3
(1998), 153–204, pp. 188–9. The numbers declined after appeals. Heras Santos, *La
justicia penal*, 298–300, says public shaming was a ceremonial way of restoring social
honor; in this case I would disagree, as there is no indication that quarantine violations in
any way injured collective honor, which in any case is an ill-defined concept. Heras
Santos does not specifically mention quarantine violations in his book.

shame.[94] His name was Andrés Alonso, and he was a *vecino* of San Martín de la Bodega, a quarter-league outside Burgos. According to the appeal, the Lt. Corregidor at the time, Dr. Pineda de Tapia, said that it had come to his attention that an inhabitant there had taken in three or four people from the pestilent city of Santander, so he sent an *alguacil*, Aguero Niño de Mercado, to investigate. Somehow, according to Niño, Alonso had run into a certain captain from Santander and had allowed him and his two companions, later referred to as his servants, to enter San Martín and Burgos draped in peasant's clothing (including a large cape) which belonged to Alonso. As a result, Alonso was sent to jail, and Pineda de Tapia on February 13, 1597, ruled that he should be "taken from jail on the back of a mule, according to justice, and suffer shame through the public streets of this city of Burgos and that he be banished from this city and its jurisdiction for four years, and if he should violate this sentence without permission from the king he shall serve on the galleys without salary." Alonso naturally appealed, but the public shame part of the sentence was carried out even though the appeal was pending; this was a judicial error on Pineda de Tapia's part that eventually led to the verdict being overturned not on matters of fact but on matters of law.

The Chancillería on May 2 restored Alonso's honor and sentenced Pineda de Tapia to two years' loss of office and ordered him to pay 20,000 maravedies to Alonso within nine days and 30,000 in legal penalties within three days. Now it was Pineda de Tapia's turn to appeal. He pointed out how grave a crime Alonso had committed by sheltering people from Santander. He had "risked the total ruin and death of the city," and had "disguised the enemy in clothing very different from what they wore when they went to his house, knowing full well that they were sick and pestilent" and were from a land "devastated by plague." He was a "traitor to the patria," Pineda's lawyer went on, and had shown malice aforethought (*dolo*) in giving refuge to the three pestilent men. In fact, he said, Alonso deserved the death penalty not only for having endangered the city but for having dissimulated; here the attorney echoes the era's frequent concern with falseness. A representative of the city council, Luis Fernández, joined Pineda's appeal, reminding the higher court of the tremendous losses the city had suffered during the plague of 1565, which was why the town criers had repeatedly called out prohibitions against

---

[94] The case, which took place before Vargas's tenure, appears in two places: ARCV Registro de Ejecutorías, Caja 1838, 8, fols. 1–67, where it is oddly captioned as concerning theft of a large cape; and AMB-HI 3653, June 2, 1597. I draw on both in the following discussion.

sheltering people from pestilent towns. Like Pineda, Fernández emphasized the duplicity of having disguised the men so they could enter the city, and he pointed out rather sensibly that "if rigor is not applied then the guards and expenses are not of much use." The city also wrote a letter about the case to the king (still Philip II), dated June 2. It too referred back to 1565, "a plague so huge that its memory will endure eternally as long as buildings stand." And, most interestingly, the city noted that it was clear by then that the infection "does not come from corrupt air but rather from contact with *ropa* [clothing and linens] and communication with people who come from those areas with illness..." Again, the notion of contagion was being empirically worked out. The city's letter also fills in some narrative gaps, explaining that Alonso's subterfuge had been uncovered by a guard at the Burgos city gate who had not believed whatever it was they were telling him. As a result, the three men fled, leaving Alonso to take the fall. He confessed he had given them disguises. Like Fernández with the Chancillería, the city emphasized to the king the critical importance of halting traffic and imposing stiff penalties. People had been fined, yes, but because "they did not cease taking in their friends and acquaintances," more rigor, not less, was required. The appeals court agreed to halve Pineda's damages award to Alonso, but the rest of the sentence was left intact.

There are many unanswered questions in this case: what was Alonso's relationship to the three men, why did he bother disguising them, why did they want to enter Burgos, and why was the case handled by the lieutenant corregidor instead of by the corregidor at the time, Gerónimo de Montalvo. (When Vargas said later in 1597 that public shame would be imposed, he was thus merely reiterating Montalvo's prior practice.) But the critical point is that the city and the lieutenant corregidor were telling the king that the royal appeals court was undercutting their authority, which could have drastic consequences for public health throughout the kingdom. The case also seems to indicate that public shame and even the gallows – visible to everyone, situated in "the most public place" of every town – were not much of a deterrent. If people were continually sheltering their friends, family, and acquaintances, as the city said, then it would seem they were willing to run that risk.

With marketplaces shuttered or very quiet and street traffic sparse, the only remaining public event that quickly comes to mind when thinking about bad times in the early modern era are religious processions. But in fact there were few until the plague finally departed, at which point processions of thanksgiving probably were universal; in northern and central Castile many were held in the summer of 1600, coinciding with the feast days of San Roque or Santa Ana. A procession of thanksgiving (sadly premature, as it turned out) took place in Bilbao already in early 1599, with people walking out to the city's Roque shrine.[95] But in general, outdoor religious gatherings were scarce before the plague lifted. For one thing, many people, including the clergy, had left, so there was no one to process. Furthermore, cities and the church had to balance the good of coming together to beg for God's mercy and honor the saints, with the bad of spreading the disease. I noted earlier that Carlo Cipolla wrote that church and secular institutions in Italy disagreed on the virtue of prohibiting large gatherings, but I have found no such disagreements in Castile; there does not seem to have been pushback from the church in this regard. That does not mean it did not happen, and indications are that Seville did opt for religious processions, both during this plague and in later ones.[96] In 1629, when Madrid was guarding against the south, the city council first agreed to tell towns within five leagues to hold religious processions. But the following day, the city withdrew the suggestion. Instead, the president of the Council of Castile, who at the time was cardinal of Málaga, told the capital city's prelates that churches, convents, and monasteries should instead organize their own private prayer sessions.[97] In a similar manner, the city council of Burgos in 1597 resolved to ask local monasteries to "make sacrifices [que hagan sacrificios] begging Our Lord to free this city of the plague."[98] In both these cases, plague had actually not yet arrived, so in theory a crowd would anyway not have posed contagion problems. The obviously thoughtful and pious Francisco Gavaldá, writing about the later plague in Valencia, considered it only logical that the devout should want to gather in such times: "the greater the danger, the more voices there are." But at the same time, he noted, if a disease is contagious, then devotion "is its own undoing." For that reason, he was of the opinion that large gatherings should not be allowed, and he added that he had observed that the sick toll always went up the day after a procession.[99]

If there were processions during the turn of the century plague, in general they took place before the full weight of the epidemic hit, and they most often seem to have had the local shrine to San Roque as their

---

[95] AFB libro 024, January 28, 1599. The caretakers of the shrine were nuns; see AFB libro 023, September 1, 1598.

[96] For example, RAH Jesuitas 9-3662/181, from June 1599; and, from 1649, Francisco Morales Padrón, ed., Memorias de Sevilla (1600–1687) (Córdoba: Monte de Piedad y Caja de Ahorros de Córdoba, 1981), 115–27, transcribed documents from the Biblioteca Capitular y Columbina.

[97] AV Secretaria 1-138-4.   [98] AMB-HI 3653, June 3, 1597.

[99] Gavaldá, Memoria de los sucesos particulares de Valencia, part 5.

destination, if there was one.[100] *Votos,* or vows dedicated to a specific saint, were more common than processions and did not require public gatherings outdoors; though contagion inside a church was more likely, increasing the danger, fewer people attended. Madrid took a vow to both Ana and Roque in 1597, but in attendance were just the civil and church authorities, not the city's inhabitants.[101] At the height of the plague, in August 1599, Segovia's city council took a vow to Roque in the cathedral, promising to venerate him and celebrate his saint's day, and again the only ones present were religious and secular authorities.[102] In Pamplona during the 1566 plague, the city council on the eve of St. Martin's day (in November, very late for plague season) resolved to hold a procession and Mass for the saint every year from then on. But given the danger of crowds under the current circumstances, which the city said could lead to even greater *daños y inconvenientes,* the council's statement proclaims that right now they would just hold a Mass, without a procession, and that "no one should attend except the city council in the name of the whole city."[103] Also in Pamplona, but at the end of the century, the new bishop, Antonio Zapata y Cisneros, called on the city's inhabitants to attend church several times a week to pray for health, marking somewhat of an exception in that he was summoning them to gather together. There was a procession in October and vows to the patron saint, Fermín, as well as to Roque and Sebastián, the third great plague saint – but again, the vows were attended only by dignitaries, with townspeople standing outside the church.[104] One exception seems to be Burgos, where the

---

[100] Burgos in April 1599 decided to hold a procession on San Roque's day, but that decision came the very week that church authorities said they wanted to leave town. AMB-LA 130, April 27, 1599.

[101] The vow is translated in William A. Christian, Jr., *Local Religion in Sixteenth-Century Spain* (Princeton, NJ: Princeton University Press, 1981), 209–10. For more on Roque and the cult of the plague saints, see Chapter 6.

[102] AMS leg. 1016; see also the articles in Paco del Caño and Miguel Ángel Clemente, eds. *San Roque, Voto de Ciudad: IV Centenario, 1599–1999* (Segovia: Parroquia de San Millán, 1999).

[103] José Luis de Orella y Unzué, "El Cardenal Diego de Espinosa, consejero de Felipe II, el monasterio de Iranzu y la peste de Pamplona en 1566," *Príncipe de Viana* 36:140–1 (1975), 565–610; the relevant documents from the Pamplona cathedral archive appear on 605–6.

[104] Baleztena, "Relación de la peste desta ciudad de Pamplona," 195–6. Bishop Zapata is one of the heroes of this plague. Though he easily could have left Pamplona, instead he stayed to organize the public health effort, apparently spending a good amount of time with the sick. He later became Archbishop of Burgos, a cardinal, an inquisitor general, and Viceroy of Naples. William Christian remarks that Sebastián was the more popular plague saint in the 1507 epidemic but was supplanted by Roque later on in the century: *Local Religion,* 42.

regidor Andrés Cañas, in his *relación*, reported the city had urged "many processions to all the churches and images in this city that are of special and great devotion. The Holy Sacrament was taken out of many churches and processed and ... there is no relic that has not been taken outside..."[105] Another odd case, in that inhabitants participated but officials did not, was recorded in Valladolid, probably around July 24, 1599, where one Sunday there was a general procession that visited Sebastián and Roque, carrying with it the Lady of San Llorente. The event ended at 9 p.m., with all the windows lit up with candles. Soon afterward, the Lady was carried once again (with martyrs) to the main church, and that march too was lit up, ending at 10 p.m. The members of the Chancillería did not attend.[106]

But in general, the rarity of processions, this diminishment of ritual, meant citizens were deprived of one of the most familiar occasions for coming together, a time when they could walk the familiar paths of faith and community with company by their side. The spectacle of prayer, the comfort of being part of the whole, gave way to more private devotion, or at least the knowledge that someone else was doing your praying for you. Scenes such as that described by William Christian from pestiferous 1507 Barcelona, where flagellating children processed as they cried out to San Sebastián for mercy, with an audience of weeping townspeople looking on, were no longer common, if they occurred at all.[107]

In addition to missing their regular markets and fairs, along with processions, the demoralized inhabitants of plague-ridden towns were deprived as well of other collective entertainment. Theatrical perform-ances (*comedias*) throughout Spain were canceled soon after the death of Philip II's daughter Catalina Micaela in November 1597, and again (or still) in 1598. A petition from Madrid to the king asking that he rescind the order suggests that bad health (and "fear in these times so poor in health") also was a factor in the cancelation. "As times get better," the city said, "there is no reason to fear the crowds that generally gather at the *comedias*." Plays' occasional, albeit reprehensible, excesses

---

[105] Brumont, "La peste de 1599," 161.

[106] RBP II-2163, doc. 87, Francisco de Villapadierna (in Valladolid) to Gondomar (in Toro), 24th of month, probably July 1599.

[107] William A. Christian, Jr., "Provoked religious weeping in early modern Spain," in *Religious Organization and Religious Experience*, J. Davis, ed. (London: Academic Press, 1982), 97–114, p. 98. On this shift toward more individual and interior religious experience throughout the sixteenth century, see the classic John Bossy, *Christianity in the West, 1400–1700* (Oxford: Oxford University Press, 1985); in a festschrift for Bossy, Simon Ditchfield refers to the new "diminished religious universe": "Introduction" to *Christianity and Community in the West: Essays for John Bossy*, Simon Ditchfield, ed. (Aldershot: Ashgate, 2001), xxii.

in no way outweighed their useful, didactic, and instructive qualities, and silencing the stages would be like killing a sick man instead of curing him, the city said. In addition, and crucially, in Madrid three or four hospitals were kept afloat by alms from *comedias*.[108] Indeed, many established (i.e. not ad hoc) hospitals in Spain subsisted through theaters' payments of alms (*limosnas*), and the logical reduction in the number of performances during these years meant hospitals had less revenue exactly when they needed it the most. Madrid's general hospital, which would not have had plague patients, sent a petition to the crown in August 1598 saying it had insufficient funds "due to the lack of *comedias*" as well as rising prices, and it begged the king for financial assistance.[109] The Antón Martín hospital, which did have plague patients, sent a similar appeal in December 1598, noting that *limosnas* were going down just as the number of patients was going up and asking that more performances be allowed throughout the kingdom so as to bring in more revenue. At the same time, the Council of Castile advised Philip III that performances should be allowed as long as women did not attend.[110] Chronicler Diego Colmenares says Segovia banned *comedias* during the plague.[111] But Valladolid took a different path, with the corregidor on July 10, 1599 – just two weeks before the Chancillería declared that things were so bad it was leaving town – telling the city council that a playwright had contacted him about obtaining a license to produce plays there. The councilors conferred on the matter and resolved that, "so as to cheer up the town and make the *vecinos* happy, it is right that the said *comedias* be produced, and thus they asked the Señor Corregidor to order that the license be granted…"[112] The same month as Valladolid authorized *comedias*, Ávila organized events known as *juegos de toros y cañas*, a team-sport of jousting on horseback that dates back to the Muslim presence.[113]

---

[108] Cristóbal Pérez Pastor, *Bibliografía madrileña; o descripción de las obras impresas en Madrid (siglo xvi)*, vol. 1 (Madrid: Tip. de los Huérfanos, 1891), 304–8; the document is undated but Pérez Pastor says it also was 1598. He also notes that Madrid's hospitals in January 1599 requested that *comedias* be allowed again, indicating they still (or again) were not; they were allowed again in April 1599 and then in February 1600. See Chapter 7 for more on Madrid's hospitals.

[109] AGS-CC leg. 800 (memoriales), August 30, 1598.

[110] AHN CS libro 2.768, fols. 149r–v.

[111] Diego de Colmenares, *Historia de la insigne ciudad de Segovia y compendio de las historias de Castilla* [1637], vol. 2 (Segovia: Academia de Historia y Arte de San Quirce, 1970), 364, according to which "First, they prohibited all gatherings, *comedias*, schools, and even sermons." Colmenares is not always reliable, however.

[112] AMVA sig. 21-0 (also 22-0), July 10, 1599.

[113] AGS-E leg. 183, doc. 332, July 28, 1599; the event was held to celebrate the feast day of Santiago, Spain's patron saint.

Even more startling, in late June 1597 the seriously afflicted town of Melgar de Fernamental, in a letter notifying Burgos about the relentless succession of disease and death there in recent days, said it had organized processions, bonfires, and bullfights, a spectacle of death of a different sort, to "cheer people up."[114]

[114] BL Eg. 356, vol. 2, fols. 366r–v.

Site 6: Town Hall

The geographic and political center of any town was the town hall, the *ayuntamiento*, generally next to or across from the main church. As its name suggests, this was where things came together, where people gathered, where all matters could and should be sorted out. Its dealings were the constant hum in the background, the machinery of good government, though the hum might now and then give way to raised voices. It was where prices were set, processions ordered, hospitals financed, communication centralized. It also was where conflicts played out between governing factions, commoners and nobles, the resentful and the undeserving. The stunned inhabitants of plague-infested villages, towns, and cities might have perceived the *ayuntamiento* as friend or enemy, but in either case it was the local manifestation of the bedrock of their social and political existence.

The history of Castile is the history of its towns and cities, which usually possessed special royal charters dating back to time immemorial granting them rights and privileges in exchange for obedience and service. Aristotelian thinkers and humanists in Spain's sixteenth century often reflected upon the virtues and excellence of the city, the source of happiness, conversation, and prosperity, the home of good vassals.[1] Histories of cities written during this era, a popular genre, stressed beautiful surroundings, clean air, abundance, wonderful fruits, spectacular royal visits, and bustling commerce. Plagues were rarely if ever mentioned.[2]

---

[1] On the political culture and discourse of Castilian cities, a good place to start is Xavier Gil, "City, communication and concord in Renaissance Spain and Spanish America," in *Athenian Legacies: European Debates on Citizenship*, Paschalis M. Kitromilides, ed. (Florence: Olschki Editore, 2014), 195–222. Two wide-ranging collections are José Ignacio Fortea Pérez, ed., *Imágenes de la diversidad: El mundo urbano en la Corona de Castilla (S. XVI–XVIII)* (Santander: Universidad de Cantabria, 1997); and José Ignacio Fortea Pérez and Juan E. Gelabert, eds., *Ciudades en conflicto (Siglos XVI–XVIII)* (Valladolid: Junta de Castilla y León, 2008).

[2] Santiago Quesada, *La idea de ciudad en la cultura hispana de la Edad Moderna* (Barcelona: Universitat de Barcelona, 1992); Richard L. Kagan, *Clio and the Crown: The Politics of*

In my discussion in Chapter 1 of how towns asked the crown and the Cortes to reduce certain tax payments once the epidemic had moved on, I briefly outlined the interlocking structures of Castilian political life. The republic, in rough terms, had four instances: king, Cortes, municipalities (large and small), and individuals (vassals, *vecinos*, petitioners). The word "city" (*ciudad*) had a specific meaning in early modern Castile, though here I use the term generically. Juridically, the king had to grant a town the privilege of calling itself "city," which entailed certain rights, possibly including representation in the Cortes.[3] The hierarchy among the instances at any given moment could shift, though of course in the last analysis the crown was the crown. Each relationship between levels embodied the trade-off between privilege or rights, on the one hand, and obedience, on the other, and by its very nature the entire system assumed and even encouraged incessant negotiation. It is worth noting, as Thompson has pointed out, that the period under discussion in this book constituted a turning point not only in the change of century, declining economic fortunes, and the person of the monarch. There also were changes in how the monarchy, kingship, and government were perceived.[4] Most notably, in the seventeenth century the Cortes's power would shrink radically.

Virtually all measures we have seen enacted thus far as the plague approached and then crossed city walls were the result of municipal decisions. The crown was kept apprised, and it had to approve most sorts of funding, but both because of the urgency and possibly because of the de facto interregnum in 1599 and its uncertainty, executive power to a large degree lay in the town hall. We also have seen that smaller towns, which also had councils and town halls, often but not always had to report to the capital of their jurisdiction. This is most obvious in the case of Burgos, where the corregidor, Diego Vargas Manrique, had particularly broad powers. But the city council minutes of all the cities I have mentioned contain reports from and decisions concerning smaller surrounding towns, and when corregidores filed their reports with Philip III in 1599, they generally included information on dependent

History in Medieval and Early Modern Spain (Baltimore, MD: Johns Hopkins University Press, 2009).

[3] José Ignacio Fortea Pérez, "Las ciudades de la Corona de Castilla en el Antiguo Régimen: Una revisión historiográfica," *Boletín de la Asociación de Demografía Histórica* 13:3 (1995), 19–59, p. 22, says that in 1591 there were around 100 towns with 5,000 or more inhabitants. This article is a superb introduction to early modern Castilian urban structures and networks during a decade of crisis.

[4] I. A. A. Thompson, "From *Reinos* to *Monarquía*: Political Association in Late 16th-Century Spain," *TEMPUS: Revista en Historia General* [Medellín] (2016), 91–110.

municipalities.[5] Towns, in turn, might have certain responsibilities over villages. They might also use the crisis as a good excuse to pull rank or gain advantage; examples we have seen include inhabitants of one plague-ridden town being prevented from using mills in other towns and towns allegedly spreading rumors that others were pestilent when they were not. Another example, possibly reproduced in other places as well, was a lawsuit filed by the town council of Alzola against the town council of Elgoibar (both in the province of Guipúzcoa) because the latter town insisted the former was obliged to help with its guard duty.[6] In any case, this vertical chain of obligation and responsibility among villages, towns, and cities, all of which had decision-making and judicial institutions, albeit small ones, meant not only that there was continual push and pull, but that all instances felt themselves to be, and acted as if they were, pieces of a sprawling political apparatus held together by the language of rights.

City councils met several times a week in the town hall. Meetings were chaired by the corregidor or his lieutenant and attended by council members, notaries, and justice officials.[7] They were supposed to be orderly and well attended, an objective they did not always meet. Reports from several cities during the plague reflect an inability at some point to reach decisions for lack of a quorum as regidores left town. During the enormous 1565 plague in Burgos, only four regidores attended meetings in July despite the (theoretical) imposition of a fifty-ducat fine, and in the end meetings began being held regularly only in November, once the plague had moved on.[8] Often important matters would be dealt with not by the full council but by committees that kept their own records, which is what happened during the 1599 plague, and probably other epidemics as well, when cities established separate juntas de salud.

"In the long run, the most important factor determining the strength of a state's sanitary defense was the emergence of ideas which associated

---

[5] For an account of how Seville tried to manage its wider jurisdiction during an earlier epidemic see Alexandra Parma Cook and Noble David Cook, *The Plague Files: Crisis Management in Sixteenth-Century Seville* (Baton Rouge, LA: Louisiana State University Press, 2009).

[6] ARCV Pleitos Civiles Pérez Alonso (Olv.) 1285–10.

[7] Lieutenants were always *letrados*. There were frequent conflicts between them and the corregidores being that lieutenants often had to purchase their posts from corregidores. The Cortes ended this practice in 1618 but it soon reappeared; Benjamin González Alonso, *El corregidor castellano 1348–1808* (Madrid: Instituto de Estudios Administrativos, 1970), 162–70. Castillo de Bovadillo, in vol. 1 part 1 of his guide for corregidores, spent a lot of space trying to sort out their respective jurisdictions, which were never clear.

[8] Francisco José González-Prieto, *La ciudad menguada: Población y economía en Burgos S. XVI y XVII* (Santander: Universidad de Cantabria, 2005), 117-8.

freedom from epidemics with good governance," Mark Harrison has written.[9] Health was important not just because one felt better and was not dying; it was also important as evidence that the republic was working. Earlier we touched on debates by both civil and religious authorities regarding the ethics and expedience of leaving rather than staying. As with everything else, balance was the theoretical goal: enough leaders had to remain to ensure that bodies and souls could be attended to, but if they could conduct their business from safer quarters, then that was permitted, or even mandated. Some regidores might need to stay to participate in guard duty or manage relief efforts, while others could leave.[10] Perhaps they cycled through, relieving each other. But if balance was the stated goal, sometimes the more pragmatic goal was simply to get out, leaving duties behind. This was not good government, and later on there were lawsuits and discipline against those who had abandoned their post, physically or otherwise, or who had made unreasonable demands.

Two such conflicts took place in La Rioja. In one, the council and *vecinos* together sued a collection of local and regional officials for having deserted the town of Pedroso during the plague. Pedroso lost in the lower courts, but the case was heard by the royal appeals court. There it was explained that suit had been filed because the defendants, "saying there was peste in the said town, had left, leaving it defenceless, and [the plaintiffs] wanted an accounting of how the town properties [*propios*] had been spent and certain amounts that had been borrowed in 1598 and 1599 to buy wheat and other things." The defendants included the mayor, at least one member of the town council, the town attorney, the man in charge of the granary, and the surgeon. The case file is over 1,000 pages and difficult to read, but it would appear that the defendants, especially the man in charge of the granary, were being accused of financial improprieties in addition to having deserted the town, where "more than 500 people died of hunger."[11] A much more important town in La Rioja, Santo Domingo de la Calzada, had its own conflict regarding desertion, though it does not seem to have ended up in court. The corregidor (along with the bishop, gone nearly a year) had left town as soon as the plague was said to be approaching and had left matters in the hands of a *vecino* who had two relatives on the town council and who, precisely because he was a *vecino*, was in any case ineligible to govern.

---

[9] Mark Harrison, *Contagion: How Commerce Has Spread Disease* (New Haven, CT: Yale University Press 2012), 12.

[10] Daniel Defoe, *A Journal of the Plague Year* (New York: Meridian Classic, 1960), 181–2, wrote that London's Lord Mayor, his aides, magistrates, and constables all stayed.

[11] ARCV Pleitos civiles Alonso Rodríguez (Olv.) 555-1, 556-1.

The remaining town councilors figured out a rotation system that promptly fell apart as certain members refused to leave their homes outside the city to come back and do their duty. The sick were wandering around unattended, there was no money, the priests had left along with the bishop, and by September 9, 1599, exactly one regidor remained. He apparently had control over certain funds which he refused to cede to the *alcalde* (the two men belonged to different political factions). Eventually that autumn the plague moved on, and the "rich *vecinos*" who had left and now wished to return were assessed fines to alleviate the suffering of the poor.[12]

Briviesca, a Burgos town leaning toward La Rioja on the route from Burgos to Bilbao and which suffered from plague fairly late, in 1600, also ended up in court the following year. Nearly all the town's notaries had fled, which in Castile amounted to a calamity. The remaining town council appointed new ones, and the escapees, displaying audacity equal to their cowardice, sued to get their jobs back.[13] Quite a bit further south, in the town of Lominchar (Toledo), the notary admirably had stayed on the job amid the devastation. Later, his son wrote to the Camara de Castilla to say that his father, Gabriel Hernández de Villorez, "had worked throughout the said illness on the last wills and testaments of the sick and other things ... and he died, and as all his belongings and papers were pestilent they were burned, and his wife and some of his children also died." As a result of all this, the surviving son, also named Gabriel, petitioned that he be awarded his father's post.[14]

In Laredo, one of the first towns to be devastated, the corregidor vanished in the autumn of 1597, leaving matters in the hands of his lieutenant, who in turn engineered a complicated handoff of responsibilities leaving just one regidor, a man named Gil de Rey, who went to nearby Ampuero, where he was assisted by a couple of appointed *vecinos*.[15] Later, in 1599, by which time Laredo was healthy and everyone else was infected, Gil de Rey wrote to the Council of War to say that now that things were back to normal, the town council of Laredo would not reimburse him for his civic efforts. He told the Council of War that the

[12] Diego Téllez Alarcia, "La peste Atlántica en Santo Domingo de la Calzada (1599)," *Berceo* 162 (2012), 85–119, based on city council minutes.

[13] Francis Brumont, *Campo y campesinos de Castilla la Vieja en tiempos de Felipe II* (Madrid: Siglo Veintiuno, 1984), 88–9, citing AHN Consejos 28.256, no. 2.

[14] AGS-CC Memoriales leg. 807 no. 107. The Cámara attended to appointments and favors. The corregidor of Toledo, Francisco de Carbajal, told the king that 168 people had died in Lominchar, and the toll may have risen; AGS-E leg. 183, doc. 310, August 27, 1599.

[15] AGS-GyM leg. 489, doc. 289, October 5, 1597.

epidemic had lingered in Laredo for eight months, killing more than 600 people. During that time, "with a desire to serve God and Your Majesty and that town, he decided to stay and help the sick and also defend the town from its enemies, being that the town was in danger because everyone had left and there was no defense. He worked to that end, putting his life and that of his family at risk, he spent his money and sought surgeons, doctors, medicines, and supplies to remedy the sick." The king, who was in Valencia, told the Council of War to pay.[16]

Sometimes the problem was not just those who left but those who stayed, as there were opportunities during epidemics for ill-gotten gains that would be foresaken if one were to flee. Often, the opportunity came with the buying and selling of grain. There was, for example, the case of *alguacil* Juan Vallejo, who had temporarily been dispatched from Estella with his wife and children to the Navarrese town of Villatuerta, from where he was supposed to ensure some sort of supply chain to Estella. But according to a subsequent criminal case against him, instead he had been "very remiss and negligent in the performance of his duties and in supplying the said city [Estella] with firewood, coal, poultry and other things." He engaged in "great bribery and fraud," the prosecutor said, supplying neither Villatuerta nor Estella but making a bundle for himself. The exact details of the operation are not clear to me, but apparently he would buy up all or most of the village's wheat and barley, saying it was for the poor of Estella, and then store it in his friend's granary. Sellers were allowed to sell only after 2 p.m., after official hours, making him the only buyer. He also allegedly used false weights and measures. The entire operation was supposed to help Estella, but that city filed papers in the case saying that in fact it had never received the grain and supplies it needed. According to one witness, Vallejo was destroying Villatuerta's twice-weekly markets, where people could neither buy nor sell as before. He was arrested and punished with six months' exile and disqualification from holding public office, which he requested be reduced on account of his own business matters which he said required him to travel throughout Navarre.[17]

The behavior of individual town leaders reflected their individual character, of course, but also the degree to which they understood or believed in the tenets of good government that were part of every law, petition, charter, and mirror book since the Middle Ages. Those who

[16] AGS-GyM leg. 553 doc. 119, August 23, 1599. The Council of War may have been involved here because Laredo had defensive functions.

[17] AGN TR Procesos 088878. The case dates from 1600; I do not know if the sentence was reduced.

stayed had to balance not only economics and health, the well-being of some while not of others, but also their own conduct. They had to decide whom to listen to, how to placate, and whether to tell the truth. Dissimulation or outright lies by corregidores who assured the outside world as well as their own residents that, really, their city was just fine, was obviously part of a strategy to ensure material survival. Here I want to revisit the matter from a more theoretical angle than the purely commercial quandaries outlined in Chapter 5. In the context of the plague, lies can be seen as a sort of additional fortification or wall protecting a town's interests, albeit temporarily, and whether or not the corregidores in the late sixteenth century were aware of it, there was a spirited debate among contemporary political theorists regarding the legitimacy of this particular construction and its furtherance or negation of good government.

Christian authorities were quite clear that there could be no excuse for lying. In Augustine's eyes it was always wrong, while Thomas de Aquinas distinguished among several types of lies, but they were all sins to varying degrees.[18] Juan Ginés de Sepúlveda, the great sixteenth-century theologian best known today for debating Bartolomé de las Casas on the justice of Spain's oppression of American natives, also took up the subject in his case inquiring on the legitimacy of withholding information in a judicial setting so as not to harm someone.[19] Machiavelli marked a shift, of course, in allowing the prince to engage in deceit and even evil if necessary: "[I]n order to maintain his state [the prince] is often forced to act in defiance of good faith, of charity, of kindness, of religion... He should not deviate from what is good, if that is possible, but he should know how to do evil, if that is necessary."[20] The degree to which plague-era corregidores knew or cared about Machiavelli and the subsequent debate, including in Spain, is unknown to me. But the behavior of these busy crown-appointed officials, who were prominent, well-connected, and often rising servants of the monarchy, nonetheless bears looking at in the context of contemporary discussions regarding what they should and should not do. All Spanish political writers believed prudence and morality had to balance one another, and that politics and Christianity

[18] Augustine's essays are "De mendacio" and "Contra mendacium"; the Aquinas reference is to *Summa Theologiae* 2a2ae q.110, arts. 1–4.
[19] Juan Ginés de Sepúlveda, *Teófilo*, in his *Obras completas*, vol. 15 (Pozoblanco: Ayuntamiento de Pozoblanco, 2010) José María Núñez González and S. Rus Rufino, eds., clxv–cxcii, 193–245. The treatise, a 19-chapter dialogue first published in Valladolid in 1538, coincided with the Inquisition trial of the Spanish Erasmist Juan de Vergara, who was accused, among other things, of keeping secret his communication with his brother, who also faced charges. My thanks to Luna Nájera for this reference.
[20] Niccolo Machiavelli, *The Prince*, trans. George Bull (London: Penguin Books 1961), 101.

were not incompatible. But though the means for ensuring a sound reason of state must be Christian, the discussions of *simulación* and *disimulación* display a recognition that things had changed and, loathsome as Machiavelli might be, that adjustments had to be made in statecraft. This clearly can be seen in the work of the great Jesuit theorist Pedro Ribadeneira, who ends up essentially admitting that deceit can be justified.

Quite nicely for our purposes, Ribadeneira called Machiavelli "pestilential."[21] Yet he ended up wandering dangerously close to the vile Italian. Ribadeneira's most famous passage on the matter is this: "It is not a lie, if great necessity or utility so demand, to utter words that are truthful in one sense even though the speaker believes that the listener, given the equivocal meaning of the words, will interpret them in a different sense. And what I am saying about words can also be said of deeds; many times, especially during war, they are performed in order that the enemy understand them to be something else entirely, even the opposite of one's intentions. And that is not a lie but rather doing things prudently for the good of the Republic. And as Doctor Navarro says, there are two arts of simulation and dissimulation, one performed by those who, with neither reason nor gain, lie and pretend that what was not, is, and the other performed by those who prudently let it be understood, when necessity or utility so require and with neither deceit nor falsehood, that one thing might be another."[22] The difference between this and Machiavelli's lies is very slight indeed, a situation that other Spanish writers also found themselves in, and Ribadeneira's advice about venturing out on such thin ice was admittedly weak: "When walking among enemies, one must go armed, using dissimulation against dissimulation; but one must be careful to not go so far as to offend God.[23]

---

[21] Pedro Ribadeneira, *Tratado de la religión y virtudes que debe tener el príncipe christiano para gobernar y conservar sus estados. Contra lo que Nicolas Machiavello y los políticos deste tiempo enseñan* ... (Madrid: P. Madrigal, 1595), 273. For an introduction to Ribadeneira's criticism of Machiavelli see J. A. Fernández-Santamaría, *Reason of State and Statecraft in Spanish Political Thought, 1595–1640* (Lanham, MD: University Press of America, 1983), 18–24. Ribadeneira (1526–1611) is also sometimes referred to as Ribadeneyra.

[22] Ribadeneira, *Tratado de la religión*, 289–90. Fernández-Santamaría, *Reason of State and Statecraft*, 92, has a slightly different translation, as he used the 1605 version of the original. According to Ronald W. Truman, *Spanish Treatises on Government, Society and Religion in the Time of Philip II: The "de regimine principum" and Associated Traditions* (Leiden: Brill, 1999), 297, the Doctor Navarro referred to is the theologian Martín de Azpilcueta, who in 1584 wrote an essay on dissimulation.

[23] Ribadeneira, *Tratado de la religión*, 285. On the approximation between Spanish writers and Machiavelli see Keith David Howard, "The Anti-Machiavellians of the Spanish Baroque: A Reassessment," *LATCH: A Journal for the Study of the Literary Artifact in Theory, Culture or History* 5 (2012), 106–19.

Just six years before Ribadeneira published *Tratado de la religión*, the Flemish humanist Justus Lipsius had published his *Politica*. Like Machiavelli, he allowed the prince to lie for the sake of the common good. Paraphrasing part 4 of the *Politica*, Fernández-Santamaría has written, "The prince, living among foxes, must on occasion resort to fox-like conduct, especially if the public good so requires it. In short, 'a little water does not alter the nature of the wine; and neither does prudence cease to be prudence because a few drops of *disimulación* or *fraude* have been added. It is understood, of course, that the amount shall be small and aimed at a good end'."[24]

Again with the caveat that Diego Vargas Manrique and his colleagues throughout Castile may or may not have been cognizant of the political and philosophical writings floating through European capitals and universities at the time, the fact is that this art of mental reservation, the art of stating lies while admitting to oneself that not only were one's words not quite true and might well be misunderstood, but that a greater good outweighed the falsity, probably was practiced by them all. The theory of mental reservation, championed especially but not only by Jesuits, "was concocted in order to reconcile the ban on lying with such duties as saving lives and preserving secrets."[25] That is exactly what corregidores were doing. I have run across just one acknowledgement, albeit tacit, that this strategy did not work in the long run, and it comes from Pamplona. The chronicle I have been relying upon states that the city resolved to "not dissimulate at all but rather admit the disease and make sure of it and *give it a name*, because [if we] hide it … it is difficult to remedy later on, and it is better to lose communication [i.e. commerce] than to suffer the damages the disease causes, and in any case secrets can get out."[26] Few if any other city councils acted as wisely.

The city council minutes (*libros de actas*) that survive in Castilian cities, towns, and even villages, are the principal source for this book, and they also must have been the principal source for town leaders as they

---

[24] Fernández-Santamaría, *Reason of State and Statecraft*, 88. Lipsius's work, which was put on the Index, is known as *Six Books on Politics or Civil Doctrine*. For more on Lipsius and these questions see Christopher Brooke, *Philosophic Pride: Stoicism and Political Thought from Lipsius to Rousseau* (Princeton, NJ: Princeton University Press, 2012), 19–20; also the superb analysis in Noel Malcolm, *Reason of State, Propaganda and the Thirty Years' War* (Oxford: Clarendon Press, 2007), 92–123.

[25] Johann P. Sommerville, "The 'New Art of Lying': Equivocation, Mental Reservation, and Casuistry," in *Conscience and Casuistry in Early Modern Europe*, Edmund Leites, ed. (Cambridge University Press, 1988), 159–84, p. 176.

[26] Ignacio Baleztena, ed., "Relación de la peste desta ciudad de Pamplona del año 1599," *Príncipe de Viana* 23 (1946), 377–94, p. 391 [Chronicle by Martín de Senosiain], my emphasis.

organized yet another public health campaign each time plague threatened. The minutes were their memory.[27] In the previous chapter I quoted J. G. A. Pocock as saying that "awareness of a past, then, is a social awareness," and I argued that repetition (I was referring to town criers, but it could have been anything else) cemented people's rooted-ness in their place, in their tradition. The very existence of minutes spoke to a place's past and testified to its methods for fighting off disruptions, injustice, or calamity. The large bound books lined up on a shelf somewhere, often in two sets when notaries worked in pairs, also spoke to continuity, to repetition. They confirmed Jerónimo Castillo de Bovadilla's widely shared opinion that it was far better that things not change. This avoidance of novelty has been interpreted, both by contem-poraries and historians, as a critical defect proving the rule of immobility. There is certainly a good argument there, but I would like to slice the question obliquely to posit that repetition also meant that each time the plague arrived, towns were not starting all over again. It would appear that they learned from mistakes and accomplishments and knew what to expect. They knew where they came from.

The *Relaciones topográficas* sometimes included pretty exact dates for plagues in the past, indicating people had a place to go and check. In 1629 in Madrid, during a period when plague threatened (but did not arrive), the city resolved to ask permission to set up a health committee, "because in the year 1600 when peste entered the kingdom there was another junta that dealt with everything concerning the health and security of this city."[28] In Seville in June 1599, when hundreds of people were dying every week, the city wrote the Council of Castile: "A very old document has been found saying that during another pestilence more than one hundred years ago the city decided to bring [the images of] the virgins Justa and Rufina, and then the pestilence ceased..."[29] Sometimes, as in the Seville case, it seems odd that a piece of paper was even necessary to remember. Other times, during the drumbeat of routine preparations in every town and city, it seems likely that living memory, "the combined memory spans of the generations with which those living at a given moment have themselves come into contact," was operating. Most places had to deal with epidemics at least every few decades; the lucky ones had longer gaps, but still they could go back to "the edge of

---

[27] I. A. A. Thompson points out, though, that the minutes might smooth out or entirely omit conflicts within the council; "Conflictos políticos en las ciudades castellanas en el siglo XVII," in Fortea Pérez and Gelabert, eds., *Ciudades en conflicto*, 37–55, p. 39.

[28] AV Secretaria 1-138-4, September 6, 1629.

[29] RAH Jesuitas 9-3662/181, June 12, 1599.

living memory."[30] One puzzling exception was Valencia, which, as we saw, seemingly had to start from scratch in 1647 despite having suffered a steady succession of plague in the sixteenth century.[31] Another case in which memory seemed to vanish can be found in a brief plague chronicle, though from a different time and place. The exact disease is not clear (it probably was not bubonic plague), but it reached Jerez de la Frontera in April 1523. The author described dozens and even hundreds of dead bodies being dug up from their shallow graves and torn apart by dogs, with the particularity that most victims had been Moors. In fact, the Moors' community was so devastated by the plague, he wrote, that they begged Christians to enslave them and thus save them. The author did not blame them for the disease; once again, scapegoating is conspicuously absent. The disaster lifted in late June, so suddenly that "when July arrived there was no *memoria* of the pestilence, though there were much fewer people and they were fatigued and amazed at the great burdens they had borne." Here *memoria* may mean trace rather than memory, but even so it is puzzling.[32]

Such exceptions aside, I believe it was the minutes and the documents inserted therein that guided each new generation, explicitly or through memory. In the case of Burgos, the *vecinos* – though not the corregidores, who were outsiders – had 1565 to look back to, roughly a generation and a half earlier, when a brutal plague devastated much of northern Spain after entering through Aragon; during that episode, towns in La Bureba, a district in northeast Burgos province, lost half their people. Francis Brumont found this information in a study by 1560s treasury officials that surely also was available in 1597.[33] Another survey of damage in 1565 were two questionnaires in December of that year undertaken by

---

[30] Geoffrey Cubitt, *History and Memory* (Manchester: Manchester University Press, 2007), 184.

[31] Fray Francisco Gavaldá, *Memoria de los sucesos particulares de Valencia y su provincia en … tiempo de peste* (Valencia, 1651), part 14. Valencia suffered plagues in 1489, 1508, 1519, 1530, 1557, and 1559. The great Castilian plague passed it by, but it frequently received epidemics from the Mediterranean; James Casey, *Early Modern Spain: A Social History* (London: Routledge, 1999), 37.

[32] Juan Daza, *Estracto de las ocurrencias de la peste que aflixió a esta ciudad (Jerez de la Frontera) en el año 1518 hasta el de 1523*, Hipólito Sancho, ed. (Jerez de la Frontera: Ayuntamiento de Jerez de la Frontera, 1938) [1523]. The account is seven pages long.

[33] Brumont, *Campo y Campesinos*, 84–5; his source was AGS-EH leg. 69, "Averiguaciones del daño de la enfermedad de peste que hubo el año de 565 y en el de 566." Burgos city council minutes during the 1565 plague were transcribed by Gonzalo Diez de la Lastra y Diez de Güemes, in "Datos curiosos para la historia de la ciudad, sacados de los Libros de Actas del Excmo. Ayuntamiento de la M. N. y M. M. L. Ciudad de Burgos, Cabeza de Castilla y Cámara de S. M.: Peste bubónica en Burgos en el año 1565," *Boletin de Estadística e Información del Excmo. Ayuntamiento de Burgos* 261 (November 1943) to 272 (October 1944).

the Chancillería of Valladolid at the behest of the cloth and wool merchants guild to decide if the epidemic really was over. Eight *vecinos* (two doctors, two surgeons, one barber, the priest of San Esteban, and two city council members) were asked seven questions on December 10, and then again on December 29 (the latter survey with fewer *vecinos* and fewer questions). The responses, briefly, said things had been terrible (the document's editors say 9,000 people died in Burgos) but the fact that churchmen and councilors had returned was proof that the disease had moved on.[34] Returning to our plague, when Burgos wrote to Philip II in August 1597, by which time it knew danger was pressing in on it from several directions (Melgar de Fernamental was already infected), it complained bitterly at not having received replies to its previous missives and reiterated that it was about to be "finished off," just as it had been "in the events we had with the peste thirty-two years ago."[35] When Burgos regidor Andrés de Cañas drew up his report on the 1599 epidemic, he consulted the paperwork from 1565; he also wrote a report, mentioned in Chapter 3, on why San Esteban's gate should be allowed to remain open, and he must have sifted through the old surveys in which San Esteban's priest figured.[36] Burgos's sense of being unfairly burdened, both in paying for other towns' health measures and having more to lose commercially than the rest, also can be found in 1565 papers; in June of that year the city council told the Camera de Castilla among other things that the city could neither buy nor sell foodstuffs or supplies in other towns or at fairs and markets, and it asked that it receive the same treatment as Soria and Logroño, whose people at least were allowed to traffic their wool. Throughout 1599 again there would be allegations that other cities were receiving preference.[37]

---

[34] José Manuel López Gómez and Esther Padriñas de Juana, "Un testimonio inédito sobre la epidemia de peste de 1565 en Burgos," *Boletin de la Institución Fernan González* 221 (2000), 227–50. The original 11-folio document is in the Archivo Diocesano de Burgos, parroquia de San Esteban, leg. 37, no. 20. The priest worked in San Esteban, probably the reason why the survey remains there; it is worth remembering that San Esteban was the first Burgos neighborhood to suffer from plague in 1599. On the death toll, González-Prieto, *La ciudad menguada*, 99 and 122, says the death toll was between 5,000 and 6,000.

[35] AMB-HI 3653, August 14, 1597. The city also memorably said that with the quarantine, "we harm ourselves with our own hands, we are killing ourselves behind walls." The city begged Philip II to order all towns up to Santander to institute controls and force towns within fifteen leagues of Burgos to share the costs, being that they derived the benefit of Burgos's efforts.

[36] This according to Francis Brumont, "La peste de 1599 en Burgos, una relación del regidor Andrés de Cañas," *BROCAR: Cuadernos de Investigación Histórica* 13 (1987), 156, citing BL Eg. 356 vol. 2 fols. 325–6.

[37] AGS-CC Diversos de Castilla leg. 40 doc. 38.

There are clear indications, then, that people either did or could consult documents to guide or warn them. Whether or not they always paid attention or, as in Valencia, could find the papers to begin with, we cannot know. But the repetition indicates internalized knowledge. Plague and its practices were in their muscle memory. They may have thought that doing what they used to do was the safest path; but there is enough pragmatism and common sense reflected in most municipal papers from this era to suggest they were learning from mistakes as well, making alterations if not the dreaded *novedades*. Aside from minutes, petitions, and correspondence, in Spain there were a multitude of medical treatises but not what we might anachronistically call historical accounts. As noted earlier, city histories, an important genre during this period, were concerned more with heroics, mythical origins, or saintly presence than with social issues; the accounts authenticated a very particular view of the present, and in fact there are histories of cities that do not mention epidemics at all despite the high death tolls.[38] In this respect, Spain seems to have differed from Italy. Writing about Florence, Samuel Cohn has suggested that the 1575–1578 plague there gave rise to a new sort of writing that marked a turning point in how plague was recorded and remembered. These accounts were chronological; narrative stepped forward for the first time as the disease's progress was traced. The authors of these new works were not just physicians, Cohn says, but also notaries, gentlemen, or humanists whose goal was to guide people in the future. With very few exceptions, these sorts of accounts are missing in Spain; notaries, who were ubiquitous in Castile, noting down every exchange, death, petition, order, and punishment having to do with the plague, did not follow the example set by their Italian colleagues.[39]

Among the most obvious memory triggers in communities were religious traditions, things people did year in, year out, always at certain times or because of certain circumstances. The moment when a town decided to make a particular saint theirs was undoubtedly a moment of great suffering or great thanksgiving. The saint was part of the reason for their attachment to that place and its landmarks, and their choosing him

---

[38] Examples of city histories (or compilations) that entirely ignore the plague are: Francisco de Ariño, ed., *Sucesos de Sevilla de 1592 a 1604* (Seville: Sociedad de Bibliófilos Andaluces, 1873); Alonso de Morgado, *Historia de Sevilla...* (Seville, 1587); and Juan Antolinez de Burgos, *Historia de la muy Noble y Rica Ciudad de Valladolid* (Valladolid, 1615, completed in 1764 by Gaspar Uriarte). Diego Colmenares' *Historia de la insigne ciudad de Segovia y compendio de las historias de Castilla* (Segovia: Academia de Historia y Arte de San Quirce, 1970 [1637]) famously mentions the plague but gets the dates wrong.

[39] Samuel K. Cohn, Jr., *Cultures of Plague: Medical Thinking at the End of the Renaissance* (Oxford: Oxford University Press, 2010), 99.

or her or them was a collective act of recognition of some gesture – preventing or halting the plague – that affected everyone. Though there may not have been many processions in honor of (or in supplication to) plague saints until the epidemic was absolutely vanquished, I think it is safe to say that they were in the back of people's minds. Their images were stored at the back of the church, waiting to be hauled out once it was all over.

An early version of Philip II's questionnaire that later became known as the *Relaciones topográficas* may have included the following question: What remedies does the town have against pestilence and other contagious diseases, both to guard against it and to cure it? Most unfortunately for us, for whatever reason the question did not make it onto the final list. But the names of locally venerated saints did, which allows us to glimpse the presence of Roque and his colleagues, along with more local saints when towns figured they would stick to the ones they knew best.[40] I have tabulated responses to the 1575 and 1578 questions regarding religious holidays and notable events. My accounts are far from scientific; not all towns responded to all questions, sections may be missing, they may have mentioned one saint and omitted others, they may have mentioned *peste* and meant locusts or typhoid (or rabies, which appears frequently in Ciudad Real), and occasionally they mentioned Roque (or Sebastián, Ana, and others) without necessarily linking the saint to the plague, though the most frequent explanation for having chosen the saint was some variation of "*por la pestilencia.*" Many towns' replies to the king reported that it was said, or they say, or it has always been known, or according to the oldest *vecinos*, or based on what I myself remember, that when the vow to San Roque (or whoever) was made, the plague ceased. Some towns remembered more or less how long ago the epidemic had struck and how few residents were left: "they have heard that just one woman survived, her name was la Paxarera, and two or three *vecinos.*"[41] Those who reported having a plague saint said they honored him or her

---

[40] The question was supposedly suggested by the bibliophile Juan Paez de Castro, who died in 1570, before the study got under way. Paez is said to have suggested to Philip II that the king build a library at El Escorial. The early lists of questions can be found in Carmelo Viñas y Mey and Ramón Paz, eds. *Relaciones de los pueblos de España ordenadas por Felipe II* [Provincia de Madrid y Reino de Toledo], 4 vols. in 3 (Madrid: Instituto Balmes de Sociología [CSIC], 1949), vol. 2 [first part of Reino de Toledo], ix. However the editor of the Cuenca surveys says Paez's notes were not a preview of the final questionaire: Eusebio Julián Zarco-Bacas y Cuevas, ed., *Relaciones de pueblos del obispado de Cuenca hechas por orden de Felipe II*, 2 vols. (Cuenca: Biblioteca Diocesana Conquense, 1927), vol. 1, p. xxiv.

[41] Viñas y Mey and Paz, eds. *Relaciones de los pueblos de España*, vol. 2, p. 174, from the town of Cabañas de la Sagra.

with special Masses, processions, going without meat that day, or carrying out special acts of charity in their honor.

Of 150 towns surveyed in the "province of Guadalajara," sixty-three mentioned peste and/or venerated one of the plague saints. Atanzón, which had 160 *vecinos* when the questionnaire was completed, had a vow to Roque, "and the reason was that he [was asked to] intercede with Our Lord to stop a pestilence that was here around fifty years ago, and as for the other vows they do not know nor have they heard precisely why they were taken."[42] Fuentelaencina, which had 700 *vecinos* and worshipped both Roque and Sebastián, said they "had heard that when the town had more than nine hundred *vecinos* during the pestilence of 1407 only eighty married men were left."[43]

In the bishopric of Cuenca, fifty-four towns responded, of which thirty mentioned plague and/or the plague saints. El Peral venerated San Cosme and San Damián (as did several other Cuenca towns) for their powers over the plague: "In this town it is said that one night one or two Valencian men spent the night in the home of a *vecino* at a time when people were dying of pestilence in the city of Valencia, and then the next day the man's daughter came down with pestilence and then they made a vow to honor the said martyrs San Cosme and San Damián and they built a shrine that even today is greatly venerated in the said town, and never again did anyone in the said town die of the said pestilence except for the said daughter of the said host in the said house, though later people died in towns a league away, or two leagues, and this is true and certain."[44] Villarubio also worshiped Cosme and Damián, explaining that "in times past there was a great pestilence in this said town that lasted from the day of Our Lady of August to the day of these martyred saints."[45] In El Castillo de Garci Muñoz the residents preferred Sebastián "because of a great pestilence in this town, and it is known, which they have heard from their ancestors, that the people went to the shrine of San Sebastián and they heard a sung Mass, and while the Mass was being said a dove flew in and sat in the transept of the said shrine and

---

[42] Juan Catalina García López, ed., *Relaciones topográficas de España. Relaciones de pueblos que pertenecen hoy a la Provincia de Guadalajara*. In *Memorial Histórico Español*, vol. 41 (Madrid: Tello, 1903–1905), 220, responding to question 41 of the 1578 survey.

[43] García López, ed., *Relaciones topográficas de España*, vol. 42, p. 47, responding to question 39 of the 1575 survey. I am assuming they meant 1507, not 1407, though it says *mil cuatrocientos*.

[44] Zarco-Bacas y Cuevas, ed., *Relaciones de pueblos del obispado de Cuenca*, vol. 1, p. 56, responding to question 52 of the 1575 survey.

[45] Zarco-Bacas y Cuevas, ed., *Relaciones de pueblos del obispado de Cuenca*, vol. 1, p. 381, responding to question 52 of the 1575 survey.

it was there throughout the whole ceremony and once the Mass was over it flew away and then the said peste ceased."[46]

Of the ninety towns in the "province of Madrid" that responded, only twenty-eight mentioned peste. The ratio is similar to that of the 181 towns in the "kingdom of Toledo," where just fifty-five made references to something that might be construed as an epidemic and a corresponding saint. Alcorcón, the present-day Madrid suburb mentioned in the previous chapter, clearly remembered the plague that had attacked "about eighty years ago more or less," which I am guessing was the enormous 1506–1508 plague, some seventy years earlier. They remembered the flight from their town and the intense hunger, information "they have been able to find out from other old people."[47] Again and again, the ways of honoring the saints are accompanied by words of certified memory: it is said the town observes the saint in this manner because of what was said to have occurred. Getafe, today another enormous Madrid suburb, reported that "around eighty-four years ago, more or less, according to what the old people say, of which we have been informed, [there was] an illness that truly was taken to be pestilent, being that in the house where it was nobody survived except by a miracle," as a result of which meat was not eaten the day before Sebastián's feast day "because of the peste, and this is what we have heard said."[48] The tiny town of Humanejos, with just seven *vecinos* and two widows, similarly backed up its assertions with old witnesses. The town honored Sebastián, "although the Church does not impose fasting on his day, and this is a vow by the town according to what they have heard from old people and ancestors on account of a certain pestilence long ago." The town used to have thirty *vecinos*, "but it diminished because it was sick, according to what they have commonly heard."[49] Hormigos y la Higuera del Campo, in Toledo, honored Sebastián and Bridget, "and the reason why they are honored is old, so old that those who are responding to this survey do not remember."[50] And the town of Velada, also in Toledo, reported that

---

[46] Zarco-Bacas y Cuevas, ed., *Relaciones de pueblos del obispado de Cuenca*, vol. 1, p. 305. Cuenca was massively affected by the 1596–1602 plague and subsequent waves; see Sara T. Nalle, *God in La Mancha: Religious Reform and the People of Cuenca, 1500–1650* (Baltimore, MD: Johns Hopkins University Press, 1992), chapter 6.

[47] Viñas y Mey and Paz, eds. *Relaciones de los pueblos de España*, vol. 1, p. 42, responding to question 37 of the 1575 survey, which they did on January 17, 1576.

[48] Viñas y Mey and Paz, eds. *Relaciones de los pueblos de España*, vol. 1, p. 291, responding to question 37 of the 1575 survey.

[49] Viñas y Mey and Paz, eds. *Relaciones de los pueblos de España*, vol. 1, pp. 333–4, responding to questions 39 and 52 of the 1575 survey.

[50] Viñas y Mey and Paz, eds. *Relaciones de los pueblos de España*, vol. 2, p. 472, responding to question 41 of the 1578 survey.

their ancestors had made a promise "according to what is said, it is not known how long ago, and this has always been observed for as long as those present can remember for more than fifty years and it is believed that it was on account of pestilence, because that is what is said..."[51] Some towns mentioned the early sixteenth-century plague specifically with the proper date, probably because they had city council minutes. Regarding their town's vow to Saint Luke the Evangelist, for example, Ballesteros said, "they say this vow was for the pestilence in the year one thousand five hundred and eight."[52] Or, they simply referred to a huge epidemic around seventy or eighty years earlier, which amounts to the same.

Though other saints appear in the *Relaciones topográficas*, the principal protector against the plague was Roque, who had himself survived plague and was widely popular throughout Europe.[53] Though he was almost always referred to as Señor San Roque, in fact he was not a proper saint at all and would never become one. His status was blurred, an excellent example of the gap between official and popular sainthood; the qualities valued in the former were not necessarily those of the latter. In any case, the processions themselves gave evidence of his sainthood. In 1590, Pope Sixtus V "hesitated between canonizing [Roque] or taking him off the list of saints, and he did neither one nor the other," Alvar Ezquerra wrote.[54] Nine years later, with plague raging in much of Spain, Roque unexpectedly left the sacred sphere briefly to step into Spain's jurisdictional morass. In July 1599, the Madrid city council resolved to ask Philip III, the Cortes, and the pope to see what they could do to ensure that Roque was properly canonized. This was an interesting move in that believers throughout Castile seemed not at all concerned that the object of their enthusiastic piety had not been officially anointed by Rome.[55] "Given

[51] Viñas y Mey and Paz, eds. *Relaciones de los pueblos de España*, vol. 3:2, p. 672, responding to question 41 of the 1578 survey.
[52] Carmelo Viñas and Ramón Paz, eds. *Relaciones histórico-geográfico-estadísticas de los pueblos de España hechas por iniciativa de Felipe II. Ciudad Real* (Madrid: Instituto de Sociología Balmes [CSIC], 1971), 122, responding to question 52 of the 1575 survey.
[53] On the life and cult of Roque see Irene Vaslef, "The role of St. Roch as a plague saint: a late medieval hagiographic tradition." PhD diss., The Catholic University of America, 1984. Also *Bibliotheca Sanctorum* (Rome: Istituto Giovanni XXIII della Pontificia Università Laterananse, 1968), vol. 11, 263–71; and *Butler's Lives of the Saints*, S. J. Herbert Thurston and Donald Attwater, eds. (New York: P. J. Kenedy and Sons, 1956) [1st pub. 1926–1938], vol. 3, p. 338.
[54] Alfredo Alvar Ezquerra, "Estructuras socioeconómicas de Madrid y su entorno en la segunda mitad del siglo XVI." PhD diss., Universidad Complutense de Madrid, 1988, p. 569n104. See also Vaslef, "The role of St. Roch as a plague saint," 138–9, on this episode.
[55] By the end of the sixteenth century Roque was included in the Roman Martyrology; see Vaslef, "The role of St. Roch as a plague saint," 143. On popular vs. official sainthood see especially Peter Burke, "How to be a Counter-Reformation Saint," in his *The*

that this city has decided to take a vow to celebrate Señor San Roque and that this vow be perpetually kept in this city and that a shrine be built" in the Vistillas de San Francisco (though, as far as I can tell, the shrine was never built), the Madrid city council met to call a meeting to approve the vow. It also resolved "to write to His Holiness begging him to canonize this most blessed Saint and to beg His Majesty to favor this effort."[56] Later that month, the matter reached the Cortes. On July 23, Don Diego de Barrionuevo, one of Madrid's representatives, said the city had asked him to convey a message: "Given the bad health throughout the kingdom, and the fact that Madrid, in order to regain its health, had called upon the blessed San Roque as its intercessor and vowed to celebrate his feast day and hold a general procession and build a shrine, and because the city had learned he was not canonized, the city had written to His Holiness begging that he be canonized, and to that end Madrid begs the Cortes [el Reyno] to also write to him," which the Cortes agreed to do.[57] But they were still talking about it the following January, when Don Alonso Suárez de Solís reminded the assembly that, given the widespread devotion of the blessed Saint Roque and the many miracles he had performed to cure Spain of peste, and the fact that he was not canonized, they should address the matter of getting him canonized, which his colleagues agreed to do tomorrow.[58] From there, things moved up a step, albeit slowly, reaching the palace (by then in Valladolid) in autumn 1600. The Cortes did indeed finally write to the president of the Council of Castile: "Given the burdens these kingdoms have borne for the past few years from the illness of peste, which is still attacking certain areas, and the many and great mercies God our lord has performed through the intercession of the most blessed San Roque," the Cortes asked for permission to ask all the member cities of the Cortes to sponsor (and pay for) the campaign to get Rome to canonize Roque. They also

---

Historical Anthropology of Early Modern Italy: Essays on Perception and Communication (Cambridge University Press, 1987), 48–62; on p. 51 he refers to Roque's "ambiguous" status. See also Kenneth L. Woodward, *Making Saints: How the Catholic Church Determines Who Becomes a Saint, Who Doesn't, and Why* (New York: Simon and Schuster, 1990).

[56] Alvar Ezquerra, "Estructuras socioeconómicas," 555, citing AV libro 25, July 12 and 21, 1599.

[57] ACC, vol. 18, p. 336, July 23, 1599. The Cortes also got involved in saintly affairs in 1627, when it voted to make Saint Teresa co-patron saint of Spain along with Santiago; see Erin Kathleen Rowe, *Saint and Nation: Santiago, Teresa of Ávila, and Plural Identities in Early Modern Spain* (University Park, PA: Pennsylvania State University Press, 2011); and I. A. A. Thompson, "Santiago *v* Santa Teresa – signifying what?," in *Historia en fragmentos: Estudios en homenaje a Pablo Fernández Albaladejo*, Julio A. Pardos, et al., eds. (Madrid: Universidad Autónoma de Madrid, 2017), 413–22.

[58] ACC, vol. 18, p. 609, January 12, 1600.

suggested that Philip III might lean a bit on His Holiness to achieve the goal.[59] What the king thought of the idea, we do not know, but Roque officially remains a non-saint.[60]

Roque's in-between status and the obstinacy of communities throughout Castile and Europe in venerating a man without a pope's seal of approval offers another reason for considering plague saints in an otherwise civic discussion. It was really only in the late twelfth century that popes assumed a monopoly over saint-making, and even then, according to Robert Bartlett, a critical mass of the people wherever the issue arose had to share the belief that indeed the dead person was a saint. Furthermore, it was accepted that a request to the papacy had to be frequently and publicly repeated; this requirement happens to be identical to one of the usual requirements for becoming a *vecino* of a town, and when city councils considered a prospective *vecino*'s application, witnesses invariably recited that the applicant had many times said he wanted to be a *vecino*. Assessment of a saint's worth was also akin to a judicial proceeding, with witnesses recounting and repeating what they knew and what they had seen; again, a procedure of establishing evidence and proof, not unlike any of the many litigious or petitionary moments we have seen. If there was evidence, public knowledge, *voz y fama*, that people regarded someone as a saint, then his or her candidacy was strengthened, though probably in the minds of the believers he was already, in fact, a saint.[61] For another angle of the same proposition, when Cardinal Robert Bellarmine, himself a Counter-Reformation saint, tried to figure out what to do with saints who had gained a following before the era of formal papal canonization, he considered that this was a matter of law vs. custom, a tandem intimately familiar to anyone thinking about early modern Castile. These so-called popular saints were venerated by custom, not law, Bellarmine argued, but as custom can acquire the force of law through the tacit consent of the prince, popular saints thus could become legitimate.[62] So the near universal recourse to the goodness and

---

[59] AGS-PR leg. 85 doc. 495, October 6, 1600.

[60] Simon Ditchfield, "Tridentine worship and the cult of the saints," in *Cambridge History of Christianity*, vol. 6, *Reform and Expansion, 1500–1660*, R. Po-chia Hsia, ed. (Cambridge University Press, 2014), 201–24, notes that after the Council of Trent canonization was more difficult; from 1558 to 1665 there were just fourteen canonizations and twenty-seven beatifications. Irene Vaslef, "The role of St. Roch as a plague saint," 138–44, debunks apocryphal accounts of Roque's canonization.

[61] This discussion is based on Robert Bartlett, *Why Can the Dead Do Such Great Things? Saints and Worshippers from the Martyrs to the Reformation* (Princeton, NJ: Princeton University Press, 2013), 59–63.

[62] E. W. Kemp, *Canonization and Authority in the Western Church* (London: Oxford University Press, 1948), 143–46.

efficacy of Roque and his colleagues involved language and practices that were not far removed from townspeople's civic engagements, a world involving adjustment, negotiation, intermediacy, and public presence.

Though townspeople during the plague years did not often gather to carry images of their saints through the streets or even to pray together for fear of contagion, at certain points during the plague town councils, or whatever was left of them, might decide to call an open meeting. All *vecinos* (including women, if they were heads of household) were summoned by town bells to these *concejos abiertos*, which generally were convoked several days earlier and loudly announced by town criers at the usual plazas and intersections. Such meetings during the plague, or at least the ones I have found, almost all concerned money, which is logical under the circumstances. (At least one non-monetary meeting was called, however: in Santander on 17 May 1597 neighbors met to decide if the ship that was the origin of this whole monstrosity, the "*Rodamundo*," whose pestilent hull still sat offshore, should be burned. The *vecinos* of Santander did not hesitate, and it went up in flames later that month.[63]) Open meetings, often held in churches for reasons of space, were an opportunity to make public moral and political issues that may have been pushed aside as people coped with survival and caring for the sick but that surely had not been forgotten. Who should pay for all this? What about the people who had fled, should they be forced to make it up to their neighbors? How much information could be made public? Maybe talking over all these questions in the company of one's neighbors might make the loss and upheaval just a bit less unbearable.

Bartolomé Bennassar wrote of one of Bilbao's *concejos abiertos* that the decision to convoke it was of a "revolutionary" nature.[64] I do not agree, though open meetings were certainly exceptional. Judging from the municipal plague documents I have seen, they were more common in the Basque Country than in the rest of Castile, not surprising given the persistence of direct democracy in Basque townships. But though the regular medieval Castilian *concejo abierto* was far less common by the 1590s, they do appear in the sixteenth and seventeenth centuries. Matters deemed appropriate for such an occasion included but were not limited to assessing new *sisas* or other collective financial burdens, deciding how to pay for levied troops, or somehow altering the way in which municipal government was structured or to which jurisdiction a

---

[63] Bartolomé Bennassar, *Recherches sur les grandes épidémies dans le nord de l'Espagne a la fin du XVIe siècle. Problèmes de documentation et de méthode* (Paris: SEVPEN, 1969), 25, citing city council minutes.

[64] Bennassar, *Recherches sur les grandes épidémies*, 99.

town would belong. Some towns called public meetings to discuss how to answer the *Relaciones topográficas*. One of the fullest descriptions we have of such a meeting is from the town of Alfaro, in the present-day province of La Rioja. The meeting was held in 1602, just after the plague had ended; there is no mention of the epidemic in the account, so the town may have escaped or the disease was simply irrelevant to the matter at hand. That matter was the town's efforts to reinstate elected town posts that had been abolished by the crown over the past century in favor of lifetime offices bought by often unscrupulous men who by 1602 apparently were riding roughshod over the town's lands, crops, and privileges for their own benefit. Close to 300 *vecinos* attended the meeting and almost unanimously agreed to ask the crown for permission to buy back the offices: one man said the current *regidores* should be thrown out "because they are absolute lords," and another said eloquently, "one king and one law is enough." Alfaro's *vecinos* were successful.[65]

We have already seen some plague-ridden towns that held similar gatherings. Badarán, also in La Rioja, held a *concejo abierto* to discuss levying a new *sisa* to pay for plague expenses. When Elgoibar for some reason insisted that Alzola help out with guard duty, in the subsequent lawsuit Alzola said that only the town's *concejo abierto*, attended by all hidalgos, which in a Basque town meant most *vecinos*, could rule on the matter. (It's worth noting that Alzola later was incorporated into Elgoibar, so the latter may have had a point.) Also in Guipúzcoa, we saw that the inhabitants of Pasajes met after Mass one Sunday in August 1597 and voted to mortgage all the town's properties and income in order to finance public health, adding their own personal property as well.[66] In the neighboring province of Vizcaya, residents of the Ispaster district of Bilbao voted, "all together, having gathered as the bells tolled," that people fleeing to their area from Lequeitio and other pestilent towns should pay a certain amount.[67] Several towns held *concejos abiertos* specifically to figure out how to pay their doctors or surgeons. One such example, also in the Basque Country, was Fontecha (Álava), which

---

[65] I. A. A. Thompson, "El concejo abierto de Alfaro en 1602: La lucha por la democracia municipal en la Castilla seiscientista," *Berceo* (1981), 307–31. The document is AGS-CC Serie XII Oficios leg. 1.

[66] José Ramón Cruz Mundet, *"El mal que al presente corre": Gipuzkoa y la peste (1597–1600)* (San Sebastián: Kutxa Fundazioa, 2003), 159–62, no source cited. Cruz Mundet says Pasajes held open meetings all that month until it decided to entrust decision-making to the town council so as to avoid the large gatherings.

[67] AFB Notarial Merindad de Busturia, escr. Aurrecoechea 23, doc. 23/0010, November 25, 1597.

conducted endless judicial maneuverings, including an open town meeting in 1616, in order not to pay its plague-era pharmacist; the man died before he got paid.[68] Further south, the inhabitants of Valdemoro, a seigneurial town in the province of Madrid, were all summoned by their corregidor in May 1599 to organize plague guards. Then, in July, they all met to decide how to hire a doctor (they expressed a preference for someone with a degree from Alcalá de Henares). After a third open meeting they chose a local man, Cristóbal de Fernández, who promptly got sick, leading to yet another meeting and a new choice.[69] A few decades later, when another ferocious epidemic arrived, townspeople in Illescas (Toledo) held a *concejo abierto* in May 1649 to discuss which security measures to impose, a matter of enormous importance given the town's location along main roads to Madrid and Toledo.[70]

The most complete example we have of the recourse to open town meetings during the plague was the city of Bilbao, which held at least two such gatherings, both concerning money. In the context of the rest of Castile, an open meeting of such a large town (around 5,000 inhabitants at the end of the sixteenth century) was unusual, but, as noted above, the Basque Country had its own traditions. Even so, this, too, was special; according to the institutional historian Gregorio Monreal Cia, "*Concejos abiertos* were a reality within towns, with the exception of Bilbao, where they were very exceptional."[71]

The first *concejo abierto* in Bilbao during the plague was in October 1598, after the summer that Bilbao had spent denying anything was wrong. On September 10 the *procurador general* had asked that the city council, most of whose officials were in Portugalete, levy a "moderate" assessment on all *vecinos* according to their economic means. To that end, the council "ordered that the *procurador general* present the said assessment to the *alcalde* and ask, given that in similar cases the rich have the obligation and can be compelled to give and assist, that they do so now, even if through loans..." Those who refused would be jailed and

---

[68] ARCV Pleitos Civiles Pérez Alonso (F) 1337-4; and ARCV Pleitos Civiles Pérez Alonso (F) 1823-5.

[69] AMVal 2547-1 fols. 45–51.

[70] Ramón Sánchez González, "Hambres, pestes y guerras. Elementos de desequilibrio demográfico en la comarca de La Sagra durante la época moderna," *Hispania* 51:2 (1991), 517–58, pp. 539–40, citing Illescas city council minutes.

[71] Gregorio Monreal Cia, *Las instituciones públicas del Señorío de Vizcaya (hasta el siglo XVIII)* (Bilbao: Diputación de Vizcaya, 1974), 215. The Bilbao population figure is from Vicente Pérez Moreda and David S. Reher, "La población urbana española entre los siglos XVI y XVIII: Una perspectiva demográfica," in Fortea Pérez, ed., *Imágenes de la Diversidad*, 129–63, p. 131n3.

their belongings would be seized and sold.[72] A community assessment of this sort was perfectly legal, though there were rules. Castillo de Bovadilla, in his guide for corregidores, wrote that the limit a city could impose without royal license was 3,000 maravedíes as long as it was unable to finance operations using city properties. But there, too, if the situation were urgent (Bovadilla mentions locusts), the city could impose a higher assessment. A city council without royal permission also could "compel the rich to lend, receiving no interest whatsoever" so the city could buy food in times of great need, a device used very rarely, he notes, "because the rich are privileged and judges rarely challenge them." Assessments might also pay for salaries of the corregidor, the town doctor, or local troops. He cites a plethora of sources who argue over whether hidalgos should be exempt and if villages were included in a city's assessment; the clergy, the very poor, judicial officials, some out-siders, and those with twelve children, among others, were exempt.[73]

So on October 26, 1598, a *concejo abierto* was held in the San Juan church of Bilbao, attended by nearly 100 *vecinos*. Considering the city's population, this was very few, and they probably all were among the city's poorest inhabitants; if they had had money, they would not have been there. The meeting was led by the lieutenant corregidor, Lic. García Pérez de Casillas, standing in for the corregidor, Juan Pardo, who was ill. (City council minutes mention the possibility that he might die.) Pérez de Casillas explained that the September assessment had proven inadequate, and the council therefore had resolved that the *vecinos* who had left the city should also contribute. He also told those present that the council had approved the distribution of bread. The *vecinos* "said they consented, that it was very just and necessary that no *vecino* who was outside the city could return without first paying the assessed amount, according to his ability and wealth … and that the assessment be general among all *vecinos*, both those who lived inside and out." They also unanimously approved giving bread to the poor. They also unanimously said (how they unanimously said anything is not explained) that they had heard that the city treasurer wished to leave the city, which should not be permitted. "He has done so much good during this calamity, so they therefore asked and required him not to abandon them, and they would compensate his expenses and his time, as was only right, in any way they

[72] AFB libro 023. Unless otherwise indicated, the following discussion is from this book of minutes, organized chronologically.
[73] Jerónimo Castillo de Bovadilla, *Política para corregidores y señores de vasallos* (Madrid: Instituto de Estudios de Administración Local, 1978) (facs. of Antwerp: Juan Bautista Verdussen, 1704) [1597], vol. 2, libro 5, chapter 5, "De las sisas y repartimientos," passim. The quote on the rich is from chapter 5 no. 22.

could, and thus the *regimiento* spoke and they asked that it be recorded."
On November 9 the city approved a second assessment among all *vecinos*,
present and absent. Further minutes in November and December indicate the city was pulling money out of the granary and taking out second
and third mortgages on its properties.

A lawsuit and subsequent cross-complaints filed soon afterwards
described in detail, probably exaggerated detail, tax-collecting methods
and the ways in which the health emergency stirred the fathomless well of
petty local resentments. The taxpayers in this case were Doña Marina
Saez de Vergara and her sister Doña Marina Pérez de Vergara, both
widows, daughters of one Doctor Vergara, who inexplicably gave them
the same name. According to the case file, the notary Juan de Olarte had
shown up at their house in the Begoña neighborhood on September
12 and "words were exchanged" and properties seized, as a result of
which law enforcement officials were told to return to the house, holding
high the staff of justice, and to take testimony from witnesses regarding
what had transpired. Olarte said in his first statement that when he
arrived the sisters had refused to pay him anything, though he insisted
several times and told them that if they did not pay he would take their
things. The widowed sisters, with the help of two servants, thereupon
threw themselves upon the poor man and hit him, ripped his clothes,
scratched his face, and beat him with sticks and called him a thief, a
traitor, a liar and other nasty things, all of which, in his opinion, made
them worthy of a most thorough investigation and exemplary punishment. Olarte sued the sisters and the servants and also a city council
member, Juan de Zamudio, who, it was said, had tried to kill Olarte with
a sword. The sisters of course also sued, presenting their suit to the
corregidor, Pardo, who was in Portugalete. Their attorney, Juan de
Arteta, on September 13 said his clients were "noble and important
persons, modest and honest widows of high quality and wealth," who
had already paid the assessment (which throughout the case file is
referred to as *limosna*, or alms), albeit as a loan, to Zamudio. (The sisters
had been assigned 300 reales and 500 reales.) But after they had shown
Olarte their receipt, Olarte responded by violently slashing bedroom
furniture and a wooden chest, thrusting his hands into the chest and
pulling out a pile of money, 2,500 reales to be exact, along with two long
gold chains and other things, and he yelled and whacked at them with his
staff of justice and dragged them along the road saying he would throw
them into jail. In the Marinas' subsequent allegations, they added that
Olarte's violence had occurred after he left and later returned with the
men who were now his co-defendants. Zamudio also sued, saying Olarte
had lied about him and that it was he, Zamudio, who was supposed to

collect the *limosna*, not Olarte. Furthermore, Olarte's witnesses were insufficient and not credible, one of them being Olarte's own son and another his own servant. Zamudio also (with Pardo's support) tried to get the case taken out of the hands of Pérez de Casillas, who was admired by the city council for his hard work and charity.[74] Zamudio added a long story about how Pérez de Casillas had falsely accused him, Zamudio, of having illicitly copied keys to one of the guard gates when in fact he had only done what was legal and appropriate for the health of the city. Pardo ordered the release of Zamudio from jail and said he was not to be bothered in the interim until the case was decided, and he ordered that Olarte also be freed, a ruling appealed by the Marinas, who said Pérez de Castillas was on Olarte's side and asked that the latter be given the death penalty. The case thus became the meeting point for a variety of complaints regarding both the initial tax-collecting and rivalries on the city council, which most assuredly had to do with rivalries among Bilbao social classes and groups. At the end of a very long and confusing array of claims and counter-claims, in 1604 Olarte was acquitted and Zamudio and the Marinas were fined. More appeals followed, and in 1605 the verdicts were upheld, though the sisters' fines were reduced.[75]

A year after the *concejo abierto* of Bilbao met to approve the assessment in September 1598, a second such meeting took place concerning related financial and legal matters, showing how plague-related expenses lay heavy on long simmering resentments among the obviously factional government, its allies, and its enemies.[76] Already in January 1599 we find the council (down several members, who refused to move back to the city with their families) commenting on the difficulty of actually getting its hands on the loans being offered in exchange for mortgages against city properties. On February 9 the city council minutes feature sudden praise for regidor Pedro de Villarreal, whose honor had been impugned by Martín Saez de Larrañaga, who said Villarreal during the plague had taken undue authority and spoken in the name of the republic, which was untrue. On February 27, Zamudio (still a regidor) said the city had been asked to side with Villarreal in the lawsuit between the two

---

[74] The city resolved that in case Pardo died it should write to the king and the Council of Castile about how Pérez de Casillas had steadfastly remained in the city throughout the epidemic, with no real obligation to do so, working night and day. AFB libro 023, November 17, 1598.

[75] ARCV Registro de Ejecutorias, Caja 1990, 6. The case was heard in the Chancillería's Sala de Vizcaya.

[76] The following discussion is from AFB libro 024, with the exception of the minutes for September 20, 1599, which are taken from Bennassar, *Recherches sur les grandes épidémies*, 92–5. Bennassar omitted many meetings from this period, but has a complete account of this day.

men concerning "certain assessments," which Zamudio did not think was right, as "it is not just that in cases like this we ally more with the defense of one party than with the other, given that both are *vecinos*." The council was torn, and the matter disappears. In March, however, the council reiterated that the assessed loans must be collected. On August 13 it emerged that one Francisco de Novia was not collecting as he should, or possibly that he had indeed collected but had not given the city the money. Either way, there was a lawsuit. Nearly twenty-five pages of minutes in September, during which the council was meeting in the San Antón church, were devoted to non-payment. Zamudio was sent to Madrid in September to tell the king about the city's dire position, made worse by the corregidor's alleged refusal to approve health-related expenses. Instead, Pardo was sequestering monies to pay salaries owed to town officials, which Bilbao later argued should be paid by the towns, not by Bilbao.

On September 17, 1599, the city reiterated the assessment, ordering "that among the richest and most wealthy *vecinos* of this town an assessment loan or *censo* be assigned in the amount of 2,000 ducats." Three days later, the minutes note that the city's two master surgeons had both fallen ill and needed to be replaced, and they enumerate a list of the city's wealthiest and most financial able *vecinos* who were being called upon to lend money (whether still or again). Twenty-four individuals were named, several of whom would appeal or otherwise get involved in legal conflicts related to the assessment, including the two Marinas, the regidor Larrañaga, and a city treasurer alleged to have escaped to San Juan de Luz, in France. In addition to the individuals, the corporate body of merchants, the Casa de Contratación was on the list.

Ten days later, Larrañaga and his allies, who by now were being held prisoner, presented an appeal to the city. The council, "trying to seek funds for its alleged needs," had unfairly focused on some people while overlooking others, they said. There were people in Bilbao who were far richer than the defendants but yet had not been assessed. This was patently illegal for a variety of reasons, it was unfair, and furthermore the city must have plenty of other resources; where were the fruits of all the past taxes? The appellants were perfectly happy to pay, the said, but only if the richer paid more. So on September 28 the council decided to call another *concejo abierto* to address this conflict between the city and its potential creditors, as well as the role of the lieutenant corregidor of Vizcaya, Pérez de Casillas, whose actions (or inactions) regarding matters "so important for the service of God and the royal majesty and the good of this republic" were causing the sick to die. The city therefore "ordered that a *pregonero* announce publicly in the plazas and the usual sites in this city that today at four in the afternoon a *concejo abierto* will be held" in the Church of the Saint Johns.

At the open meeting, attended by around ten city officials and more than sixty-five *vecinos*, the council accused the corregidor (whether Pardo or his lieutenant, Pérez de Casillas, is not clear) not only of having allowed the plague to enter but also of encouraging his friends not to pay the assessment. The *alcalde*, a sworn enemy of Larrañaga and associates, reminded the crowd of the city's dire situation and explained why it had called for the assessment. "And all the said *vecinos*, anxious as they were, unanimously and together … said they had approved the reply given by the council," that is, the assessment, given that they were all on the brink of collapse. "And the intention of the said Sr Corregidor, speaking with all due respect, has been and is that the said city should be ruined and lost," according to the minutes. The reason "the said illness had entered the said city was that he had left it defenseless without wanting to give the slightest remedy or assistance, and had delivered the said orders [instructing non-payment] knowing full well that the said city had no money it can get its hands on." The city then asked the corregidor to allow it to move forward with the assessment, which was in the king's best interest, adding rather imprudently that the other side were "trouble-makers in the republic, harming it in the extreme, friends of the said Corregidor" who were calling upon other *vecinos* to join them in not paying. Nearly two months later, on November 19, the council resolved that there should be yet another assessment among the rich, which would not include those who had been asked to loan money previously.

As Helen Nader pointed out years ago, everyone in Castile lived in a municipality.[77] You could live nowhere else. You might inhabit a little shack up on a hill or out in the woods, you might spend part of the year traveling with your sheep or on the road selling your fish, but you belonged to a town. You wanted to be a *vecino*. It was the town council (or perhaps the *concejo abierto*) that determined who would guard, who would pay, when people would gather to pray, that fought (through the corregidor) for the king's attention, that set prices and supply, ordered *pregoneros* to cry out the news, and that lied or bargained to ensure that outsiders might think the walls really had protected it from disease. Minutes literally enacted towns' memory, offering guidance and lessons. And the omnipresent notary – dispatched by officials to the gate, hearings, sickbed, plaza, gibbet, home – ensured that whatever act was

---

[77] Helen Nader, *Liberty in Absolutist Spain* (Baltimore, MD: Johns Hopkins University Press, 1990).

ensuing was duly recorded and thus had actually happened in proper legal fashion. The experience and the landscape of the plague; the degree to which the common good managed to survive the onslaught; the measure of people's sense of where they were in relation to everything else, both physically and more abstractly, these were questions largely defined and possibly resolved at the meeting tables in the ayuntamientos. If the councilors had upstairs offices, they looked over the plaza and the steeple out to the gates, to the excluded rabble milling around, the guards controlling passage in and out; and they gazed beyond to the fields and down along the roads that brought them visitors, news, supplies, orders from Madrid, lies from elsewhere – and maybe plague.

Site 7: Sickbed

And while all of this was going on – while taxes were renegotiated, walls fixed, goods smuggled in and out, fairs canceled, supplies delivered, clothes burned, orders issued, and meetings held – people were getting sick and dying. They died at home, in a hospital, or somewhere in-between, usually just a few days after suddenly becoming feverish, delirious, nauseous, wracked with pain, and suffering from buboes. I began the long, meandering and jumbled passage of the great Castilian plague in the Palace. It ends by the sickbed or, more probably, by a mattress.

As many as half a million people died during the roughly five years the plague lasted. Some towns lost one-fifth or more of their population to illness and part of the rest to emigration or displacement, at least temporarily. Madrid had developed plague already in 1597, probably owing to the constant traffic in and out, but it still had cases in late 1599. Madrid's corregidor, Mosen Rubí de Bracamonte, was one of the few to send regular reports to the king starting in May 1599 as per the latter's request.[1] The arithmetic is never clear, but he tallied the sick, the convalescent, discharges, admissions, deaths, those who died of this, those who died of that, those who were shifted from sick wards to recovery wards. By August around 100 people were dying per week in the capital city, and the following month the curve finally began shifting. Rubí de Bracamonte's colleague in Valladolid, Antonio de Ulloa, on the job since just June 1599, sent similarly relentless numbers to the king that summer, though he had started off by reassuring Philip III that things were not as bad as they were said to be and that the illness was not really plague. By the end he had to order the construction of no fewer than six hospitals and witness the departure of the Chancillería from his city. In mid-July, Ulloa wrote to his friend the corregidor of Toro saying he had

---

[1] AGS-E leg. 183, scattered documents throughout. Rubí de Bracamonte had a lesser role than corregidores elsewhere owing to the crown's direct intervention in Madrid's anti-plague campaign, though by fall 1599 the court was edging toward moving to Valladolid.

lots of work, what with 800 patients in the hospital. Speaking of the dead, he said, "It is mostly their own fault for not wanting to get care or getting it late. May God give us strength."[2] Valladolid may have been making up for lost time, but we have seen that other towns and cities throughout Castile had been implementing measures since early 1597 to fend off death and avoid the expense and hardship of actually having to deal with doctors and patients. At some point, however, they all had to switch their attention from guard duty and prophylactic municipal sanitation to medicine. In most cases, the shift came too late.

Not every town had a doctor or even a barber or surgeon. Larger cities may have had one on salary, but the scramble for medical personnel once plague passed through city gates makes it clear that staffing was held to a minimum unless needed. After that, it was a sellers' market. The town of Socuéllamos (Ciudad Real) said it had been devastated during the terrible 1565 plague, losing most of its population ("especially pregnant women") and could not find a doctor, surgeon, or barber "who dared to be in this town."[3] And if doctors were present, in Socuéllamos or anywhere else, there was no general rule as to how they would get paid. Some were paid by patients, others from city properties, others with funds reserved from a particular tax, generally a *sisa*. Castillo de Bovadilla's guide for corregidores allowed for a general head tax from which to pay doctors' salaries; but he also said that the Council of Castile had once ordered the town of Requena to pay 300 ducats among all the *vecinos* and they had refused, so the doctor had to treat the poor for free. He also cited older sources saying sick patients should pay only once they were cured and only if the doctor was not allowed to leave the town and was obligated to treat contagious diseases.[4]

According to reforms put into place by Philip II toward the end of his reign, strictly speaking doctors had to have a university education and then would be licensed by the Protomedicato, a quasi-judicial and professional entity first established by Isabel and Ferdinand and revamped

---

[2] On Valladolid: AGS-E leg. 183, docs. 264–5, and AGS-E leg. 184, docs. 288–9. Ulloa to Gondomar in RBP II-2163, doc. 22.

[3] Carmelo Viñas and Ramón Paz, eds. *Relaciones histórico-geográfico-estadísticas de los pueblos de España hechas por iniciativa de Felipe II. Ciudad Real* (Madrid: Instituto de Sociología Balmes [CSIC], 1971), 474.

[4] Jerónimo Castillo de Bovadilla, *Política para corregidores y señores de vasallos* (Madrid: Instituto de Estudios de Administración Local, 1978), 2 vols. (facs. of Antwerp: Juan Bautista Verdussen, 1704). [1597], vol. 2, pp. 606–7. Anastasio Rojo Vega, *Enfermos y sanadores en la Castilla del Siglo XVI* (Valladolid: Universidad de Valladolid, 1993), 20–8, says towns usually paid doctors with *propios*, generally from 40,000 to 50,000 maravedíes a year.

by Philip II after 1588.[5] Barbers and surgeons did not go to university but had to present evidence of having worked for four years in a hospital. However there were plenty of surgeons who in fact had gone to university and were far more skilled than the ignorant bleeder depicted in literature, and many of them were referred to as doctors. *Boticarios* (apothecaries or pharmacists) also had to spend a certain number of years studying and then pass an examination. But just as doctors often devised recipes for cures, *boticarios* in small towns essentially practiced medicine, as did veterinarians (*albéitares*), and the distinctions between all these various categories, which were not, in fact, categories, are often blurred.[6] Towns that did not have semi-permanent medical staff might rely upon traveling doctors, certified or not, though I have not found that Castile in this regard was similar to Venice, where the phenomenon was frequent enough that William Eamon writes that by the mid-sixteenth century, "the image of the itinerant healer had already evolved into a well-defined literary trope."[7] I have found just one case of an obvious non-professional who either claimed to be able to cure plague or was thought to do so. He was Blas Díez, a 60-year-old *vecino* of the town of Acevedo, in León, who was called before a judge, probably for the second time, for allegedly claiming to cure "*la enfermedad de las bubos.*" He had been working in Extremadura and seems to have been approached by sick people there who knew of his abilities. In his statement, he told the judge that he told them that he "did not know anything" about medicine, but it appears he might have given them some sort of medication or remedy.[8]

---

[5] Michele L. Clouse, *Medicine, Government and Public Health in Philip II's Spain: Shared Interests, Competing Authorities* (Farnham: Ashgate, 2011); María Soledad Campos Díez, *El real tribunal del protomedicato castellano (siglos XIV–XIX)* (Cuenca: Universidad de Castilla-La Mancha, 1999); José María López Piñero, "Los orígenes de los estudios sobre la salud pública en la España renacentista," *Revista española de salud pública* 80:5 (September–October 2006), 445–56. Several of the medical experts named in this book, among them Pérez de Herrera, Mercado, and Zamudio de Alfaro, were *protomédicos*.

[6] María Luz López Terrada, "Médicos, cirujanos, boticarios y albéitares," in José María López Piñero, ed., *Historia de la ciencia y la técnica en la Corona de Castilla*, vol. 3 (Valladolid: Junta de Castilla y León, 2002), 161–85. The contents of a good pharmacist's medicine cabinet can be found in the scrupulous Charles Davis and María Luz López Terrada, "Protomedicato y farmacia en Castilla a finales del siglo XVI: Edición crítica del *Catálogo de las cosas que los boticarios han de tener en sus boticas*, de Andrés Zamudio de Alfaro, protomédico general (1592–1599)," *Asclepio* 62:2 (July–December 2010), 579–626. Once the worst of the plague had passed, the Council of Castile instructed cities to restock their pharmacies: AMB-LA 131, fols. 23r–23v, January 22, 1600.

[7] William Eamon, "The Canker Friar: piety and intrigue in an era of new diseases," in *Piety and the Plague: From Byzantium to the Baroque*, Franco Mormando and Thomas Worcester, eds. (Kirkesville, MO: Truman State University Press, 2007), 156–76, p. 170.

[8] AHN Nobleza, Frias, C. 1626, doc. 3. The 3-page document dates from 1601.

The city of Burgos in 1561, when it was at the peak of its importance, had seven doctors, five surgeons, fifteen barbers (the two categories were sometimes separate, sometimes combined), six *boticarios*, and just one midwife (*partera*).[9] It is likely, given the city's prominence, that few if any cities had more than that, though it is worth pointing out that once plague arrived, medical professionals were reluctant to serve.[10] Madrid in 1600 seems to have had five doctors and around seventy-five surgeon-barbers, plus eight midwives (*comadres*), both men and women.[11] But by around 1627 a city as important as Bilbao said it had no doctor worth the title (*médico alguno que sea de consideración*) and therefore wished to impose a new *sisa* on wine so as to hire one.[12]

Valladolid had a medical school, a considerable advantage when it came to hiring, and on June 23, 1599 – a bit late in the game – the city council there decided to ask the medical faculty for names of a doctor and surgeon willing to help out at the San Lázaro hospital. A week later, as things quickly got worse, the city council agreed that no doctors, surgeons, or graduates of the medical school could leave the city, but if they did leave they would be fined 200 ducats to be given to the hospital (though if they left, it is unclear how they would or could pay a fine.) By July 14, by which time the surgeon had fallen ill, the city was urgently appointing more personnel and resolved that if those appointed did not wish to help out, the city could take whatever measures it thought necessary to ensure compliance.[13]

Other cities had an even harder time. In July 1599 Santo Domingo de la Calzada frantically cast about for a doctor. The city council managed to get assurances from a Dr. Montoya, who had worked in San Sebastián, that he would work for an "honest salary" for a period of four years. But even what turned out to be an immense salary, hammered out after

---

[9] Manuel Fernández Álvarez, "Burgos en el siglo XVI," in *La Ciudad de Burgos: Actas del Congreso de Historia de Burgos. MC Aniversario de la fundación de la ciudad, 884–1984* (León: Junta de Castilla y León, 1985), 221–32, p. 225, citing the Censo de Calle Hita, in Simancas.

[10] Francis Brumont, "Le Coup de Grace: la peste de 1599," in *La Ciudad de Burgos: Actas del Congreso de Historia de Burgos* (Valladolid: Junta de Castilla y León, 1985), 335–42," pp. 338–9, quotes regidor Andrés de Cañas remarking that the city had to seek doctors elsewhere "because none in Burgos were willing to help" at the Rebolleda hospital.

[11] AV Secretaría, 1-138-4, report at the end of the *legajo*. This was just before the capital moved to Valladolid.

[12] AFB Consulado 0281/001/079, probably from 1627.

[13] AMVA sig. 22-0, June 23 and 30, 1599; AMVA sig. 21-0, July 14, 1599. In his musings on whether or not one should leave a pestilent town, Cellorigo, in Valladolid, wrote that physicians should be compelled to serve; Martín González de Cellorigo, *Memorial de la política necesaria y util restauración a la Republica de España* (Madrid: Instituto de Cooperación Iberoamericana, 1991 [1st ed. 1600]), 28.

several round of talks, proved insufficient to attract the doctor, who was afraid of getting sick. So the city council sent one of its members to Valladolid, and then to Salamanca, in search of help, which they found, though at a steep price. They also tried to poach a surgeon from Bilbao, Bartolomé Masón, more on whom below.[14] The Segovian village of Carbonero el Mayor in July 1599 hired a surgeon named Andrés Gutiérrez, who came all the way from Madrid and charged 100 ducats for twenty days of work. Yet when a doctor inspected the town in October, he reported that 273 people had died since July, two-thirds of them children.[15] In Villalón de Campos after the doctor fled and his assistant died, the town managed to find a replacement from Villada, who charged 1,500 maravedies per day and refused to actually sleep in Villalón. Then he, too, got sick and was replaced by someone from the province of Cuenca, who charged 1,200 maravedies *per patient*.[16] And in nearby Valladolid, where Santo Domingo eventually found its man, a report was drawn up at around the same time showing that of twenty-four towns in its jurisdiction, just two had doctors, though several had surgeon-barbers. Interestingly enough, fifteen had hospitals, though obviously no medical care was offered there. So either doctors or surgeons had to be hired, or the already stressed personnel in the cities would be sent out to the villages.[17]

The struggles of the town of Olmedo, though occurring before the plague, are of interest in understanding how medical appointments, particularly during epidemics, cut across matters of finance and municipal relations. The dispute there started in September 1574 when Olmedo told the crown that it had lost its copy of the license permitting it to hire and pay a surgeon out of its *propios*, and it asked for a copy. Instead of simply sending a copy (which perhaps did not exist), Philip II, eager as always to collect information, asked Olmedo to hold open town meetings

---

[14] Diego Téllez Alarcia, "La peste Atlántica en Santo Domingo de la Calzada (1599)," *Berceo* 162 (2012), 85–119, pp. 99–101. Téllez makes the excellent point that officials were racing against the speed of news; as with today's pre-existing conditions *avant la lettre*, the worse the rumors were of a town's bad health, the scarcer the resources to cure it and the higher the price.

[15] Manuela Villalpando Martinez, "Tres noticias de la Segovia antigua: Un brote de peste en la Segovia de 1653," *Estudios Segovianos* 95 (1997), 17–26, pp. 21–5; the author does not cite the source.

[16] Elena Maza Zorrilla, "Villalón de Campos y la peste de 1599," *Cuadernos de investigación histórica* 2 (1978), 363–86, p. 381.

[17] Anastasio Rojo Vega, "La caridad, factor de mortalidad en la epidemia de peste de 1599 en Valladolid," *Medicina y Historia* 30 (1989), 1–16. Rojo Vega cites AHPV Prot. leg. 1023, from the king to the city, and says the city responded with the report, though he gives no citation for the latter. The two towns with a doctor were Tudela de Duero (582 *vecinos*) and Olivares de Duero (305).

to gather evidence. *Vecino* after *vecino* then testified that ever since they could remember Olmedo had paid its doctor/surgeon (both appear in the record) out of *propios* and that the missing license allowed for this practice. A new round of testimony took place in early November, perhaps because Philip wanted more or perhaps because villages were now protesting. The first question was, "If they know that for the past ten twenty thirty forty sixty a hundred and more years, so long ago that no man's memory could contradict it, the council of this town, with permission from His Majesty, has had the custom of using its *propios* to pay the salaries of the doctors and surgeons who have resided in the said town, and the *vecinos* of the said town and its jurisdiction have always paid their doctors." Another question asked, "If they know that the *vecinos* have no other *propios* from which to pay the said salaries except the common properties of the town and its lands, from which they have always been paid, and that each town council [*concejo*] of the villages has its own ... from which [Olmedo] neither asks nor expects payment for the said salaries." Olmedo's ability to hire a doctor appears to have encountered opposition from several of its subject towns (Valdastillas, Matapozuelos, Hornillos, La Nava, and Serranos), which persuaded the king's advisers to recommend in April 1575 that Olmedo's license not be granted (or renewed). Olmedo found this to be preposterous, as villages stood to gain if the larger town had a doctor. The five opposing towns were far away and therefore should not care, it said, and a sixth, Alcazaren, anyway had its own doctor. Olmedo had seventeen villages with a total of 2,000 *vecinos* who needed medical care, and it therefore asked permission to summon open town meetings in each one to gauge support. Given that the named villages lie between Olmedo and Valladolid, one has to assume they were affected by plague in 1599.[18]

Virtually all requests to impose *sisas* in order to pay medical expenses during or after the plague mention salaries, which were onerous. For that reason, towns were anxious to get the staff off the payroll as quickly as possible. Madrid, for example, in August 1599 asked the *junta de la salud*, the crown entity overseeing the anti-plague campaign there, to remove "midwives, doctors, surgeons, and barbers who are curing *secas*, given the great improvement in the city, thanks be to God." The junta evidently was more cautious, and so in late November the city had to ask again that medical staff, along with the notary and the police officer

---

[18] AHN Consejos leg. 24.640, doc. 25, escr. Escariche. The corregidor of Olmedo told the king in April and May 1599 that the town was fine and that Valladolid's Dr. Ponce de Santa Cruz had visited, but the epidemic only really landed in the following months; AGS-E leg. 183, docs. 257, 298, and 299.

guarding the guards, all be dismissed, "because it is not necessary for salaried people to be doing this."[19] Just as towns took down their guards too early, they dismissed their doctors, and in many cases both measures ended up costing far more than the salaries.

An easier way to save money was to promise a salary and then not pay it, and the archives are littered with lawsuits and complaints for non-payment long after the last patient had died or recovered. (Although, the reverse could also be true: when the present-day town of Bidaurreta [Navarre] was sued by a surgeon for non-payment, the town countered that he had cured no one because the town had not fallen ill.[20]) The best documented case I have found is that of the above-mentioned Bartolomé Masón, a surgeon who was a *vecino* of San Sebastián and whom Bilbao decided to hire in September 1598, having heard he had done a good job in Lequeitio. Bilbao hired him for an optimistic thirty-day spell, for which he would be paid 200 ducats. A week later Masón was joined by a Flemish surgeon, who was to receive fifty reales a day for thirty days.[21] Thirty days came and went, and still Masón was on the job. A new contract was drawn up in early January 1598, with the city council being unusually prudent; yes, the disease had abated, the minutes state, but nonetheless they thought it a good idea to keep Masón around to deal with convalescents and just in case things took a turn for the worse, and a new contract was approved. On March 4 it emerged that Masón had been sued by a certain captain whose house apparently had been requisitioned and where objects had been damaged. On March 11, Masón was dismissed as of March 5 (sic) and was owed (according to city council minutes) his salary from November to March, showing he had never been paid at all.[22]

Masón sued both Bilbao and Lequeitio, the latter having followed similar accounting practices as its larger neighbor. In 1600 Lequeitio authorized a city notary to settle with Masón. It did exactly the same thing in February 1608, meaning, of course, that nothing had transpired. Later that same year, in September, a sales contract appears granting Masón 300 trees in the Balastegui mountains worth 400 ducats. According to the contract, "the said surgeon had sued the said town for nonpayment of professional services during the time of the plague and

---

[19] AV Actas, August 30 and November 26, 1599.

[20] AGN TR Procesos 040215. The town, which could have been lying, also said he had quarantined a six-year-old boy who had merely suffered a swelling after a bad fall.

[21] AFB libro 023 starting September 26, 1598.

[22] AFB libro 024, January 7–8, March 4, 11, 1599.

had won a *carta ejecutoria*," an appeals decision by the Chancillería. The document adds, Masón "did a great service to this town."[23] So Masón had had to wait a decade, but he at least he got some satisfaction and 300 trees. He would not be so lucky in Bilbao, where his initial thirty-day tenure had reached 436 days, meaning either that he had been rehired at some point after the dismissal or that the calculation included fines. According to a brief presented by a city official in 1618 – twenty years later – Masón had won rulings in his favor not only for back wages but for legal costs and other expenses, reaching well over 10,000 reales, which the city would have had to mortgage all its properties and income in order to pay. The suits had been "very expensive and of dubious purpose," the official admitted. So the city proposed paying Masón 600 ducats at a rate of 100 ducats per year for six years and asked the official for his legal opinion. The sensible man, probably very relieved, said the offer was a good one for the city, as it was far less than the surgeon was owed and would put an end to the matter once and for all. Before finalizing the deal, however, he suggested the city convoke a *concejo abierto* so all the vecinos could be informed.[24]

Many doctors and surgeons, then, were hired too late and dismissed too early. But there were other medical professionals, usually those on the city or royal payroll to begin with, whose early investigations and reports were essential in helping officials sense what it was that surrounded them. Toledo in spring 1599, when its population was around 9,000 *vecinos*, appears to have had at least five doctors at its disposal, including one borrowed from the Inquisition, and Corregidor Francisco de Carbajal sent them all out to surrounding towns.[25] Diego Vargas de Manrique, the overworked corregidor of Burgos, spent much of the fall of 1597 shuffling medical workers back and forth among Melgar de Fernamental, Revilla del Campo, Cogollos and the other pestilent towns in his region, borrowing at least one, named Pedro López, from Valladolid.[26] The following year he summoned a group of doctors to determine if Melgar really was safe, and he also

---

[23] AFB Notarial Lequeitio, escr. Amezqueta; the documents are 15/0640, 18/0199, and 18/0294. The higher ruling appears to have been for 1,014 ducats plus eight reales, which the town must not have had. Balestegui mountains appear nowhere on current maps.

[24] AFB, Bilbao Antigua 0312/001/004/014.

[25] AMT Libros no. 176, unfoliated, roughly April to August. Population from Julián Montemayor, *Tolède entre fortune et déclin (1530–1640)* (Limoges: PULIM, 1996), 147. Carbajal's correspondence is scattered in AGS-E leg. 183.

[26] AMB-HI 3651, September 22, 1597, instructions for López, "que va a curar la peste de Melgar y Padilla de Abajo y de Arriba y Arenillas de Río Pisuerga."

asked the city of Vitoria to gather testimony from doctors, surgeons, *boticarios*, and priests to confirm their city was healthy.[27]

The successor of his successor, Gonzalo Manuel, paid the price for optimism, carelessness, or both, when a new wave of plague swept through in spring 1600. In December he sent one of his officials out to the seigneurial town of Torquemada (today in the province of Palencia) to interview the local medical staff. Dr. Diego de la Puebla, 33, said he had been salaried in Torquemada for the past seven years and had begun noticing patients with buboes in spring, but he did not judge them to be serious. Then they became "malignant," he said, "though not enough to call it peste or pernicious illness." He had treated around 800 patients, he said, and the proof that the disease was not peste was that most of his patients had not died; he put the death toll at around fifty, most of them children. A barber, Sebastián de la Puerta, who was sixty years old, who had been a *vecino* there for the past forty years, agreed that the buboes were "benign" and not really plague. His colleague Juan de Herrero, said the same thing, as did the *boticario*. The priest, Tomás García, had been there for just three years, and he deferred to the doctor regarding the medical aspects, adding that "he has not heard of nor knows of any town in Castile guarding against this town except the city of Burgos, and also the town of Baltanás for a while, but he also heard that those from Baltanás were now entering this town [Torquemada] and were grinding their grain, and this is true."[28]

A good number of the hundreds of messengers, spies, and scouts on the road were doctors or other medical practitioners. They gathered information, and it was they (occasionally with priests) who determined what was true and what was false. They told a story, often a chronological one; one thing led to another, and there were reasons for that.[29] Doctors were not universally liked or trusted. Some left their post or refused to visit sick towns, pretended to be licensed when they were not, or made a bad situation worse. In Pamplona during an earlier plague, doctors took advantage of the city's open-gate policy and fled en masse.[30] The word *matasanos* does not appear, but even an accomplished doctor, Valentín

---

[27] On Melgar, AMB-HI 3650, March 23, 1598; on Vitoria, AMB-HI 3650, September 16, 1598, but referring back to a request in January 1598, when Vitoria was still healthy. By September it was not, and Vargas wanted new testimony.

[28] AMB HI-3652, "Informaciones sobre el estado de la salud pública..." He also visited Los Balbases and Revilla Vallejera. The corregidor confronted yet another episode of plague in 1601.

[29] On doctors' medical accounts in general see Nancy G. Siraisi, *History, Medicine, and the Traditions of Renaissance Learning* (Ann Arbor, MI: University of Michigan Press, 2007).

[30] José Luis de Orella y Unzué, "El Cardenal Diego de Espinosa consejero de Felipe II, el monasterio de Iranzu y la peste de Pamplona en 1566," *Príncipe de Viana* 36:140–1

de Andosilla, griped about "pseudo doctors with tyrannical interests and vile earnings committing a thousand idiocies and reckless acts with patients, hitting the nail once for every hundred swings of the hammer."[31] In a similar vein, Cristóbal Soares de Figueroa remarked on the number of homes in which people wept over the doctors' habit of "ignorantly trying out idiotic things with the lives of others."[32] Doctors often scorned their own peers, ridiculing them for overlooking the obvious or using faulty methods; though Dr. Juan Ximénez Savariego began his treatise by saying, "Friends and those of my profession have asked me to write my opinions down," a reader of one extant copy jotted down in the margin, "because he has few [friends] in his profession."[33]

When Sancho Panza became governor of Barataria, the post came equipped with a doctor with a medical degree from the University of Osuna (Seville), Pedro Recio, whose salary was paid by the *insula* and whose only apparent task was to control what Sancho ate. At their first meeting he ordered plate after plate of food to be removed from in front of Sancho for questionable and confusing dietary reasons, finally prompting the hungry new ruler to expel him and threaten to throw a chair at him. If called before a judge, Sancho announced, he would say he had "done God's work by killing a bad doctor, *verdugo de la república.*"[34] Contemporaries could and did complain about the medical profession, but doctors' knowledge and skill (assuming they were for real), particularly during emergencies, obviously made them indispensable. As Soares de Figueroa acknowledged, medicine was a *ciencia utilísima.* Yet even with all that skill, they still could not agree. As with any other situation of truth-testing, whether to determine the veracity of a plaintiff's story or the poverty level of an overtaxed town that had buried many of its inhabitants, a multitude of statements were required.

(1975), 565–610, p. 585. On physicians' moral responsibilities, including whether to stay or to flee, see Patrick Wallis, "Plagues, morality and the place of medicine in early modern England," *The English Historical Review* 121:490 (February 2006), 1–24, which also discusses the views of Luther and other Protestants mentioned in Chapter 5.

[31] Valentin de Andosilla Salazar, *Libro en que se prueba con claridad el mal que corre por España ser nuevo y nunca visto: su naturaleza, causas, pronosticos, curacion, y la prouidencia que se deue tener con él* ... (Pamplona: Mathias Mares, 1601), 109v.

[32] Cristóbal Soares de Figueroa, *Plaza Universal de Todas Ciencias y Artes*... (Madrid: Luis Sánchez, 1615), 68r–71r.

[33] Juan Ximénez Savariego, *Tratado de peste, donde se contienen las causas, preservación, y cura*... (Antequera: Claudio Bolan, 1602), chapter 1. This particular copy is held by the Real Academia de España; the one held by the Biblioteca Nacional does not contain the same margin note. The book's author was *protomédico* of the galleys, a job previously held by Cristóbal Pérez de Herrera.

[34] *Don Quijote* II:47.

We have seen that everybody was questioned, interrogated, and asked to present proof again and again, and medicine was no different. Medical debates, the determination of truth, was often a collective affair that took place in public with the public. Doctors and officials relied on the observations of *vecinos* and local medical staff and listened carefully (or carefully read) their responses to the batteries of questions put to them. When did the disease first arrive? What were the symptoms? How did the illness move? How many had died? What sort of people were they? As if they were dealing with a matter of law, officials used evidence, the more the better, to reconstruct events so as to arrive at the truth. Falsity was a frequent concern; in this account we have seen false keys, disguised travelers, false doors, false plague, deceptions of all sorts. How was one to know if things were true or false? The ubiquitous notaries helped somewhat as they recorded testimony, assured the safe routes of objects and people, and verified the hand-off of goods and money. But even there, deception might sneak into the record. The wide-open space of the public sphere, featuring as many responsible voices as possible, was a better guarantee. The disease, after all, was a public matter, and *vecinos* were in effect participating as health officials; they stopped or allowed traffic, oversaw cleaning campaigns, watched over sick houses, carried the dead, probably spied on their neighbors and certainly spread rumors. This was what Andrew Mendelsohn has called "knowing in common."[35]

I am assuming that most if not all the patients and victims of this epidemic had bubonic plague, caused by the *Yersinia pestis* pathogen. Bubonic plague today moves according to well-established vectors and hosts; it may have moved differently in late-sixteenth-century Spain, and that is of enormous importance in evaluating the measures that contemporaries took. I mentioned briefly in the Introduction and in Chapter 3 that the past couple of decades have been a time of vivid debate among historians of medicine on this point. I am not a historian of medicine and remain somewhat agnostic on the point, but all evidence points to bubonic plague.

The symptoms generally were these: people developed hot, painful buboes in the groin or axilla which could last several days and then rupture, giving off pus and/or blood. Extremities developed gangrene. Other lesions, caused by hemorrhages, appeared throughout the body, and they might turn black and swell up and burst and then dry out; these were what were called *secas* and/or *carbuncos*. Patients suffered high fevers

---

[35] From a talk Mendelsohn, of Queen Mary University of London, delivered at Stanford University on November 18, 2016, "Learning in Public: Physicians, Barber-Surgeons, Lawyers, Housewives, Councilors, Neighbors in Early Modern Germany Communities."

and blisters and generally died three to seven days after infection, though some died more quickly and some lasted longer. It was believed that they might have acquired the disease from cloth, from another person, from the air (or misalignment of heavenly spheres), or from a combination of these, and that they might not have fallen ill, or might have survived, had they been healthier and better fed to begin with. Some said it was peste, others said it was not, some thought it was an entirely new disease, or maybe a combination of known diseases. The corregidor of Guipúzcoa, Diego Fernández de Arteaga, who seemed to think it was peste, told Philip II that in his opinion "the doctor was mistaken in saying that what he found in the groin, under arms, and behind ears were buboes, because there is another more dangerous name."[36] According to what Burgos corregidor Francisco de Valencia wrote to the king in April 1599, despite the slight increase in cases, "The doctors believe that, as the illness has not become widespread or common, it cannot be called peste, because in order that it be such it is necessary that many more be sick and that most of them die, because that is the definition of peste."[37]

Virtually all city councils summoned doctors to give their opinion in gatherings known as *juntas de médicos*. The president of the Chancillería in Valladolid assured Philip III that at the first "suspicion of illness" he had ordered such a junta to meet and figure out what to do and which medicines to order.[38] This obligatory move by all city leaders may have been regarded as prudent and professional, but the physicians' dithering and arcane disputes inspired impatience and ridicule. Dr. Nicolás Bocángel, who served the royal family and had little regard for his fellow professionals, devoted an entire chapter of his medical treatise to the "diversity of opinions" among doctors regarding this *enfermedad de secas*.[39] The seventeenth-century Jesuit writer Baltasar Gracián, in his allegorical novel *El Criticón*, described a dying man being besieged by teams of doctors from Heaven and Earth, each of whose questionable advice directly contradicted the other's.[40] With all the usual caveats for introducing a fictional episode from another time period entirely, it is worth thinking about Camus's dialogue among the members of his latter-day junta:

[36] AGS-GyM leg. 489, doc. 227, September 20, 1597.
[37] AGS-E leg. 183, doc. 267, April 22, 1599.   [38] AGS-E leg. 184, doc. 290.
[39] Nicolás Bocangel, *Libro de las enfermedades malignas y pestilentes, causas, pronósticos, curación y preservación* (Madrid: Luis Sánchez, 1600), 58–66. Bocangel, sometimes called Bocangelino, came from a Genovese family; his father had worked for Charles V and his son was a distinguished poet.
[40] Baltasar Gracián, *El Criticón, tercera parte, en el invierno de la vejez* (Antwerp: Verdussen, 1669), 284–5.

Richard hesitated, then fixed his eyes on Rieux.

"Please answer me quite frankly. Are you absolutely convinced it's plague?"

"You're stating the problem wrongly. It's not a question of the term I use; it's a question of time."

"Your view, I take it," the Prefect put in, "is this. Even if it isn't plague, the prophylactic measures enjoyed by law for coping with a state of plague should be put into force immediately?"…

The doctors confabulated. Richard was their spokesman:

"It comes to this. We are to take the responsibility of acting as though the epidemic were plague."

That way of putting it met with a general approval.

"It doesn't matter to me," Rieux said, "how you phrase it. My point is that we should not act as if there were no likelihood that half the population would be wiped out; for then it would be."[41]

The best known of the *juntas de médicos* during our plague epidemic was in Madrid, starring Luis Mercado, doctor to both Philip II and his son. Once the plague made its presence known, the old king had summoned a junta of his personal physicians and *protomédicos*, among them Cristóbal Pérez de Herrera, Andrés Zamudio de Alfaro, and Mercado, who agreed that unsanitary conditions were the cause of the disease but could not agree on the best treatment. Philip III's council on April 13, 1599 summed up the opinion of Mercado and his colleagues, which was that the *secas* were not plague because not enough people were dying.[42] But they were definitely pestilent and very bad news (*de mala calidad*). Philip III, who was in Martorell, gave Mercado an order dated July 14, that was later included with the subsequent treatise, to reissue in the vernacular what would become the best-known plague tract, first published in Latin in 1598. The objective was that everyone "understand and know with certainty which disease it is and how they should protect themselves," and the king gave the author 2,000 ducats for printing expenses. In addition, when the book was published it was to be distributed throughout the kingdom by delegates to the Cortes. No need for a book tour or publicists.[43] The hyper-competent crown official who

[41] Albert Camus, *The Plague*, trans. Stuart Gilbert (New York: The Modern Library, 1948), 47.

[42] AGS-E leg. 183, doc. 11, consulta.

[43] On the 2,000 ducats, Bartolomé Bennassar, *Valladolid au siècle d'or: Une ville de Castille et sa campagne au XVI siècle* (Paris: Mouton, 1967), 363. The king's letter says he wanted the book "to be printed as I have ordered and then distributed without delay by the *procuradores de Cortes* throughout my kingdoms." The letter also appears in Cristóbal Pérez Pastor, *Bibliografía madrileña; o descripción de las obras impresas en Madrid (siglo xvi)*, vol. 1. (Madrid: Tip. de los Huérfanos, 1891), 336. In a conversation with me, Fernando Bouza pointed out another unusual advantage: Mercado's treatise was not subject to censorship.

oversaw the clean-up of Alcalá de Henares gratuitously mentioned him in his report: "everything that Doctor Mercado ordered with such erudition and prudence was put into effect to the degree possible."[44] The head of Ávila's health commission, Luis Pacheco, also went out of his way to mention Mercado as the guiding light of health measures.[45] In January 1600, as Burgos was waiting for the Council of Castile to declare the city pest-free following a visit by Mercado, it received a shipment of his book, by then in its third or fourth edition, to distribute among "the doctors of this jurisdiction."[46] Nicolás Bocangel referred to him as "doctísimo" and "sapientíssimo."[47]

Mercado also oddly found his way into the city council minutes of Valladolid, at whose university he was a professor of medicine. In January 1600, the council met in a full session to discuss a request by Mercado that the city transfer to him (by purchase or swap) six *cargas* of grain (a *carga* is around 300 pounds) which somehow were linked to a *censo* and perpetual revenue stream that the city had on the village of Viana. Mercado promised to pay whatever the city asked, probably because the operation was financially beneficial to him. A highly unusual secret vote was taken, the result being that fifteen of the seventeen council members present voted to accept Mercado's offer.[48] During the plague he had abandoned his house in Valladolid, and eight people left behind died. After the city cleared out the building, the widow of one of his dead renters, Rodrigo de Astudillo, stopped paying rent, believing (as did the city) that she had no obligation to do so. The good doctor thought differently, sued, and won.[49] Yet another odd anecdote about the prolific Mercado was that he was later accused of having poisoned Queen Margaret in 1611, the year he himself died, an alleged crime for which Philip III's closest aide, Rodrigo Calderón, was executed. A play by Tirso de Molina, "La Prudencia en la Mujer," includes a Calderón-type character, Infante Don Juan, who conspires with a Jewish doctor to poison the child king. The queen discovers the evil doctor with a glass of poison in his hand and forces him to drink it.[50]

---

[44] RAH Jesuitas 9-3662/182.   [45] AHMA libro no. 25, fol. 28v.
[46] AMB-HI 3653, January 5, 1600; AMB LA 131, fols. 23v–24r. It was probably distributed among the residents of other cities as well. Mercado's treatise was also mentioned in the Burgos *junta de médicos* report of April 22, 1599 as the city prepared itself for the onslaught; AGS-E leg. 183, doc. 267.
[47] Bocángel, *Libro de las enfermedades malignas*, 69 and 239.
[48] AMVA sig. 23-0, January 9, 1600. According to Bennassar, Mercado held municipal bonds worth 259,282 maravedies; *Valladolid*, 257.
[49] Narciso Alonso Cortés, "Gómez Pereira y Luis Mercado," in *Miscellanea Vallisoletana*, vol. 5 (Valladolid: Emilio Zapatero, 1930), 65–117, p. 15.
[50] My thanks to Ted Bergman for hunting down information on this and other plays.

Already in 1586 Mercado had published something on pestilence, followed by the treatise on the subject in Latin in 1598 commissioned by Philip II. Presumably he was in Madrid in 1597, when many witnesses said the capital suffered mightily from peste, but his presence on the front lines is not detected. Mercado's exalted status is a bit hard to figure out. He misidentified the disease (other less famous physicians got it right, or at least got close) and at one point opined that the best way of fighting it was to pray, process, and do good works.[51] His insistence on the key function of air as host and vector went beyond that of local officials, who prudently kept that possibility open but whose measures spoke to a more grounded understanding of the epidemic. Even hagiographer Nicasio Mariscal had to admit that parts of the treatise were taken from Dr. Juan Tomás Porcell's 1565 practical treatise on plague, which Mercado does not cite.[52]

His famous treatise begins with a feverish attempt to determine if the disease is true peste, if peste amounts to *secas y carbuncos* or is something else, and if it is contagious, the idea being that only once one has positively identified the disease may one proceed. Ordinarily this would make sense, in that treatment follows diagnosis, and not the other way around, but here the gap between his ruminations on the true cause of the Santander calamity and his knowledge of (or interest in) what actually happened there is noteworthy. He also lays out the obligatory theoretical basis for his treatise: Why is the peste called a contagion? he wonders in a more lexical than medical register. What is contagion, anyway? Is it popular and pernicious? How should the various lesions be called? What are the types and sub-types of each of these categories? Later on in the volume he provides what were surely useful recipes and detailed instructions on such techniques as lancing sores and using purgatives. But once he leaves the bedside, his advice seems less useful. Telling officials that once plague threatened they should start guarding their town or city and prohibit the presence of outsiders was stating the obvious, while suggesting to towns battling depopulation and bad harvests to stock up on "wheat, barley, wine, meat, poultry, sugar, preserves and other foodstuffs necessary for patients" and to make sure that medicine cabinets were full to the brim was adding insult to injury at a time when many towns had no doctor, surgeon, or *boticario*, much less the ability to stock up on food.[53] Perhaps towns sprang into action only after

---

[51] Luis Mercado, *El libro de la peste del Dr. Luis Mercado* … (Madrid: Imp. de Cosano, 1921), 217. This is the 1599 Spanish translation.

[52] See Mariscal's 150-page introduction to Mercado, *El libro de la peste del Dr. Luis Mercado*.

[53] Mercado, *El libro de la peste del Dr. Luis Mercado*, 221.

reading his guide, but I doubt it. Other measures he proposes are like a wish list: wouldn't it be nice if old people in every town named one of their own to act as their representative? Or if no cost were spared in taking care of the sick?

Dozens of similar plague treatises were written during these years in Spain. The historian Luis Granjel found seventy-three for the seventeenth century (he began counting in the 1590s, during this plague).[54] They follow a similar pattern, including discussions of the cause of the disease, parsing of its various components and symptoms, and remedies and treatment instructions, occasionally drawn from examples from the author's own experience. Most sneer at other doctors for ignoring the obvious, misunderstanding their sources, or being clumsy. The way in which these books were actually used is an important question for establishing the relationship between theory and practice, and it is a question I cannot answer to my satisfaction. There are references to Mercado's book in municipal records, but I suspect they are due to his rank and to the crown's obvious interest in publicising it, not necessarily to its utility. Most treatises were in Latin, though several of the authors whose books I have examined, including Mercado, deliberately state at the start that they are writing in Spanish to ensure wider distribution. The books are formulaic, tedious, laden with references to classical sources and the hidden ways of God, and generally bereft of current examples. I would tentatively propose that, though there may have been exceptions, most treatises responded not to actual conditions or even to a public health project but rather to a tradition of scientific debate and competition. These men were writing for each other. Prevailing notions of cause and remedy are far more easily apparent in municipal documents than in treatises, which were an art form. The only exception to this are the recipes, which indeed were useful and were likely to have been followed carefully, probably by women.

Among the other more prominent authors, Miguel Martínez de Leyva (or Leiva) was a *natural* of Santo Domingo de la Calzada, according to the title page of his treatise, and if he were a doctor the title page surely

---

[54] Luis S. Granjel, "Las epidemias de peste en la España del siglo XVII," *Asclepio* 29 (1977), 17–36. For lists of treatises see Antonio Carreras Panchón, *La peste y los médicos en la España del Renacimiento* (Salamanca: Universidad de Salamanca, 1976); Randal P. Garza, *Understanding Plague: The Medical and Imaginative Texts of Medieval Spain* (New York: Peter Lang, 2008); Juan Ballesteros Rodríguez, *La Peste en Córdoba* (Córdoba: Diputación Provincial, 1982); and José María López Piñero, "Los orígenes de los estudios sobre la salud pública en la España renacentista," *Revista española de salud pública*, 80:5 (September–October 2006), 445–56. Around a dozen are listed in the bibliography of this book, and the obvious search terms in the Biblioteca Nacional catalog will lead to dozens more.

would have mentioned that. The Cortes in December 1597 gave him 200 reales for publication costs, so clearly he knew someone, a connection made obvious, too, by the presence of his book today at the palace library.[55] Martínez de Leyva had worked in a Seville hospital during an epidemic in the 1580s that probably was influenza, not plague, which he himself suggests by noting that practitioners were "veterinarians and idiots" looking for buboes that did not exist. Doctors did not know very much, in his opinion, and had little practical experience. The book contains the usual chapters on pestilent air, wind, fire and earth; recipes and medical techniques; and a closing section on the "cruel, perfidious, and malignant envy" he had suffered when he was a doctor, indicating that, sadly, he no longer was one.[56] A similarly bitter assessment came from Rodrigo de Cabrera, who began by noting in his 1599 self-published volume that Seville had asked the city's doctors for their suggestions, "and although I was not among those thus called, I would be violating my desire to serve" were he to remain silent.[57]

Several prominent practitioners wrote plague treatises. One was the *protomédico* and royal physician Andrés Zamudio (or Çamudio) de Alfaro, who first published his work in Seville in 1568 and, once the great plague arrived in the late 1590s, brought it out again, sending 100 copies to the city of Toledo.[58] He also appeared as the author of a 1599 response to a plague treatise by Cristóbal Pérez de Herrera, another *protomédico* whom we saw earlier advocating poor reform.[59] Antonio Ponce de Santa Cruz, the University of Valladolid medical professor

---

[55] ACC vol. 15, p. 564. His hometown suffered terribly in the plague; see Téllez Alarcia, "La peste Atlántica en Santo Domingo de la Calzada (1599)," 85–119.

[56] Miguel Martínez de Leyva, *Remedios preservativos y curativos para en tiempo de la peste; y otras curiosas experiencias* (Madrid: Viuda de Bartholomé de Nágera, 1597), 54v and 145r.

[57] Rodrigo de Cabrera, *Avisos Preservativos y declaraciones de los remedios para el contagio pestilente … Dirigido a la insigne Ciudad de Sevilla e impresos por su mandado* (Seville: el autor, 1599). A bound manuscript of three little treatises at the Biblioteca Nacional (ms. 11233) is probably from this same call for papers from the city.

[58] Julián Montemayor, "Una ciudad frente a la peste: Toledo a fines del XVI," in *La ciudad hispánica durante los siglos XIII al XVI: actas del coloquio celebrado en La Rábida y Sevilla del 14 al 19 septiembre de 1981*, 3 vols., Emilio Sáez, et al., eds. (Madrid: Universidad Complutense, 1985), 1113–31, p. 1124. The treatise is *Regimiento curativo y preservativo de pestilencia* (Madrid, 1599). The book may have been sent elsewhere as well, and I do not know if, as in Mercado's case, the crown was covering the expense. On Zamudio's life and publications see Davis and López Terrada, "Protomedicato y farmacia en Castilla."

[59] Andrés Zamudio de Alfaro, *Orden para la cura y preservación de las secas y carbuncos…* (Madrid: Luis Sánchez, 1599). Zamudio opines in this little pamphlet (in octavo) that Mercado had already said all there was to say about plague and there was no need for more; see fol. 2r. A total of eleven professionals seem to have contributed to this report.

who discovered Valladolid's first plague patient and was not believed by the city council, dedicated his own treatise to Mercado. (The facts in Valladolid spoke for themselves, he remarked bitterly in the introduction.)[60] Porcell, a pioneer in anatomical pathology, wrote an important medical handbook about the 1564–1565 plague in Zaragoza and his autopsies of victims.[61] Another distinguished professional, whose work is outside the geographic scope of this book, was Alonso de Freylas, a physician for the duke of Lerma's brother, Cardinal Bernardo de Rojas Sandoval, and who described the experience that Jaén underwent in 1602.[62] The treatise by Bocangel, one of Philip III's doctors, mainly concerned all the varied opinions about the nature of the disease.[63] A royal surgeon and doctor, Antonio Pérez, dedicated his treatise on the plague in Madrid to Zamudio; the book was published in 1598, making it once again obvious that the capital had been affected in 1597: "The diseases at present affecting Madrid and its region, though not entirely pestilent, being that they do not arise from corrupted air, are nevertheless malignant and pernicious and have the appearance of peste and the same signs, except that they are not as malignant nor as easily caught nor do they kill as many people …"[64] Dr. Valentin de Andosilla's meticulous observations about his time working in Navarre and La Rioja have appeared regularly throughout this book; as have those of Father Francisco Gavaldá, who was not a doctor but whose descriptions of hospitals during the 1647 plague in Valencia are among the best I have found.[65]

[60] Antonio Ponce de Santa Cruz, *Tractado de las causas y curacion de las fiebres con secas pestilenciales que han oprimido a Valladolid y otras ciudades de España* (Valladolid: Pedro de Merchan Calderón, 1600).

[61] Juan Tomás Porcell, *Información y curación de la peste de Zaragoza, y preservación contra peste en general* (Zaragoza, 1565).

[62] Alonso de Freylas, *Conocimiento, curación y preservación de la peste…* (Jaen: Fernando Díaz de Montoya, 1606). For more on Freylas's treatise see Gregorio García Sedeño, "La epidemia de peste que padeció la ciudad de Jaén en el año 1602," *Seminario médico* 2 (1953), 86–93.

[63] Bocángel, *Libro de las enfermedades malignas y pestilentes.*

[64] Antonio Pérez, *Breve tratado de peste, con sus causas, señales y curación…* (Madrid: Luis Sánchez, 1598), 7–8. Pérez formed part of the group of professionals, along with Zamudio, who upon the crown's request responded to Pérez de Herrera's treatise. On him see Alfredo Alvar Ezquerra, "Madrid reflejo de los problemas sanitarios de la peninsula: La peste de 1596 vista por un galeno de la corte," *Anales del Instituto de Estudios Madrileños* 20 (1983), 203–18. Doctor Pérez is not to be confused with the above-mentioned Antonio Pérez who was Philip II's disgraced secretary.

[65] Andosilla Salazar, *Libro en que se prueba con claridad el mal que corre por España*; Fray Francisco Gavaldá, *Memoria de los sucesos particulares de Valencia y su provincia en … tiempo de peste* (Valencia: Silvestre Esparsa, 1651).

Doctors made house calls. Two of Burgos corregidor Francisco de Valencia's staff members, Dr. Secada and the surgeon Lucas Vázquez, left behind notes on their rounds through town: María, married to Morales, had a dangerous *seca* in her axilla and should be taken out of the city along with her bed; Joan de la Eruz, who lived behind San Martín, had fever but no *secas* and probably could stay in his house; Melchor de Nieba's wife had a fever but she, too, could stay home because she had no *seca*; a servant of Gaspar Martínez's wife had a *seca* on her groin and should be removed from her house along with the linens; María Torres was all by herself and should be moved; while in the poorhouse a mother and daughter refused to be moved.[66]

Most patients were transferred from their homes into hospitals, which might mean a building for sick people but also for pilgrims, travelers, or poor people. Part of Philip II's medical reforms had included the consolidation of hospitals. Throughout the sixteenth century the Cortes had supported the effort to reduce the number of such institutions, though by 1598, amid the plague emergency, they had changed their mind and were now asking that new hospitals be established.[67] Before the reforms, there were more than 100 hospitals of one sort or another in Seville, reduced to eighteen in 1587.[68] Madrid in 1566 had fifteen, but in 1587 in theory (though not for long) was down to four.[69] There were no pre-existing

---

[66] BL Eg. fols. 350–1v, April 16, 1699, also transcribed in Francis Brumont, "La peste de 1599 en Burgos, una relación del regidor Andrés de Cañas," *BROCAR: Cuadernos de Investigación Histórica* 13 (1987), 155–66, p. 166.

[67] ACC vol. 16, p. 652, Capítulos Generales de las Cortes de [1592] fenecidas en [1598] y publicadas en [1604]; cap. 41: "Que se puedan fundar hospitales."

[68] Alexandra Parma Cook and Noble David Cook, *The Plague Files: Crisis Management in Sixteenth-Century Seville* (Baton Rouge, LA: Louisiana State University Press, 2009), 28. Some of the 100 "hospitals" may just have been a room with a few beds belonging to confraternities.

[69] Teresa Huguet-Termes, "Madrid hospitals and welfare in the context of the Hapsburg Empire," *Medical History* 29 (2009), 64–85. She refers to the General Hospital as a "thousand-headed dragon" (71) and describes more confusion and duplication than consolidation. See also J. Álvarez-Sierra, *Los hospitales de Madrid de ayer y de hoy*, vol. 3 (Madrid: Beneficiencia Municipal, 1952); José Luis de los Reyes Leoz, "Madrid, Laboratorio de Pobres: Asistencia y Control Social en la Corte de los Austrias," PhD diss., Universidad Autónoma de Madrid, 2003, chapter 5; Julio Gutiérrez Sesma, *La Beneficencia Municipal Madrileña: Un recorrido por su historia* (Madrid: Ayuntamiento de Madrid, 1994); and Luis Ortega Lázaro, "Antón Martín: el Hermano Antón Martín y su Hospital en la Calle Atocha de Madrid, 1500–1936." *Boletín Informativo Hermanos Hospitalarios*, supplement, no. 73 (February 1981). Madrid further had infirmaries for foreigners, and a women's hospital, La Pasión, later absorbed by the General Hospital. There is huge confusion in archival documents and the secondary literature between two alleged hospitals in Madrid: San Antón and Antón Martín. No archivist or historian has been able to resolve this question for me, and the Antón Martín archives burned during the Spanish Civil War. Cortes minutes and municipal documents refer to both,

plague hospitals. Rather, every time contagion swept through, normal hospitals were repurposed, with non-contagious patients being moved elsewhere, and additional buildings and facilities were requisitioned. There were separate buildings for the sick and the convalescent, patients being moved from the former to the latter, and medical staff resided in buildings outside the city walls. (Pamplona placed one of its city council members outside the wall so he could supervise the hospital.[70]) Locking the sick in their homes seems to have been the exception, and I am guessing that when that occurred it was because there was a shortage of hospital beds or the patients absolutely refused to be moved; in Madrid there were special quarantined houses on specific streets reserved for the sick except for "people of quality," who should not be sent there.[71] But clearly, there were times when people were not moved from their homes to hospitals: for example, after Miguel de Aspiroz's wife died in the couple's home in Pamplona, everyone who had been with her also was confined, and the wife's brother, who had arrived on the woman's third sick day, eventually also died after thirty-seven days indoors.[72]

Not everyone thought hospitals were a good idea. Alonso de Freylas, the cardinal's doctor, thought that even if the hospital were extramuros, which they all were, they were still liable to spread infection. Patients' terror of being dragged off to such places "full of confusion and bad smells" would lead them to conceal their illness, he argued, making the problem even worse. Instead, everyone should be allowed to stay in their houses, which should be marked and where they could be visited by physicians.[73] Juan de Silva, in a letter to his friend the Marquis of Velada, described Lisbon's hospital as being called "*la casa que llaman de la salud.*"[74]

But in fact most surviving descriptions are not of filth and chaos, though it is likely that no one reading this book would want to be a

---

sometimes interchangeably in the same entry. A hospital called San Antón was founded in 1438 at the end of Calle Hortaleza after an episode of plague; Álvarez-Sierra and Gutiérrez Sesma also refer to the Hospital del Fuego Usagroso, or San Antonio Abad, also on Calle Hortaleza, probably the same place. Antón Martín, meanwhile, was founded in 1552 by followers of Juan de Dios at the intersection now occupied by the Metro station of the same name. (All that's left is part of the Cine Doré, on Calle Santa Isabel.) It was sometimes referred to as Amor de Dios, as it faced onto that street. The two institutions may have merged administratively at some point, or maybe the old name was used for the newer one.

[70] Ignacio Baleztena, ed., "Relación de la Peste desta Ciudad de Pamplona del año 1599," *Príncipe de Viana* 22 (1946), 191.
[71] RAH Salazar leg. 23 carpeta 4 no. 11, fol. 386r.
[72] Baleztena, ed., "Relación de la peste desta ciudad de Pamplona," 377.
[73] Freylas, *Conocimiento, curación y preservación de la peste*, 174r–82r.
[74] BN ms. 6.198, fol. 129v, August 21, 1599.

patient in a 1599 hospital and that sanitary objectives probably were not always met. In Valladolid in January 1599, before the plague arrived, there were five hospitals (Niños de la Doctrina, Viejos de San Juan, Santa Barbara, Resurrección, and Desamparados), none of which was equipped to care for plague patients. They probably were housing the poor, whose illnesses began causing problems in spring, so the city council decided to put all the sick people in San Lázaro and San Bartolomé, both extramuros. Beds, either built or requisitioned, should be taken there, along with menial staff (nurses, litter bearers, clothesburners), who would be paid with the *sisa* on wine and meat. A few days later the councilman in charge of this job realized the poor patients could not all fit in San Lázaro, so they began requisitioning nearby inns at the same time as they hired medical staff. A month later they were overwhelmed and resolved to ask the king for permission to spend an additional 8,000 ducats on the sick patients (who were in what they referred to as the general hospital) and also to create a convalescent hospital, which they hoped could be financed with donations from guild members and with judicial fines from the Chancillería.[75] Bilbao waited even longer than Valladolid, and as late as August 1599 the city council minutes remark on the need to establish a hospital where *mal contagioso* patients could be confined and treated.[76] At least in theory, in most places patients were picked up upon the orders of neighborhood or parish bosses, checked in, relieved of their clothing and linens (though sometimes they arrived with their own bed), fed, and monitored. If they got better, they were moved to the convalescent hospital. A Segovia document remarks that children "cannot be picked up," so possibly they remained in their houses; Gavaldá describes mothers who tried to bribe officers in order to stay home with their children, but in that case it was the mothers being taken, not the children.[77]

A description of Madrid's plague hospital states that lamps were lit all night, men were separate from women, and there should be just one person per bed: "A doorman ensures that no one may enter except those who work in the hospital, even if they be parents, siblings, wife, husband, children, or relatives, given the risk that they might be infected and to avoid possible harm to patients with their presents and gifts of food that they might secretly bring in and give them."[78] The Zaragoza surgeon José

---

[75] AMVA sigs. 21-0 and 22-0, May 24, 28, June 18, 1599. It is possible that the city dropped the plan to solicit from the guilds.

[76] AFB libro 024, August 28, 1599.

[77] AGS-E leg. 184 doc. 183; Gavaldá, *Memoria de los sucesos particulares de Valencia*, part 8.

[78] RAH Salazar leg. 23 carpeta 4 no. 11, fols. 388v–90v. This refers to the Hospital of San Antón (sic).

Estiche was quoted in Chapter 4 as recommending a long and varied list of food for patients, who were fed several times a day.[79] Gavaldá described patients' beds in Valencia: "They were two feet [wide?] with four strips of wood instead of panels. On them there was a straw mattress, which was emptied and refilled with new straw, and every time a patient died the cloth was washed. [Most other places burned or buried the linens of the dead.] There was a pillow and two sheets, which were carefully sewn by Valencian nuns, the city having given them linen, which was often washed and mended." Gavaldá despaired thinking of the loneliness of those who died at home, unable to turn themselves over in their beds to reach the bit of chicken or mutton that a parish priest or a kindly neighbor might have left for them, standing at a distance, using a stick to poke the food closer to the bed. "Those who died in Hospitals did not suffer such grief," he wrote, "because they died in a bed, with a doctor and a surgeon, attended by a confessor, attended upon with love and charity and, once they died, piously buried."[80]

Around fifty years separated the great plague and the time Estiche and Gavaldá worked, so possibly things were more advanced in their day, though their descriptions more or less match the intentions of the earlier episode. Certainly the royal official overseeing the campaign in Alcalá de Henares in 1599 expressed similar attitudes regarding separation of sick from convalescent and men from women, food, and cleanliness.[81] Burgos city councilman Andrés Cañas, in his subsequent report, described the Nuestra Señora de Rebolleda hospital, which opened its doors in late January 1599, as a place with considerable organization, though eventually it would be inundated. At first it was staffed by just one woman and a man (un pícaro) who fed patients, along with four pícaros more who lived nearby at a shrine and carried the sick back and forth, with donkeys and draft horses carrying meals and medicines. The doctor whom Burgos had appointed to be in charge refused the honor, had a change of heart when the salary was increased, but then backed out again. His colleague Lic. Haro ended up taking charge of Rebolleda in exchange for 1,000 ducats a year. The staff grew to thirty people, and even that proved insufficient.[82]

The beds that Gavaldá described sound as if they were all the same and thus provided specifically to or by the hospital, but as has been mentioned several times, requisitioning was common. Already in fall 1597,

---

[79] José Estiche, *Tratado de la peste de Çaragoça en el año 1652* (Pamplona: Diego de Zabala, 1655), 53r–v.

[80] Gavaldá, *Memoria de los sucesos particulares de Valencia*, part 22.

[81] RAH Jesuitas 9-3662/182.   [82] Brumont, "La peste de 1599," 158–9.

during the early days of the administration of Diego Vargas Manrique in Burgos, properties were being seized. He told the disobedient town of Melgar to pick "the houses that you judge most suitable for treating the sick, and take them from their owners, who should go someplace else, and block the street or streets where the houses are located so that no one enter or leave the streets and houses … And I will give you the money with which to pay rent for the said houses and to close off the streets and pay the guards …"[83] Later, in April 1599, the Burgos city council ordered that bed linens and beds be taken from taverns in the city. Their value would be assessed by an official so owners could be properly paid. (Actual payment was another matter.) In this particular case, the linens were to be taken to "the house called San Martín de la Bodega," which had been taken over for convalescents once Rebolleda began overflowing. A cart was made and a draft horse purchased to move patients to this new site, which in time would also be overflowing and its director dead of plague.[84]

The house called San Martín de la Bodega turned out to be a complicated matter. It was owned by a noble family who were currently renting it out, along with its attached lands and meadows. The noblewoman Ana de la Torre, the wife of Francisco de Mena Vallejo, speaking on her own behalf and that of her daughter, Ana de Mena Vallejo, widow of Lope de Quevedo, wrote to the city of Burgos explaining that their father [probably Ana de la Torre's husband] was in jail "negotiating his lawsuit." The women had been hoping any day to move to the country house "to flee the horrendous and pestilential illness that is about and to take advantage of the said country house like they did in the year 1565, when many people died in the city, and more than that have died in this year of '99," adding that no one had died in the country house in 1565. But their plans were upset when the city council sent men to the country house to evict renters along with their wives, children, and servants, forcing them all to go to Burgos, where they lived in great fear of falling ill and dying. And indeed, Ana de la Torre wrote, most of them did lose their lives. The family owned a variety of larger and better houses in far more suitable places for a hospital, she pointed out. They were empty, no one would have had to be evicted, and all these irretrievable ills could have been avoided. Proving that she had contacts elsewhere, de la Torre pointed to the example of Madrid, which she said had established the San Antón hospital in a requisitioned building.[85] But Burgos did not listen, despite

---

[83] AMB-HI 3651, September 1597, fol. 33v.
[84] AMB-LA-130, March 27, April 6, 1599; AMB-HI 3653, July 4 (?) and July 30, 1599.
[85] She referred to "San Antón," and there is no indication it was requisitioned.

her and her daughter's pleas "for the love of God not to destroy them, to see that they were poor and had no wealth and no other refuge." Once the renters had been thrown out, Burgos established a hospital there for plague patients ("setting up loads of beds for the sick"[86]), and apparently the house and the property had been severely damaged, which was what led to the appeal. Pestiferous linens had been draped from trees and strewn throughout the fields, while silos, orchards, and woodpiles were depleted. As a result of all this, the surviving renters were suing the family, which in the meantime had suffered the terrible loss of Ana Vallejo y Mena (sic), who had died of plague along with two of her servants.[87]

Every city took over private dwellings and establishments to turn them into sick houses, and the ensuing legalities could go on for years. In the Basque Country, Bilbao seized a dwelling it owned on the Arenal that was being used as a storage depot by private citizens, who were told they had two days in which to move their belongings.[88] Pasajes de San Juan rented a three-story house owned by one Lorenzo Echabe; patients had to bring their own beds and leave them with the hospital once they left, dead or alive.[89] Fuenterrabia held a *concejo abierto* at which it decided to take over two private houses just outside the town, one to house the sick, the other to house the surgeons.[90] There are many examples in Pamplona: for example, the extramuros establishment where cloth was dyed (*la casa de los tintes*) was used as an infirmary.[91] The owner of another requisitioned extramuros house there, in the Magdalena neighborhood, sued the city after fire had devoured the entire building. The lawyer for plaintiff Juana de Sarasa, a widow, complained that the city had been negligent in responding to petitions and had managed to misplace documentation regarding the initial agreement between the parties. The city replied that the fire had been fortuitous, and if indeed linens and furniture had been lost, that was the result of Sarasa's

---

[86] Brumont, "La peste de 1599," 159; "se pusieron el mundo de camas para los enfermos..."

[87] BL Eg. 356, "Papeles tocantes a la ciudad de Burgos," vol. 2, fols. 360r–1v, memorial, nd.

[88] AFB libro 023, September 26, 1598. The building was to be used as a hospital where Bartolomé Masón could work, according to the minutes, though later the city still did not seem to have a proper facility.

[89] José Ramón Cruz Mundet, *"El mal que al presente corre": Gipuzkoa y la Peste (1597–1600)* (San Sebastián: Kutxa Fundazioa, 2003), 72–3.

[90] Cruz Mundet, *El mal que al presente corre*, 73–4, citing AMHondarrabia sec. A, neg. 1, leg. 20.

[91] Santiago Lasaosa Villanua, *El "Regimiento" municipal de Pamplona en el siglo XVI* (Pamplona: CSIC, 1979), 253.

carelessness in having left them there. Sarasa responded that sick patients had been streaming into her building and it was all she could do to stuff her belongings into a storage bin and get out. All her renters died. When the fire broke out, thirteen beds (holding seventeen patients) were salvaged, but neighbors would not approach the burning building with water because they were afraid. She sued for losses, she won, Pamplona appealed, and she won again.[92]

Valladolid also saw complaints over damages incurred during the long summer of 1599. A building near the Vitoria convent had been taken over and turned into a hospital called San Agustín, but the units had never been cleaned up; among other things a garden had been dug up and pestilent bodies buried there. As a result, no one would rent it anymore. The complainant, Melchor de Velasco, said he had spent more than 200 ducats trying to repair the apartments, which now had a bad name "and were regarded for a long time as horrendous." The city – by then the capital – apparently had agreed to pay forty ducats so that the plaster could be washed down but had never honored this commitment because, according to the city, at this point it was unclear who the legitimate owner actually was.[93] Another Valladolid building taken over during the plague was the *casa pública*, or the brothel. Originally it was taken in June 1599 to house the city's poor suffering from any disease; by July the city council minutes reflect that doctors, surgeons, barbers, and pharmacists were hired there, making it likely that by then it was a plague hospital, though there was discussion over whether it was for the sick or the convalescent.[94] Gavaldá reported that the *casa pública* of Valencia also was turned into a convalescent hospital for men.[95] The one in Burgos may well have too, given that in 1597 Melchor de los Reyes asked the city council to reduce the fee he paid to run it, given the alarming lack of clientele.[96]

---

[92] AGN TR Procesos 013101. A similar case concerning a burned house in Ganuza (Navarre) was heard by the same royal court in Pamplona; AGN TR Procesos 253319. Magdalena was a poor neighborhood, and probably for that reason was where most of the sick houses were; chronicler Martín de Senosaian blamed women there for having brought the disease in the first place after a marketing trip to Estella; Baleztena, ed., "Relación de la Peste desta Ciudad de Pamplona," 190.

[93] The incoming corregidor, Diego Sarmiento de Acuña, took care of the payment in May 1603; AMVA-CH 145-3 (ant. leg. 264).

[94] AMVA sigs. 21-0 and 22-0, June 3, July 15, 16, 1599.

[95] Gavaldá, *Memoria de los sucesos particulares de Valencia*, part 23.

[96] Paul Hiltpold, "Política paternalista y orden social en la Castilla del Renacimiento," *Cuadernos de Investigación Histórica BROCAR* 13 (1987), 129–40, p. 135, citing AMB actas, July 1, 1597, fol. 207.

If a city was looking to requisition large buildings that could be turned into infirmaries, religious establishments were the obvious place to start. Shrines, we have seen, served as supply depots and clearinghouses. Some also housed the sick, town officials, or hospital staff. But cities also had their eye on much larger structures, and the regular and secular clergy owning or inhabiting them were not always enthusiastic. During the 1580 influenza epidemic, when Seville considered setting up a new hospital in Triana, the Carthusians, whose real estate the city coveted, protested that their monastery "is a most principal house where they offer much hospitality, and such a multitude of people frequent it," including the papal legate, currently a guest, that the hospital should most definitely be housed elsewhere. The city appears to have ended up requisitioning a building owned by one Juan Pardo Tavera, who also complained and later sued.[97] Later on, when the great Castilian plague made its way down to Jerez de la Frontera, just south of Seville, the clergy first refused to pay extra taxes to fight the plague (they were already praying for the city's good health, the Archbishop of Seville pointed out, so there was no need to tax them as well, which in any case would have violated their privileges[98]). But additionally, they refused to cede buildings once the city's plague hospital became over-crowded. With virtually every neighborhood reporting plague victims and no place to put them other than in requisitioned homes and inadequate facilities that baked in the relentless summer heat, the city proposed a swap: the extramuros convent of Nuestra Señora del Carmen, also known as San Benito, would be vacated, and in exchange the city offered the Dominican friars what it said was a most desirable location inside the city, a place referred to as the *carpintería*.[99] The existing situation was untenable, the city said, with doctors, clergy, and staff besieged with patients and themselves dying, and the city also wished to separate the convalescent from the newly ill, who would now be moved to Nuestra Señora del Carmen. In fact, that same building had been used as a hospital during the epidemic of 1580–1582, though on that occasion there had been no polite negotiations, the city itself admitted; instead, officials had "violently and forcibly expelled the religious from their houses and monastery through one door while the newly sick entered through another." Then, too, the religious had been resettled within the city walls. Perhaps with the unpleasant earlier experience in mind, a variety of secular and regular

---

[97] Cook and Cook, *The Plague Files*, 81–2.
[98] RAH Jesuitas 9/3678/6, letter to the city of Jerez, April 18, 1600.
[99] The Carmen church was new, having been founded in 1587, initially in the San Benito shrine, and later moved.

clergy, the latter including the nuns of la Victoria, opposed the proposal even though, as the city pointedly told the archbishop, in seeking his support, "the friars of the said convent are our *vecinos.*" The corregidor, Antonio Montesinos, asked the archbishop for his assistance, telling him that he was spending more time on this dispute than on the plague itself. The situation had further been complicated, he said, by the fact that the Augustinian friars, "with the aim of preventing and twisting our intention," had decided to rent the very building where the city wanted the occupants of Carmen to go, possibly a preemptive move on behalf of their Dominican brethren, threatening to make the conflict truly endless. By the end of July, the archbishop somehow arranged the move in accordance with the beleaguered and grateful city's wishes.[100]

But for a good number of the patients who found their way to a hospital, it was all useless. They died quickly and painfully – though not alone, as Gavaldá pointed out. Receiving the sacraments from a priest or a friar, ensuring that theirs would be a good death, was obviously of the utmost importance to sixteenth-century Castilians.[101] Churches and religious orders throughout Castile, as we have seen, frequently argued in favor of keeping certain gates open at certain times to allow their members to visit outlying villages and infirmaries so they could kneel at bedsides, straighten the linens, touch patients' burning skin, recite the prayers, and send them on their way. Not all men of God were willing to risk their lives, though. Some orders withdrew part of their personnel so as to allocate resources where they were most needed, while fearful individual priests and friars sometimes simply vanished or refused to visit certain places. The noble exceptions are mentioned often: the Jesuit fathers who nearly all died in Burgos in 1565[102]; the Bishop of Pamplona, who remained when everyone else left; the secular and regular clergy in Alcalá de Henares. Less lucky places had to cast around for replacements once their clergy left. During the 1580 influenza epidemic in Seville, Discalced Carmelites came from Alcalá de Henares to lend a hand.[103] Burgos had to pay priests from elsewhere to administer last rites

---

[100] RAH Jesuitas 9/3680/117, a bundle of correspondence from June–July 1600. The description of friars being pushed out the door came from the city itself, June 14.

[101] Carlos M. N. Eire, *From Madrid to Purgatory: The Art and Craft of Dying in Sixteenth-Century Spain* (Cambridge University Press, 1995), 26–34 on the art of dying well and the multitude of published instructions during precisely these years.

[102] Francisco José González-Prieto, *La ciudad menguada: Población y economía en Burgos S. XVI y XVII* (Santander: Universidad de Cantabria, 2005), citing Lic. Joaquín de Villalba, *Epidemiología e historia cronológica de las pestes, contagios, epidemias y epizootias ...* (Madrid: Imprenta de D. Fermín Villalpando, 1803, vol. 1), 100. That human toll may have prompted the order to evacuate more places after 1597.

[103] Cook and Cook, *The Plague Files*, 100.

and hear confessions at the hospital, where the shortage was such that the admirable and hardworking archbishop himself had to visit every day. Nearby Dominicans, once they heard of the need, came to Burgos in April 1599 to help out not only in the hospital but to make house visits.[104]

The dead were recorded, one after another, in hospital after hospital, city after city. This is one aspect (the most important of all, one could argue) in which notaries are invisible, though they must have been nearby. When corregidores wrote to Philip III throughout the spring of 1599 with their weekly death tolls, the grim accounts most probably came to them via the notaries, who somehow got them from the hospitals and churches: "The list of those who have died in the city of Valladolid from June 1 and who were buried in the parish churches and monasteries and those who died in hospitals established to cure *secas*: In the month of June, 455 people were buried in the parishes and monasteries of Valladolid. There is no account of those who died that month in the hospitals. From July 1 to July 10 noon, 338 people died in the parishes and were buried there and in the monasteries. In that time 37 people died in the hospitals where *secas* are cured. From the 10th to the 16th, 345 people died in the parishes and were buried there and in the monasteries. In the hospitals 149 died of this illness. From the 17th to the 23rd of July, 509 died in the parishes. Eight died in the hospitals. From the 23rd to the 30th of the said month of July, 509 died in the parishes. In the said period 286 died in the hospitals. From July 31 to August 6, inclusive, 542 have died. In the hospitals 105 died."[105] That same summer, a Seville church official reported to his superior about the dire situation in Triana, attaching fifteen pages of weekly lists of admissions, deaths, and transfers to convalescent centers: "On Sunday, August 1, 11 people entered, 4 died. On Monday, August 2, 10 entered, 4 died. On Tuesday, August 3, 9 entered, 6 died. On Wednesday, August 4, 10 entered, 9 died … It appears that on the said days, 67 people entered and 54 died"[106] (Figure 7.1).

Few people other than doctors described any particular death or had occasion (or time) to record their losses. Miquel Parets, the Barcelona tanner, famously wrote of the death of his wife and three of his four

---

[104] Brumont, "Le coup de grace," 340; also in Brumont, "La Peste," 158–61.

[105] AGS-E leg. 184, doc. 288, mid-August 1599. Given the paucity of good records, it is difficult to draw comparisons to "normal" times in Valladolid, as explained by Bennassar, *Valladolid*, 193–5. Bennassar extrapolated from AGS documents and parish papers to conclude that Valladolid lost 17–18 percent of its population to the plague in 1599, or around 6,600 people; *Valladolid*, 202–5.

[106] RAH Jesuitas 9-3662/180 and 181; the writer was don Luis de Melgarejo, elsewhere identified as a church judge; the recipient might have been the archbishop. The numbers do not add up exactly.

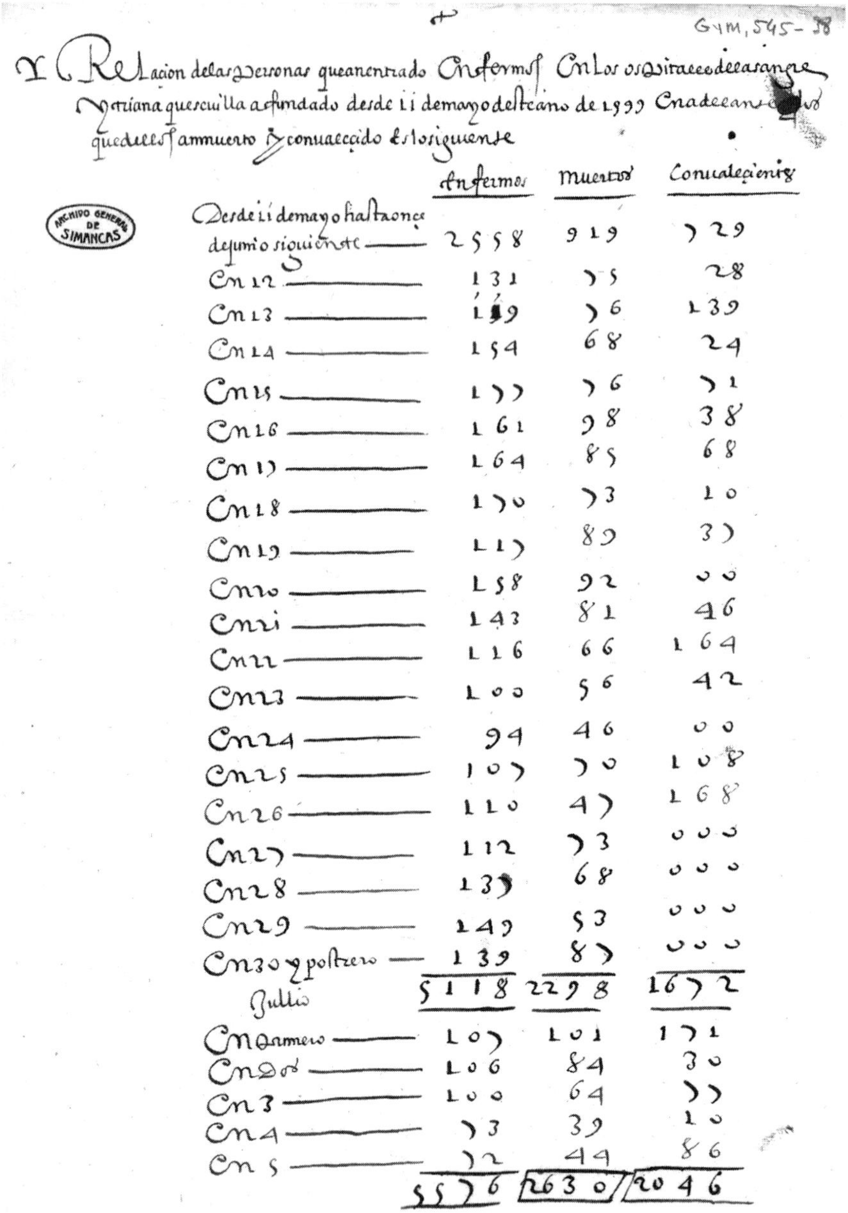

GYM, 545-58

Relacion delas personas que an entrado enfermos en los ospitales dela sangre y de sancta mariana que se cilla a fundado desde 11 de mayo del año de 1599 en adelante con declaracion delas que dellos an muerto y convalecido es lo siguiente

	enfermos	muertos	convalecientes
Desde 11 de mayo hasta once de junio siguiente	2558	919	729
En 12	131	75	28
En 13	189	76	239
En 14	154	68	24
En 15	177	76	71
En 16	161	98	38
En 17	164	85	68
En 18	170	73	10
En 19	117	89	37
En 20	158	92	00
En 21	143	81	46
En 22	116	66	164
En 23	100	56	42
En 24	94	46	00
En 25	107	70	108
En 26	110	47	168
En 27	112	73	000
En 28	133	68	000
En 29	149	53	000
En 30 y postrero	139	87	000
Julio	5118	2298	1672
En primero	107	101	171
En 2do	106	84	30
En 3	100	64	77
En 4	73	39	10
En 5	72	49	86
	5576	2630	2046

ARCHIVO GENERAL DE SIMANCAS

Figure 7.1 List of patients, the dead, and the convalescent in two Seville hospitals in May 1599.

children.[107] His sorrow surely was immense, but he did not waste many words on his loss. The man from Lominchar who requested his deceased father's job as notary said in passing that his father's wife and several children had been felled; those were the petitioner's mother and siblings. Nothing more was said. The upper classes had both more time and more words, but, again, it would be anachronistic to expect much expression of feeling. One of the future count of Gondomar's correspondents in Madrid, Gonzalo de Monroy, provided one description of a particular death, but it was more a question of news than of sorrow: "Sr. D. Juan Ramírez and I visited Sr. [Juan Sarmiento de] Valladares on Monday on business concerning the city gate, and we gave him a letter and he was fine and healthy, and the next day, Tuesday, he arose ill and lasted until yesterday, Saturday, when he died in the morning and they buried him in the afternoon. Some say he died of a side ache, others say it was *tabardillo*, and others *secas* … that attack the throat and the groin, and many people are dying, and they are shocked because they say it is known peste and those who have it do not last long. I did not go to his burial, but I heard that neither the president [of the Council of Castile] nor the other councillors dared enter the house, which is not a good sign."[108]

Sometimes, though rarely, tabulations of deaths throughout Castile and the occasional city council minutes included names. I will end this tour through pestilent plazas, streets, roads, town halls, social gatherings, deathbeds, and gravesites not by describing how guard posts and ad hoc hospitals were demolished, how bills were settled, or how treatises were reread and rewritten as towns awaited the next visitation, but rather by naming some of the hundreds of thousands of victims. I can do so at length for just one place, Pamplona, thanks to a brave chronicler who, as if a latter-day Homer reciting the names of the 240 fallen Trojan and Greek warriors, thought to take us, parish by parish and block by block, through the blasted wreckage of his city[109]:

In the fifth house [of the block in the Barrio de la Magdalena] Tripon and his wife died, also another woman named María Ordoque with three small children and a girl who was the dead Tripon's daughter, she was seven, she got sick and recovered, but in the Burlada infirmary a field worker named Gorriaran and his

[107] James S. Amelang, ed. and trans., *A Journal of the Plague Year: The Diary of the Barcelona Tanner Miquel Parets, 1651* (New York: Oxford University Press, 1991), 59–66.

[108] *Tabardillo* is typhus. RBP II-2145, doc. 9, Monroy, in Madrid, to Gondomar, in Toro, March 28, 1599. It is remarkable that the writer did not know that peste was certainly in Madrid and had been there since 1597. Sarmiento de Valladares had been a member of Philip II's council, was an inquisitor, and may have been *asistente* (corregidor) in Seville. Monroy may have been a councilman in Toro.

[109] Baleztena, ed., "Relación de la peste desta ciudad de Pamplona."

wife died, and a servant of theirs named María de Elia got sick and recovered …
In the first house around the corner from the Descalzos, Pedro de Sola, a farmer,
died with his three small children, his wife got sick but recovered… In the
Descalzos monastery a novice friar named Fray Miguel de San Miguel, from
the town of Echalar, died… And in another house that is a wall and a half away
from Galfasoro's house a man named Íñigo died and his wife, Graciana de
Erasso, got sick and recovered, and in the house of the said Galfasoro two of
his children got sick and died, on October 14 and 15 … On the 9th of October, in
the village of Osacayn, Mase Sancho de Cilveti, a surgeon, died, he was a *vecino* of
[Pamplona] and when the disease started he went down to the Barrio de la
Magdalena to heal the pestilent and then he withdrew to the said village, where
he died … And four gravediggers died, named Lejela and Mugorre and Montoya
[it is unclear which of the surnames is composite] and another came from Puente
de la Reina, he died on October 10, and in another house next to the basilica of
the Magdalena two disinfectors who had come from Puente de la Reina died …
Around the corner, in the home of *Relator* Elizondo, on October 4 Catalina de
Legassa got sick, she was the wife of Joanes de Uterga, a skinner, she had two
carbuncos on both breasts, she went to the Burlada infirmary, where she was
cured, and six days before she got sick her child whom she was nursing died
just a few days after getting sick … In the same street, across from the Monastery
of Carmen, in a house belonging to the General Hospital, on November 29 María
Martín de Eugui, the wife of Martín de Arrechea, a tailor, went to the Prado
infirmary along with two small children, all of them sick with peste; one of the two
children, Beltrán de Arrechea, died on November 29, and the other, named
Graciosa, died on November 30, and the said María Martín died on December
15 … And in another house next to the Jesuit school a woman named María de
Usechu got sick, with her two small children, they were taken to the infirmary
where they all died, and a few days later the wife of Sebastián de Aranalde, a
soldier, died, they said she had died in childbirth and later they saw that she had
died of Peste, because all the people in the said house were taken to a house
outside and four of her children got sick and were taken to the infirmary, where
they died, and another woman named María de Mongelos got sick and died in
the said infirmary, and another woman named Cathalina de Orsinaga died on
November 1 with an eight-year-old child and another one of six, also both sick
but they recovered, and María de Sorauren and they all lived in that
same house …

After it was all over, the survivors and the unscathed prayed, they gave
thanks, and – we are in Spain – they celebrated. August 1599 was a
nightmarish month in Valladolid, with hundreds dying every week. Yet
the following month, with carts still making their rounds picking up
bodies, the city council met to discuss "when we should hold the procession of thanksgiving."[110] In early October the council was still talking
about what to do with patients lingering in the hospital, but a week later

---

[110] AMVA sig. 22-0. The surviving minutes do not include an account of the procession
itself.

changed its tone now that the city was "entirely healthy" and went back to the much more pleasant subject of the procession. It was supposed to be held later that month, but one correspondent noted on the 23rd that the bishop was delaying because of a tiff with the corregidor, and the president of the Chancillería had canceled a bullfight scheduled for that same week, also apparently because of something the corregidor had done.[111] At long last on December 16 councilors held a special meeting devoted to the festivities at which they decided on the order of procession participants: first would come the musicians, then the police, then the city hall porters, wearing red velvet and silver insignias, and then the chief notary of the city, presumably clearing the way for the distinguished councilors themselves, with everyone on horseback. And they ordered, with more than a hint of wild jubilation, that town criers be sent out to all the squares and the usual places to summon everyone in Valladolid to the great celebration "with trumpets and drums – even if it's at night."

[111] RBP II-2138-6, Francisco de Vera (in Valladolid) to Gondomar, October 23, 1599.

Postmortem

The plague would return to Spain, of course, but less frequently as the years went by. The most infamous instance came in 1647–1651, when the disease coincided with fierce hunger, tremendous hardships, and social tumult, especially in Andalusia. Again the figure of a half-million deaths is often used. There was one final sweep in the early 1680s, and then, like most of the rest of Europe, the Iberian Peninsula was at long last left alone.[1]

The aftermath of each episode and of the entire monstrosity was not merely a time of stunned disbelief at having survived chaos and madness, and relief at now being able to get on with the business of social recovery and normality. As I began this book by saying, logic continued operating throughout. The political culture and institutional foundations that existed at the start of the cycle existed at the end of the cycle. They were tattered, they may have been temporarily altered, but they were there. Each round of disease provided new information, new chronologies, new confirmations. The repetition, the circularity, gave people tools. Though they might still harken back to Thucydides's images of parents and children abandoning one another, and though there might have been occasional language about thunderbolts from heaven, those familiar words do not signal immobility. Rather, they provided markers. When a member of the Cortes for Burgos, Jerónimo de Salamanca, wrote in 1597, "It was the peste of the year 1565 when all this city's troubles began, because twelve thousand people died then, and that is when its decline began," he was constructing a history of his town. Regardless of the fact that his genealogy quite conveniently omitted the crown's foreign and domestic policies, which surely bore more of the blame for the once great city's collapse, still, the past was both repetition and change, and that was useful.[2]

---

[1] The best-known work on the troubles in Andalusia is Antonio Domínguez Ortiz, *Alteraciones andaluzas* (Madrid: Narcea, 1973).

[2] Francisco José González-Prieto, *La ciudad menguada: Población y economía en Burgos S. XVI y XVII* (Santander: Universidad de Cantabria, 2005), 114.

Among the many insufficiently explored facets of plague in the early modern era, silence is particularly intriguing. It is true that epidemics might have been mentioned in seventeenth-century treatises proposing remedies for all of Spain's ills, often as a convenient metaphor. But in general, as I have said, plagues do not appear in contemporary city histories, which were annals of accomplishments, gifts, and beauty; and if the epidemics are by chance mentioned it is only as the exception that proved the rule, the interruption and denial of the true and glorious essence of whatever place the chronicler was extolling. Why did contemporaries not linger on these dreadful moments? I would like to tentatively suggest that, from their perspective, there was nothing much to say. The plague was cyclical, it was known, and it was no more awful than famine; in fact, maybe less so, because it was rarer and more selective. From our point of view, the coming of the plague was a spectacular occasion; from theirs, not so much, not because they did not care if their families and neighbors were felled or scarred but rather because it was familiar. It was part of their memory. They knew what to do. They inhabited a space between memory and expectation, a space in which practices and reasoning continued to function and change in accordance with need and knowledge. The structures that surrounded them – the monarchy, the interlocking ties among municipalities and the Cortes, the harvests, the taxes, the town meetings, judicial procedure – all would perdure.

By pointing to the virtual absence of written accounts, along with the occasional recourse to rhetorical flourish, I do not wish to suggest that language and literature were insignificant frills atop the solid fortress of social and economic relations. Rather, I want to call attention to that relative silence and respect it so as to better understand it. Word and event are not necessarily reflective, as they are often mistakenly represented in works of history in our own day, but nor is the former mere decoration. Words, along with silence, all made sense, they meant something, they served a purpose. They were part of the political and social culture that remained intact, and that is true beyond the plague and beyond the Iberian Peninsula. It was all of a piece, and it all lay within the vast landscape observed by that wheeling swallow with which I opened this tour of death and destruction, of words and deeds, of wiliness and survival.

Glossary

alcabala:	sales tax, a lump sum generally negotiated by the crown and the Cortes
alcalde:	judicial official
alcalde mayor:	local appellate judge, but also frequently a sort of mayor
alguacil:	constable, police
alhóndiga:	public granary
arrendador:	leasee, usually of a tax
arroba:	liquid measure of around sixteen liters
azumbre:	liquid measure of around two liters
boticario:	apothecary, pharmacist
calenturas:	fever
carbunco:	a sore, possibly a bubo; almost always appears with *secas*
celemín:	dry measure equal to around 4.6 liters, or one-twelfth of a fanega
censo:	annuity, mortgage loan (the word also means census)
cerca:	barrier
concejo abierto:	open town meeting
consejo:	council
corregidor:	royal governor
ducat:	gold coin worth 375 maravedies or 11 reales
fanega:	variable dry measure divided into 12 celemines; approximately 1.5 bushels or an English bushel. Also refers to the land on which a fanega of grain was sown.
forastero:	outsider, foreigner
hidalgo:	a person with noble status exempt from certain taxes
landres:	tumors or swellings in lymph glands
legua:	league, 5.5 kms

limosna:	alms
maravedi:	basic unit of currency, smallest unit of account
mesón:	inn
millones:	extraordinary negotiated grants by the Cortes to the crown
morisco:	baptized former Muslim
muro:	wall
natural:	native-born
oidor:	civil judge
pechero:	taxpayer
posada:	rooming house
pósito:	public granary
pregón:	public announcement cried aloud
pregonero:	town crier
propios:	municipal properties
procurador general:	elected municipal official representing the interests of the commons before municipal councils
protomedicato:	medical advisory board established by the king
protomédico:	crown-appointed physician, usually prominent, who had medical, administrative, and/or didactic responsibilities
real:	silver coin worth 34 maravedíes
regidor:	city council member
renta:	rents, here generally revenues on particular royal taxes
ropa:	clothing, bed linens
seca:	growth or swelling under arms, neck, groin that was drained. *Secas y carbuncos* was the general euphemism for buboes.
señorío:	lordship, seigneurial estate or jurisdiction; the term was also used to address cities and Basque provincial governments
sisa:	local excise tax, usually on foodstuffs
sobras:	excess amounts from alcabalas collection
tabardillo:	typhus
tapia:	wall, barrier
vara:	staff or scepter
vecino:	citizen, neighbor, resident

Bibliography

Accampo, Elinor and Jeffrey H. Jackson. "Introduction," *French Historical Studies* 36:2 (Spring 2013), 165–74.

Actas de las Cortes de Castilla [ACC] vols. 15, 16, 17, 18, 19. Madrid, various years.

Adelman, Jeremy. *Worldly Philosopher: The Odyssey of Albert O. Hirschman.* Princeton, NJ: Princeton University Press, 2013.

Álamos de Barrientos, Baltasar. *Discurso político al Rey Felipe III al comienzo de su reinado.* Barcelona: Anthropos, 1990.

Alfani, Guido. *Calamities and the Economy in Renaissance Italy: The Grand Tour of the Horsemen of the Apocalypse,* trans. Christine Calvert. New York: Palgrave, 2013.

Alfani, Guido and Tommy E. Murphy. "Plague and lethal epidemics in the pre-industrial world," *The Journal of Economic History* 77:1 (March 2017), 314–43.

Alfonso X, Rey. *Las siete partidas,* 3 vols. [facs. of version edited by Lic. Gregorio López, Salamanca: Andrea de Portonariis, 1555]. Madrid: Boletín Oficial del Estado, 1974.

Alonso Cortés, Narciso. "Gómez Pereira y Luis Mercado," in his *Miscelánea Vallisoletana,* vol. 5, pp. 65–117. Valladolid: Emilio Zapatero, 1930.

"Médicos vallisoletanos," in his *Miscelánea Vallisoletana,* vol. 3, pp. 133–46. Valladolid: Cuesta, 1921.

Alvar Ezquerra, Alfredo, "Castilla, 1590: Tres historias particulares," *Studia Historica. Historia Moderna* 17 (1997), 121–43.

"Espacios sociales del Madrid de los Austrias," in *El Madrid de Velázquez y Calderón: Villa y Corte en el siglo XVII,* vol. 1, Miguel Morán and Bernardo J. García, eds. Madrid: Ayuntamiento de Madrid, 2000, 151–68.

"Estructuras socioeconómicas de Madrid y su entorno en la segunda mitad del siglo XVI." PhD diss., Universidad Complutense de Madrid, 1988.

"Madrid reflejo de los problemas sanitarios de la peninsula: La peste de 1596 vista por un galeno de la corte," *Anales del Instituto de Estudios Madrileños* 20 (1983), 203–18.

"Viajes, posadas, caminos y viajeros," in *La Vida Cotidiana en la España de Velázquez,* José N. Alcalá-Zamora, ed. Madrid: Temas de Hoy, 1989, 109–26.

Álvarez González, María Isabel. "Historia y evolución del voto de la ciudad al Señor San Roque," in *San Roque voto de la ciudad: IV centenario, 1599–1999,*

Paco del Caño and Miguel Angel Clemente, eds. Segovia: Parroquia de San Millán, 1999.

Álvarez-Sierra, J. *Los hospitales de Madrid de ayer y de hoy*, vol. 3. Madrid: Beneficiencia Municipal, 1952.

Amelang, James S., ed. and trans. *A Journal of the Plague Year: The Diary of the Barcelona Tanner Miquel Parets, 1651*. New York: Oxford University Press, 1991.

Andosilla Salazar, Valentin de. *Libro en que se prueba con claridad el mal que corre por España ser nuevo y nunca visto: su naturaleza, causas, pronósticos, curacion, y la prouidencia que se deue tener con él ...* Pamplona: Mathias Mares, 1601.

Appleby, Andrew B. "The disappearance of plague: a continuing puzzle," *The Economic History Review* 33:2 (May 1980), 161–73.

"Disease or famine? Mortality in Cumberland and Westmorland 1580–1640," *The Economic History Review* 26:3 (1973), 403–32.

"Epidemics and famine in the Little Ice Age," *Journal of Interdisciplinary History* 10:4, *History and Climate: Interdisciplinary Explorations* (Spring 1980), 643–63.

Aram, Bethany. *Juana the Mad: Sovereignty and Dynasty in Renaissance Europe.* Baltimore, MD: Johns Hopkins University Press, 2005.

Aranda de, Juan. *Lugares comunes de conceptos, dichos, y sentencias, en diversas materias.* Seville: Juan de León, 1595, fol. 25.

Arazuri, José Joaquín. "La peste en Pamplona en tiempos de Felipe II," *Príncipe de Viana* 35:134–5 (1974), 179–92.

Arrizabalaga, Jon, John Henderson and Roger French. *The Great Pox: The French Disease in Renaissance Europe.* New Haven, CT: Yale University Press, 1997.

Artola, Miguel. *La hacienda del Antiguo Régimen.* Madrid: Alianza Editorial, 1982.

Azero y Aldovera, Fr. Miguel de. *Tratado de los funerales y de las sepulturas, que presenta al excelentísimo señor Conde de Floridablanca.* Madrid: Imprenta Real, 1736.

Bailey, Gauvin Alexander, et al., eds. *Hope and Healing: Painting in Italy in a Time of Plague, 1500–1800.* Worcester: Clark University, et al., distr. University of Chicago Press, 2005.

Baleztena, Ignacio, ed. "Relación de la peste desta ciudad de Pamplona del año 1599," *Príncipe de Viana* 22 and 23 (1946), 186–201 and 377–94. [Chronicle by Martín de Senosiain].

Ball, Rachael. "'Beautiful serpents' and 'cathedras of pestilence': antitheatrical traditions, gendered decline, and political crisis in early modern Spain and England," *Sixteenth Century Journal* 46:3 (2015), 541–63.

Ballesteros Rodríguez, Juan. *La peste en Córdoba.* Córdoba: Diputación Provincial, 1982.

Bamji, Alexandra. "Health passes, print and public health in early modern Europe," *Social History of Medicine* (December 2017), https://doi.org/10.1093/shm/hkx104 (accessed January 2019).

Bartlett, Robert. *Why Can the Dead Do Such Great Things? Saints and Worshippers from the Martyrs to the Reformation.* Princeton, NJ: Princeton University Press, 2013.

Belmonte Diaz, José. *La Ciudad de Ávila: Estudio histórico*, 2nd ed. Ávila: Caja de Ahorros, 1987.

Bennassar, Bartolomé. "Organisation municipale et communautés d'habitants en temps de peste: L'exemple du nord de l'Espagne et de la Castille a la fin du XVIe siecle," *Annales de la Faculté des Lettres et Sciences Humaines de Nice* 9–10 (December 1969), 139–43.

Recherches sur les grandes Épidémies dans le nord de l'Espagne a la fin du XVIe siècle. Problèmes de documentation et de méthode. Paris: SEVPEN, 1969.

Valladolid au siècle d'or: Une ville de Castille et sa campagne au XVI siècle. Paris: Mouton, 1967.

Bernaldez, Andrés. *Historia de los reyes católicos Don Fernando y Doña Isabel*. [Biblioteca de Autores Españoles, vol. 70.] Madrid: Atlas, 1953, 567–773.

Bernardos Sanz, José Ubaldo. *Trigo castellano y abasto madrileño: Los arrieros y comerciantes segovianos en la Edad Moderna*. Valladolid: Junta de Castilla y León, 2003.

Bianucci, Raffaella, et al. "Quinto Tiberio Angelerio and new measures for controlling plague in 16th-century Alghero, Sardinia," *Emerging Infectious Diseases*, September 2013 (open access journal published online monthly by the Centers for Disease Control and Prevention). http://wwwnc.cdc.gov/eid/article/19/9/12-0311_article (accessed January 2019).

Bilinkoff, Jodi. *The Avila of Saint Teresa*. Ithaca, NY: Cornell University Press, 1989.

Biraben, Jean-Noël. *Les hommes et la peste en France et dans les pays Européens et Méditerranéens*, 2 vols., Paris: Mouton and École des Hautes Études en Sciences Sociales, 1975.

Bocángel [also Bocangelino], Nicolás. *Libro de las enfermedades malignas y pestilentes, causas, pronósticos, curación y preservación*. Madrid: Luis Sánchez, 1600.

Boccaccio, Giovanni. *The Decameron*, trans. G. H. McWilliam. London: Penguin Books, 1972.

Boeckl, Christine M. *Images of Plague and Pestilence: Iconography and Iconology*. Kirksville, MO: Truman State University Press, 2000.

Bossy, John. *Christianity in the West, 1400–1700*. Oxford: Oxford University Press, 1985.

Bowers, Kristy Wilson. "Balancing individual and communal needs: plague and public health in early modern Seville," *Bulletin of the History of Medicine* 81:2 (Summer 2007), 335–58.

Plague and Public Health in Early Modern Seville. Rochester, NY: University of Rochester Press, 2013.

"Tradition and innovation in Spanish medicine: Bartolomé Hidalgo de Agüero and the *Vía Particular*," *Sixteenth Century Journal* 41:1 (2010), 29–47.

Brett, Annabel S. *Changes of State: Nature and the Limits of the City in Early Modern Natural Law*. Princeton, NJ: Princeton University Press, 2011.

Brooke, Christopher. *Philosophic Pride: Stoicism and Political Thought from Lipsius to Rousseau*. Princeton, NJ: Princeton University Press, 2012.

Brozzi, Mario. *Peste, Fede e Sanita in Una Cronaca Cividalese del 1598*. Milan: Dott. A. Giuffrè, 1982.

Brumont, Francis. *Campo y Campesinos de Castilla la Vieja en Tiempos de Felipe II.* Madrid: Siglo Veintiuno, 1984.

"Le coup de grace: la peste de 1599," in *La Ciudad de Burgos: Actas del Congreso de Historia de Burgos.* Valladolid: Junta de Castilla y León, 1985, 335–42.

"Le pain et la peste: Épidémie et subsistances en Vieille-Castille a la fin du XVIe siècle," *Annales de Démographie Historique.* Paris: EHESS, 1989, 207–20.

"La peste de 1599 en Burgos, una relación del regidor Andrés de Cañas," *BROCAR: Cuadernos de Investigación Histórica* 13 (1987), 155–66.

Burke, Peter. "History of events and the revival of narrative," in *New Perspectives on Historical Writing*, 2nd ed., Peter Burke, ed. Cambridge: Polity, 2001, 283–300.

"How to be a counter-reformation saint," in *The Historical Anthropology of Early Modern Italy: Essays on Perception and Communication.* Cambridge: Cambridge University Press, 1987, 48–62.

Butler, Alban. *Butler's Lives of the Saints*, Herbert Thurston and Donald Attwater, eds. New York: P. J. Kenedy and Sons, 1956, 4 vols.

Butler, Thomas. "Review article: plague gives surprises in the first decade of the 21st century in the United States and worldwide," *American Journal of Tropical Medicine and Hygiene* 89:4 (October 2013), 788–93.

Cabrera, Rodrigo de. *Avisos preservativos y declaraciones de los remedios para el contagio pestilente … dirigido a la insigne ciudad de Sevilla e impresos por su mandado.* Seville: el autor, 1599.

Calvi, Giulia. *Histories of a Plague Year: The Social and the Imaginary in Baroque Florence*, trans. Dario Biocca and Bryant T. Ragan, Jr. Berkeley, CA: University of California Press, 1989.

Campos Díez, María Soledad. *El Real Tribunal del Protomedicato Castellano (Siglos XIV–XIX).* Cuenca: Universidad de Castilla-La Mancha, 1999.

Camps Clemente, Manual, et al. "La peste de 1599 en Loporzano (Huesca)," in *Actas del IX Congreso Nacional de Historia de la Medicina*, vol. 2. Ayuntamiento de Zaragoza, 1991, 459–73.

Camus, Albert. *The Plague*, trans. Stuart Gilbert. New York: The Modern Library, 1948.

Caño, Paco del and Miguel Ángel Clemente, eds. *San Roque, voto de ciudad: IV centenario, 1599–1999.* Segovia: Parroquia de San Millán, 1999.

Carabias Torres, Ana-María. "Estudiantes burgaleses y colegios mayores (siglo XVI), in *La Ciudad de Burgos: Actas del Congreso de Historia de Burgos.* León: Junta de Castilla y León, 1985, 33–60.

Carmichael, Ann G. "Contagion theory and contagion practice in fifteenth-century Milan," *Renaissance Quarterly* 44:2 (Summer 1991), 213–56.

Plague and the Poor in Renaissance Florence. Cambridge University Press, 1986.

"Plague persistence in Western Europe: a hypothesis," *The Medieval Globe* 1:1 (2014), 159–92.

Carreras Panchón, Antonio. "Dos testimonios sobre la epidemia de peste de 1599 en Valladolid," *Asclepio* 25 (1973), 351–57.

La Peste y Los Médicos en la España del Renacimiento. Salamanca: Universidad de Salamanca, 1976.

Casado Alonso, Hilario. *Señores, mercaderes y campesinos: La Comarca de Burgos a Fines de la Edad Media.* Valladolid: Junta de Castilla y León 1987.

Casey, James. *Early Modern Spain: A Social History.* London: Routledge, 1999.

"'Queriendo poner mi ánima en carrera de salvación': la muerte en Granada (siglos xvii–xviii)," *Cuadernos de Historia Moderna Anejos* (2001), 17–43.

"Spain: a failed transition," in *The European Crisis of the 1590s*, Peter Clark, ed. London: George Allen and Unwin, 1985, 209–28.

Castillo de Bovadilla, Jerónimo. *Política para corregidores y señores de Vasallos.* Madrid: Instituto de Estudios de Administración Local, 1978, 2 vols. [facs. of Antwerp: Juan Bautista Verdussen, 1704). [1597]

Cavallo, Sandra and Tessa Storey. *Healthy Living in Late Renaissance Italy.* Oxford: Oxford University Press, 2013.

Cavillac, Michel. "El Madrid 'utópico' (1597–1600) de Cristóbal Pérez de Herrera," *Bulletin Hispanique* 104:2 (2002), 627–44.

Ceccarelli, Giovanni. "Risky business: theological and canonical thought on insurance from the thirteenth to the seventeenth century," *Journal of Medieval and Early Modern Studies* 31:3 (Fall 2001), 607–58.

Cervantes, Miguel de. *El ingenioso hidalgo don Quijote de la Mancha*, 2 vols., Luis Andrés Murillo, ed. Madrid: Clásicos Castalia, 1978.

Champion, Justin. "Epidemics and the built environment in 1664," in *Epidemic Disease in London*, J. A. I. Champion, ed. London: Centre for Metropolitan History, 1993, 35–52.

Chase, Marilyn. *The Barbary Plague: The Black Death in Victorian San Francisco.* New York: Random House, 2003.

Chaves Martín, Miguel Angel. *Apuntes para una historia de la medicina en Segovia.* Segovia: Colegio Oficial de Médicos de Segovia, 1998.

Christian, William A. Jr. *Local Religion in Sixteenth-Century Spain.* Princeton, NJ: University Press, 1981.

"Provoked religious weeping in early modern Spain," in J. Davis, ed., *Religious Organization and Religious Experience.* London: Academic Press, 1982, 97–114.

Christensen, Peter. "'In These Perilous Times': plague and plague policies in early modern Denmark," *Medical History* 47 (2003), 413–50.

Cipolla, Carlo M. *Faith, Reason, and the Plague in Seventeenth-Century Tuscany.* New York: W. W. Norton & Company, 1979.

Clark, Peter, ed. *The European Crisis of the 1590s.* London: George Allen and Unwin, 1985.

Clouse, Michele L. *Medicine, Government and Public Health in Philip II's Spain: Shared Interests, Competing Authorities.* Farnham: Ashgate, 2011.

Cobb, Richard. *The Police and the People: French Popular Protest, 1789–1820.* Oxford: Clarendon Press, 1970.

Cohn, Samuel K., Jr. "The Black Death: end of a paradigm," *American Historical Review* 107:3 (June 2002), 703–38.

Cultures of Plague: Medical Thinking at the End of the Renaissance. Oxford: Oxford University Press, 2010.

Cohn, Samuel K., Jr. and Guido Alfani, "Households and plague in early modern Italy," *Journal of Interdisciplinary History* 38:2 (Autumn 2007), 177–205.

Colmenares, Diego de. *Historia de la insigne ciudad de Segovia y compendio de las historias de Castilla*. [1637], 2 vols. Segovia: Academia de Historia y Arte de San Quirce, 1970.

Cook, Alexandra Parma and Noble David Cook. *The Plague Files: Crisis Management in Sixteenth-Century Seville*. Baton Rouge, LA: Louisiana State University Press, 2009.

Covarrubias Orozco, Sebastián de. *Tesoro de la lengua castellana o española*, Felipe C. R. Maldonado, ed. Madrid: Editorial Castalia, 1995 [Madrid 1611].

Crawshaw, Jane L. Stevens. *Plague Hospitals: Public Health for the City in Early Modern Venice*. Farnham: Ashgate, 2012.

Cruz, Anne J. *Discourses of Poverty: Social Reform and the Picaresque Novel in Early Modern Spain*. Toronto: University of Toronto Press, 1999.

Cruz Mundet, José Ramón, *"El mal que al presente corre": Gipuzkoa y la peste (1597–1600)*. San Sebastián: Kutxa Fundazioa, 2003.

Cubitt, Geoffrey. *History and Memory*. Manchester: Manchester University Press, 2007.

Cummins, Neil, M. Kelly and C. O' Grada. "Living standards and plague in London, 1560–1665," *Economic History Review* 69:1 (2016), 3–34.

Davis, Charles and J. E. Varey. *Los corrales de comedias y los hospitales de Madrid, 1574–1615. Estudio y documentos*. Madrid: Támesis, 1997.

Davis, Charles and María Luz López Terrada, "Protomedicato y farmacia en Castilla a finales del siglo XVI: Edición crítica del *Catálogo de las cosas que los boticarios han de tener en sus boticas*, de Andrés Zamudio de Alfaro, protomédico general (1592–1599)," *Asclepio* 62:2 (July–December 2010), 579–626.

Daza, Juan. *Estracto de las ocurrencias de la peste que aflixió a esta ciudad (jerez de la frontera) en el año 1518 hasta el de 1523*, Hipólito Sancho, ed. Ayuntamiento de Jerez de la Frontera, 1938 [1523].

Dean, Katharine R., et al. "Human ectoparasites and the spread of plague in Europe during the Second Pandemic," *PNAS [Proceedings of the National Academy of Sciences]* 115(6), February 2018, 1304–9, http://doi.org/10.1073/pnas.1715640115 (accessed January 2019).

Defoe, Daniel. *A Journal of the Plague Year*. New York: Meridian Classic, 1960.

Diaz, José Simón. "Otro romance sobre desgracias logroñesas," *Berceo* 23 (1952), 241–52.

Diez de la Lastra y Diez de Güemes, Gonzalo, "Datos curiosos para la historia de la ciudad, sacados de los Libros de Actas del Excmo. Ayuntamiento de la M. N. y M. M. L. Ciudad de Burgos, Cabeza de Castilla y Cámara de S. M.: Peste bubónica en Burgos en el año 1565," *Boletin de estadística e información del Excmo. Ayuntamiento de Burgos*, no. 261 (November 1943) to no. 272 (October 1944).

Díez Sanz, Enrique. *La Tierra de Soria: un universo campesino en la Castilla oriental del siglo XVI*. Madrid: Siglo Veintiuno, 1995.

Ditchfield, Simon. "Introduction," in *Christianity and Community in the West: Essays for John Bossy*, Simon Ditchfield, ed. Aldershot: Ashgate, 2001.

"Tridentine Worship and the Cult of the Saints," in *Cambridge History of Christianity*, vol. 6, *Reform and Expansion, 1500–1660*, R. Po-chia Hsia, ed. Cambridge University Press, 2014, 201–24.

Ditrich, Hans. "The transmission of the Black Death to Western Europe: a critical review of the existing evidence," *Mediterranean Historical Review* 32:1 (June 2017), 25–40.

Domínguez Ortiz, Antonio. *Alteraciones andaluzas*. Madrid: Narcea, 1973.

The Golden Age of Spain, 1516–1659, trans. James Casey. New York: Basic Books, 1971.

Eamon, William. "The Canker Friar: piety and intrigue in an era of new diseases," in *Piety and the Plague: From Byzantium to the Baroque*, Franco Mormando and Thomas Worcester, eds. Kirkesville, MO: Truman State University Press, 2007, 156–76.

"Plagues, healers and patients in early modern Europe," *Renaissance Quarterly* 52:2 (Summer 1999), 474–86.

Einbinder, Susan L. *After the Black Death: Plague and Commemoration Among Iberian Jews*. Philadelphia, PA: University of Pennsylvania Press, 2018.

Eiras Roel, Antonio, "Migraciones internas y medium-distance en España en la Edad Moderna," in *Migraciones internas y medium-distance en la Península Ibérica, 1500–1900*, Antonio Eiras Roel and Ofelia Rey Castelao, eds. Santiago de Compostela: Xunta de Galicia, 1994, vol. 2, 37–84.

Eire, Carlos M. N. *From Madrid to Purgatory: The Art and Craft of Dying in Sixteenth-Century Spain*. Cambridge University Press, 1995.

Elliott, J. H. "The decline of Spain," in J. H. Elliott, *Spain and Its World, 1500–1700*. New Haven, CT: Yale University Press, 1989, 217–40.

"Self-Perception and Decline in Early Seventeenth-Century Spain," in J. H. Elliott, *Spain and Its World, 1500–1700*. New Haven, CT: Yale University Press, 1989, 241–61.

Enciclopedia General Ilustrada del País Vasco, vol. 53. San Sebastián: Editorial Auñamendi, 2001.

Ermus, Cindy. "The Spanish plague that never was: crisis and exploitation in Cádiz during the *peste* of Provence," *Eighteenth-Century Studies* 49:2 (Winter 2016), 167–93.

Escobar, Manuel. *Tratado de la essencia, causas y curacion de los bubones y carbucos pestilentes … Dirigido al Doctor don Alonso de Agreda del Supremo Consejo y Comisario general de las cosas tocantes a la salud del Reyno*. Alcalá de Henares: Justo Sánchez Crespo, 1600.

Escudero de Cobeña, Matías. *Relación de casos notables ocurridos en la Alcarria…* [1582], Francisco Fernández Izquierdo, ed. Guadalajara: Ayuntamiento de Almonacid de Zorita, 1982.

Estiche, José. *Tratado de la peste de Çaragoça en el año 1652*. Pamplona: Diego de Zabala, 1655.

Fernández Albaladejo, Pablo. *Fragmentos de Monarquía*. Madrid: Alianza Universidad, 1992.

Fernández Álvarez, José Manuel. *Peste y supervivencia en Oviedo (1598–1599)*. Oviedo: KRK, 2003.

Fernández Álvarez, Manuel. "Burgos en el siglo XVI," in *La ciudad de Burgos: Actas del congreso de historia de Burgos. MC aniversario de la fundación de la ciudad, 884–1984*. León: Junta de Castilla y León, 1985, 221–32.

Fernández Hidalgo, María del Carmen and Mariano García Ruipérez, *Los pósitos municipales y su documentación*. Madrid: Abad, 1989.

Fernández-Santamaría, J. A. *Reason of State and Statecraft in Spanish Political Thought, 1595–1640*. Lanham, MD: University Press of America, 1983.

Feros, Antonio. *Kingship and Favoritism in the Spain of Philip III, 1598–1621*. Cambridge University Press, 2000.

Flynn, Maureen. *Sacred Charity: Confraternities and Social Welfare in Spain, 1400–1700*. Ithaca, NY: Cornell University Press, 1989.

Fortea Pérez, José Ignacio. "Las ciudades de la Corona de Castilla en el Antiguo Régimen: Una revisión historiográfica," *Boletín de la Asociación de Demografía Histórica* 13:3 (1995), 19–59.

"Entre dos servicios: La crisis de la Hacienda Real a fines del siglo XVI. Las alternativas fiscales de una opción política (1590–1601)," *Studia Historica, Historia Moderna* 17 (1997), 63–90.

"Hacienda real y haciendas locales en la crisis del siglo XVII: el ejemplo de Castilla," in *Le crisi finanziarie: Gestione, implicazione e conseguenze nell'età preindustriale*. Florence: Firenze University Press, 2016, 109–32.

"Impuestos o Servicios? Las Cortes de Castilla y la política fiscal de Felipe II (1573–1598)," in his *Las Cortes de Castilla y León bajo los Austrias: una interpretación*. Valladolid: Junta de Castilla y León, 2008, 161–90.

Monarquía y Cortes en la Corona de Castilla: las ciudades ante la política fiscal de Felipe II. Valladolid: Cortes de Castilla y León, 1990.

Fortea Pérez, José Ignacio, ed. *Imágenes de la diversidad: El mundo urbano en la Corona de Castilla (S. XVI–XVIII)*. Santander: Universidad de Cantabria, 1997.

Fortea Pérez, José Ignacio and Juan E. Gelabert, eds. *Ciudades en conflicto (Siglos XVI–XVIII)*. Valladolid: Junta de Castilla y León, 2008.

Freylas, Alonso de. *Conocimiento, curación y preservación de la peste...* Jaén: Fernando Diaz de Montoya, 1606.

Fuentenebro Zamarro, Francisco. *Cantalejo: Aldea, villa, ciudad*, 3 vols. Segovia: Caja de Segovia, 2007.

Gage, Kenneth L. and Michael Y Kosoy, "Natural history of plague: perspectives from more than a century of research," *Annual Review of Entomology* 50:1 (2005), 505–28.

Gallagher, Catherine and Stephen Greenblatt. *Practicing New Historicism*. Chicago, IL: University of Chicago Press, 2000.

García Arenal, Mercedes. *Ahmad al-Mansur, The Beginnings of Modern Morocco*. Oxford: One World, 2009.

García España, Eduardo. "Censos de población españoles," *Estadística española* 33:128 (1991), 441–500.

García España, E. and Annie Molinié-Bertrand, *Censo de Castilla de 1591: Estudio analítico*. Madrid: Instituto Nacional de Estadística, 1986.

García López, Juan Catalina, ed. *Relaciones topográficas de España. Relaciones de pueblos que pertenecen hoy a la Provincia de Guadalajara*. In *Memorial Histórico Español*, vols. 41–3, 45–7. Madrid: various publishers, 1903–1915.

García Sanz, Angel. "Auge y decadencia en España en los siglos XVI y XVII: Economía y sociedad en Castilla," *Revista de Historia Económica* 3:1 (1985), 11–27.

Desarrollo y crisis del Antiguo Régimen en Castilla la Vieja: Economía y sociedad en tierras de Segovia de 1500 a 1814. Madrid: Akal, 1986.

"Castile 1580–1650: economic crisis and the policy of 'reform'," in *The Castilian Crisis of the Seventeenth Century: New Perspectives on the Economic and Social History of Seventeenth-Century Spain*, I. A. A. Thompson and Bartolomé Yun Casalilla, eds. Past and Present Publications, Cambridge University Press, 1994, 13–31.

García Sedeño, Gregorio. "La epidemia de peste que padeció la ciudad de Jaén en el año 1602," *Seminario médico*, 2 (1953), 86–93.

Garriga, Carlos. *La audiencia y las chancillerías castellanas (1371–1525). Historia política, régimen jurídico y práctica institutional.* Madrid: Centro de Estudios Constitucionales, 1994.

Garza, Randal P. *Understanding Plague: The Medical and Imaginative Texts of Medieval Spain.* New York: Peter Lang, 2008.

Gavaldá, Fray Francisco, de la Orden de los Predicadores. *Memoria de los sucesos particulares de Valencia y su provincia en … tiempo de peste.* Valencia: Silvestre Esparsa, 1651.

Gelabert, Juan E. *La bolsa del rey: Rey, reino y fisco en Castilla (1598–1648).* Barcelona: Crítica, 1997.

Giginta, Miguel de. *Tratado de remedio de pobres*, Félix Santolaria Sierra, ed. Barcelona: Ariel Historia, 2000 [Coimbra 1579].

Gil, Xavier, "City, Communication and Concord in Renaissance Spain and Spanish America," in *Athenian Legacies: European Debates on Citizenship*, Paschalis M. Kitromilides, ed. Florence: Olschki Editore, 2014, 195–222.

Gómez Nieto, Leonor. *Ritos funerarios en el Madrid medieval.* Madrid: Ak-Mudayna, 1991.

Gómez-Rivero, Ricardo. "La superintendencia de construcción naval y fomento forestal en Guipúzcoa (1598–1611)," *Anuario de Historia del Derecho Español* 56 (1986), 591–636.

González, Nazario, S. J. *Burgos: La ciudad marginal de Castilla.* Burgos: Aldecoa, 1958.

González Alonso, Benjamin. *El corregidor castellano 1348–1808.* Madrid: Instituto de Estudios Administrativos, 1970.

González de Cellorigo, Martín *Memorial de la política necesaria y util restauración a la República de España.* Madrid: Instituto de Cooperación Iberoamericana, 1991 [1600].

González Monjarrés, Miguel Angel. *Andrés Laguna y el humanismo médico.* Salamanca: Junta de Castilla y León, 2000.

González Navarro, Ramón. *Felipe II y las reformas constitutionales de la Universidad de Alcalá de Henares.* Madrid: Sociedad Estatal para la Conmemoración de los Centenarios de Felipe II y Carlos V, 1999.

González-Prieto, Francisco José. *La ciudad menguada: Población y economía en Burgos S. XVI y XVII.* Santander: Universidad de Cantabria, 2005.

Goodman, David. *Spanish Naval Power, 1589–1665: Reconstruction and Defeat.* Cambridge University Press, 1997.

Gracián, Baltasar, *El criticón, tercera parte, en el invierno de la vejez.* Antwerp: Verdussen, 1669, 284–5.

Grafe, Regina. *Distant Tyranny: Markets, Power, and Backwardness in Spain, 1650–1800.* Princeton, NJ: Princeton University Press, 2012.

Granjel, Luis S. "Las epidemias de peste en la España del siglo XVII," *Asclepio* 29 (1977), 17–36.

Greene, Monica H. "Editor's introduction," *The Medieval Globe* 1:1 (2014), 27–62.

Guerrero Mayllo, Ana. *Familia y vida cotidiana de una élite de poder: Los regidores madrileños en tiempos de Felipe II.* Madrid: Siglo Veintiuno, 1993.

Gutiérrez Nieto, Juan Ignacio. "El pensamiento económico, político y social de los arbitristas," in *Historia de la Cultura Española 'Menéndez Pidal',* José María Jover Zamora, ed. vol. 1, *El Siglo del Quijote.* Madrid: Espasa Calpe, 1996, 329–465.

Gutiérrez Sesma, Julio. *La beneficencia municipal madrileña: Un recorrido por su historia.* Ayuntamiento de Madrid, 1994.

Harrison, Mark. *Contagion: How Commerce Has Spread Disease.* New Haven, CT: Yale University Press, 2012.

Heras Santos, José Luis de las. *La justicia penal de los Austrias en la Corona de Castilla.* Salamanca: Universidad de Salamanca, 1991.

Hernando, Máximo Diago. "Pastores, carreteros, y arrieros," in *El mundo social de Isabel la Católica: La sociedad castellana a finales del siglo XV,* Miguel Angel Ladero Quesada, ed. Madrid: Editorial Dykinson, 2004, 219–27.

Herrero Martínez de Azcoitia, Guillermo. "La población palentina en la Edad Moderna," in *Historia de Palencia, vol. II: Edades Moderna y Contemporánea.* Exma. Diputación Provincial de Palencia, 1984, 62–82.

  "La población palentina en los siglos XVI y XVII," *Publicaciones de la Institución Tello Téllez de Meneses* 15 (1956), 5–30.

Herzog, Tamar. *Defining Nations: Immigrants and Citizens in Early Modern Spain and Spanish America.* New Haven, CT: Yale University Press, 2003.

  "Los Naturales de España: Entre el Viejo y Nuevo Mundo," in *De la Republica Hispaniae: Una vindicación de la cultura política en los reinos ibéricos en la primera modernidad,* Francisco José Aranda Pérez and José Damião Rodriguez, eds. Madrid: Silex Universidad, 2008, 409–22.

Hibberd, Robert and J. B. Owens. "Before highway maps: creating a digital research infrastructure based on sixteenth-century Iberian places and roads." *Bulletin for Spanish and Portuguese Historical Studies* 40:1 (December 2015).

Hillgarth, J. N. *The Mirror of Spain, 1500–1700: The Formation of a Myth.* Ann Arbor, MI: University of Michigan Press, 2000.

Hiltpold, Paul Jacob. "Burgos in the Reign of Philip II: The Ayuntamiento, Economic Crisis, and Social Control, 1550–1600." PhD diss., University of Texas at Austin, 1981.

Hiltpold, Paul. "Política paternalista y orden social en la Castilla del Renacimiento," *Cuadernos de Investigación Histórica BROCAR* 13 (1987), 129–40.

"The price, production, and transportation of grain in early modern Castile," *Agricultural History* 63:1 (Winter 1989), 73–91.

Hirschman, Albert O. *Exit, Voice, and Loyalty: Responses to Decline in Firms, Organizations and States.* Cambridge, MA: Harvard University Press, 1970.

Howard, Keith David. "The anti-Machiavellians of the Spanish baroque: a reassessment," *LATCH: A Journal for the Study of the Literary Artifact in Theory, Culture or History* 5 (2012), 106–19.

Huguet-Termes, Teresa. "Madrid hospitals and welfare in the context of the Hapsburg Empire," *Medical History* 29 (2009), 64–85.

Hutton, Patrick H. *History as an Art of Memory.* Hanover, NH: University Press of New England, 1993.

Imízcoz, José María, "Hacia nuevos horizontes: 1516–1700," in *Historia de Donostia-San Sebastián,* Miguel Artola, ed. San Sebastián: Nerea, 2004, 37–63.

Jones, Colin. "Plague and its metaphors in early modern France," *Representations* 53 (Winter 1996), 97–127.

Jütte, Daniel. *The Strait Gate: Thresholds and Power in Western History.* New Haven, CT: Yale University Press, 2015.

Kagan, Richard L. *Clio and the Crown: The Politics of History in Medieval and Early Modern Spain.* Baltimore, MD: Johns Hopkins University Press, 2009.

  Lawsuits and Litigants in Castile, 1500–1700. Chapel Hill, NC: University of North Carolina Press, 1981.

  Students and Society in Early Modern Spain. Baltimore, MD: Johns Hopkins University Press, 1974.

  "A world without walls: city and town in colonial Spanish America," in *City Walls: The Urban Enceinte in Global Perspective,* James D. Tracy, ed. Cambridge University Press, 2000, 117–52.

Kemp, E. W. *Canonization and Authority in the Western Church.* London: Oxford University Press, 1948.

Laguna, Andrés, *Discurso breve sobre la cura y preservacion de la pestilencia* [1556], ed. and introduction by Juan Riera Palmero. Segovia: Diputación Provincial, 1999.

Laqueur, Thomas W. *The Work of the Dead: A Cultural History of Mortal Remains.* Princeton, NJ: Princeton University Press, 2015.

Lasaosa Villanua, Santiago. *El "Regimiento" municipal de Pamplona en el siglo XVI.* Pamplona: CSIC, 1979.

Lázaro Ruiz, Mercedes "La peste de 1600 en la ciudad de Calahorra" in *Calahorra: Bimilenario de su fundación.* Madrid: Ministerio de Cultura, 1984, 367–86.

León Pinelo, Antonio de. *Anales de Madrid (desde el año 447 al de 1658),* ed. Pedro Fernández Martín. Madrid: Instituto de Estudios Madrileños, 1971.

  Anales de Madrid de León Pinelo. Reinado de Felipe III, años 1598 a 1621, Ricardo Martorell Téllez-Giron, ed. Madrid: Estanislao Maestre, 1931.

Lerner, Robert E. "Fleas: some scratchy issues concerning the Black Death," *Journal of the Historical Society* 8:2 (June 2008), 205–28.

Little, Lester K. "Plague historians in lab coats," *Past and Present* 213 (November 2011), 267–90.

Longrigg, James. "Epidemic, Ideas and Classical Athenian society," in *Epidemics and Ideas: Essays on the Historical Perception of Pestilence*, Terence Ranger and Paul Slack, eds. Past and Present Publications, Cambridge University Press, 1992, 21–44.

Lorenzo Pinar, Francisco Javier. *Muerte y ritual en la edad moderna: El caso de Zamora*. Salamanca: Universidad de Salamanca, 1991.

López Ferreiro, Lic. P. Antonio. *Historia de la Santa A. M. Iglesia de Santiago de Compostela*, vol. 8. Santiago: Seminario Conciliar Central, 1905.

López Gómez, José Manuel and Esther Pardiñas de Juana, "Un testimonio inédito sobre la epidemia de peste de 1565 en Burgos," *Boletín de la Institución Fernán González* 221 (2000/2), 227–50.

López Gurpegui, Félix-Tomás, "Valentín de Andosilla Salazar: *El mal nuevo nunca visto*. Año 1601," *Berceo* 164 (2013), 41–68.

López Piñero, José María, "Los orígenes de los estudios sobre la salud pública en la España renacentista," *Revista española de salud pública* 80:5 (September–October 2006), 445–56.

López Terrada, María Luz. "Médicos, cirujanos, boticarios y albéitares," in *Historia de la ciencia y la técnica en la Corona de Castilla*, vol. 3, José María López Piñero, ed. Valladolid: Junta de Castilla y León, 2002, 161–85.

Machiavelli, Niccolo. *The Prince*, trans. George Bull. New York: Penguin Books 1961.

MacIntyre, Ben. "Blitz spirit dates back to the Black Death," *The Times*, December 23, 2017.

MacKay, Ruth, *The Baker Who Pretended to be King of Portugal*. Chicago, IL: University of Chicago Press, 2012.

   The Limits of Royal Authority: Resistance and Obedience in Seventeenth-Century Castile. Cambridge University Press, 1999.

Malcolm, Noel. *Reason of State, Propaganda and the Thirty Years' War*. Oxford: Clarendon Press, 2007.

Manetsch, Scott M. *Calvin's Company of Pastors: Pastoral Care and the Emerging Reformed Church, 1536–1609*. Oxford: Oxford University Press, 2013.

Manzoni, Alessandro, *The Betrothed*, trans. Bruce Penman. London: Penguin Books, 1972.

Marcos Martín, Alberto. "Medina del Campo 1500–1800: an historical account of its decline," in *The Castilian Crisis of the Seventeenth Century: New Perspectives on the Economic and Social History of Seventeenth-Century Spain*, I. A. A. Thompson and Bartolomé Yun Casalilla, eds. Past and Present Publications, Cambridge University Press, 1994, 220–48.

Mariscal, Nicasio. *El doctor Juan Tomas Porcell y la peste de Zaragoza de 1564*. Madrid: Instituto de España, Real Academia Nacional de Medicina, 1945, 2nd ed. [1st. ed. 1914].

Marshall, Louise. "Manipulating the sacred: image and plague in renaissance Italy," *Renaissance Quarterly* 47:3 (Autumn 1994), 485–532.

Martin, A. Lynn. *Plague? Jesuit accounts of epidemic disease in the 16th century*. Kirksville, MO: Sixteenth Century Journal Publishers, 1996.

Martin Galindo, José Luis, "Arrieros leoneses," *Archivos leoneses* 19 (January–July 1956), 153–79.

Martín García, Gonzalo, "Las murallas en la Edad Moderna: obras de manteni-miento y nuevas construcciones," in *La Muralla de Ávila*. Madrid: Funda-ción Caja Madrid, 2003, 115–82.

Martínez Gil, Fernando. *Muerte y sociedad en la España de los Austrias*. Madrid: Siglo Veintiuno Editores, 1993

Martínez Hernández, Santiago. *El Marqués de Velada y la Corte en los Reinados de Felipe II y Felipe III: Nobleza cortesana y cultura política en la España del Siglo de Oro*. Salamanca: Junta de Castilla y León, 2004.

Martínez de Leyva, Miguel. *Remedios preservativos y curativos para en tiempo de la peste; y otras curiosas experiencias*. Madrid, 1597.

Martorell Téllez-Girón, Ricardo. *Aportaciones al estudio de la población de Madrid en el siglo XVII*. Madrid: Estanislao Maestre, 1930.

Martz, Linda. *Poverty and Welfare in Habsburg Spain: The Example of Toledo*. Cambridge University Press, 1983.

Maza Zorilla, Elena. "Villalón de Campos y la peste de 1599," *Cuadernos de investigación histórica* 2 (1978), 363–86.

Méndez Nieto, Juan. "Sobre cierta pestilencia del año 1558 y sus remedios médicos," [1607], in *Los siglos XVI–XVII: cultura y vida cotidiana*, Luís Enrique Rodríguez-San Pedro Bezares and José Luis Sánchez Lora, eds. Madrid: Síntesis, 2000, 265–68.

Meneses, Alonso de. *Repertorio de caminos*. Madrid: Ministerio de Educación y Ciencia, 1976 [Alcalá de Henares, 1576].

Mercado, Luis. *El libro de la peste del Dr. Luis Mercado con un estudio preliminar acerca del autor y sus obras por el Dr. Nicasio Mariscal*. [Biblioteca Clásica de la Medicina Española, vol. 1] Madrid: Imp. de Cosano, 1921.

Molénat, Jean-Pierre. "Chemins et ponts du Nord de la Castille au temps des Rois Catholiques," *Mélanges de la Casa de Velázquez* 7 (1971), 115–62.

Molina Piñedo, Ramón. "La epidemia de peste de 1599 en Yunquera de Henares y el voto que se hizo a la Virgen de la Granja," *Wad-al-Hayara: Revista de Estudios de Guadalajara* 7 (1980), 241–56.

Molinié-Bertrand, Annie. *Au siècle d'or l'Espagne et ses Hommes. La Population du Royaume de Castille au XVI siècle*. Paris: Economica, 1985.

Monreal Cia, Gregorio. *Las instituciones públicas del Señorío de Vizcaya (hasta el siglo XVIII)*. Bilbao: Diputación de Vizcaya, 1974.

Monsalvo Antón, José María, "Poder municipal y mercado urbano precapitalista: Una introducción a las ordenanzas de la renta del peso mayor del concejo de Salamanca," *Salamanca: Revista Provincial de Estudios* 8 (April–June 1983), 63–76.

Montáñez Matilla, María. *El Correo en la España de los Austrias*. Madrid: CSIC, 1953.

Monteano, Peio J. *La ira de Dios: Los navarros en la era de la peste (1348–1723)*. Pamplona: Pamiela, 2002.

Montemayor, Julián. *Tolède entre fortune et déclin (1530–1640)*. Limoges: PULIM, 1996.

"Una ciudad frente a la peste: Toledo a fines del XVI," in *La ciudad hispánica durante los siglos XIII al XVI: actas del coloquio celebrado en La Rábida y Sevilla del 14 al 19 septiembre de 1981*, 3 vols., Emilio Sáez, et al., eds. Madrid: Universidad Complutense, 1985, 1113–31.

Morales Padrón, Francisco, ed. *Memorias de Sevilla (1600–1687)*. Córdoba: Monte de Piedad y Caja de Ahorros de Córdoba, 1981.

Moxó y Ortiz de Villajos, Salvador. "La venta de alcabalas en los reinados de Carlos I y Felipe II," *Anuario de historia del derecho español* 41 (1971), 487–554.

Munkhoff, Richelle. "Searchers of the dead: authority, marginality, and the interpretation of plague in England, 1574–1665," *Gender and History* 11:1 (April 1999), 1–29.

Muñoz Garrido, Rafael and Carmen Muñiz Fernández, eds. *Fuentes legales de la medicina española (Siglos XIII–XIX)*. Salamanca: Universidad de Salamanca, 1969.

Murugarren Zamora, Luis, "La peste en Guipuzcoa (1597–1599)," *Boletin de la Real Sociedad Bascongada de Amigos del Pais* 40:1–2 (1984), 247–69.

Nadeau, Carolyn A. *Food Matters: Alonso Quijano's Diet and the Discourse of Food in Early Modern Spain*. Toronto: University of Toronto Press, 2016.

Nader, Helen. *Liberty in Absolutist Spain*. Baltimore, MD: Johns Hopkins University Press, 1990.

Nakajima, Satoko. "Breaking ties: marriage and migration in sixteenth-century Spain." PhD diss., University of Tokyo, 2011.

Nalle, Sara T. *God in La Mancha: Religious Reform and the People of Cuenca, 1500–1650*. Baltimore, MD: Johns Hopkins University Press, 1992.

Naphy, William G. "Plague-spreading and a magisterially controlled fear," in *Fear in Early Modern Society*, William G. Naphy and Penny Roberts, eds. Manchester: Manchester University Press, 1997, 28–43.

Naphy, William G. Plagues, *Poisons and Potions: Plague-Spreading Conspiracies in the Western Alps c. 1530–1640*. Manchester: Manchester University Press, 2002.

Nirenberg, David. *Communities of Violence: Persecution of Minorities in the Middle Ages*. Princeton: NJ: Princeton University Press, 1996.

Odriozola Oyarbide, Lourdes, *Construcción naval en el País Vasco, siglos XVI–XIX: Evolución y análisis comparativo*. San Sebastián: Diputación Foral de Gipuzkoa, 1997.

Orella y Unzué, José Luis de. "El Cardenal Diego de Espinosa, consejero de Felipe II, el monasterio de Iranzu y la peste de Pamplona en 1566," *Príncipe de Viana* 36:140–41 (1975), 565–610.

Ortega Lázaro, Luis, "Antón Martín: el Hermano Antón Martín y su Hospital en la Calle Atocha de Madrid, 1500–1936," supplement 73 of *Boletín Informativo Hermanos Hospitalarios* (February 1981).

Ortego Gil, Pedro. "La pena de vergüenza pública (siglos XVI–XVIII): Teoría legal castellana y práctica judicial gallega," *Anuario de derecho penal y ciencias penales* 51:1–3 (1998), 153–204.

Parker, Geoffrey. *Felipe II: La biografía definitiva*. Barcelona: Planeta, 2013.

"La crisis de la década de 1590 a debate: Felipe II, sus enemigos y el cambio climático," in *Hacer historia desde Simancas: Homenaje para José Luis Rodríguez de Diego*, Alberto Marcos Martín, ed. Valladolid: Junta de Castilla y León, 2011, 643–70.

Global Crisis: War, Climate Change and Catastrophe in the Seventeenth Century. New Haven, CT: Yale University Press, 2013.

Pepys, Samuel. *London's Great Plague*. Stroud: Amberly Publishing, 2014.

Pérez, Antonio. *Breve tratado de peste, con sus causas, señales y curación…* Madrid: Luis Sánchez, 1598.

Pérez de Herrera, Cristóbal. *Amparo de Pobres*, ed. and introduction by Michel Cavillac. Madrid: Espasa-Calpe, 1975.

Pérez Moreda, Vicente. *Las crisis de mortalidad en la Espana interior (Siglos XVI–XIX)*. Madrid: Siglo Veintiuno, 1980.

"The plague in Castile at the end of the sixteenth century and its consequences," in *The Castilian Crisis of the Seventeenth Century: New Perspectives on the Economic and Social History of Seventeenth-Century Spain*, I. A. A. Thompson and Bartolomé Yun Casalilla, eds. Past and Present Publications, Cambridge University Press, 1994, 32–59.

"La poblacion de la ciudad de Segovia en las épocas moderna y contemporanea," in *Segovia 1088–1988: Congreso de Historia de la Ciudad. Actas*. Segovia: Junta de Castilla y León, 1988, 721–36.

Pérez Moreda, Vicente and David S. Reher, "La población urbana española entre los siglos XVI y XVIII: Una perspectiva demográfica," in *Imágenes de la Diversidad: El mundo urbano en la Corona de Castilla (S. XVI–XVIII)*, José Ignacio Fortea Pérez, ed. Santander: Universidad de Cantabria, 1997, 129–63.

Pérez Pastor, Cristóbal. *Bibliografía madrileña; o descripción de las obras impresas en Madrid (siglo xvi)*, vol. 1. Madrid: Tip. de los Huérfanos, 1891.

Phillips, Carla Rahn and William D. Phillips, Jr. *Spain's Golden Fleece: Wool Production and the Wool Trade from the Middle Ages to the Nineteenth Century*. Baltimore, MD: Johns Hopkins University Press, 1997.

Phillips, William D., Jr., "Spain's northern shipping industry in the sixteenth century," *The Journal of European Economic History* 17:2 (Fall 1988), 267–301.

Pimoulier, Amaia Nausia. *Virgines o putas? 500 años de adoctrinamiento femenino (1512–2012)*. San Sebastián: Haran 7, 2012.

Pocock, J. G. A. *The Machiavellian Moment: Florentine Political Thought and the Atlantic Republican Tradition*. Princeton, NJ: Princeton University Press, 2003.

"The origins of study of the past: a comparative approach," *Comparative Studies in Society and History* 4:2 (1962), 209–46.

Ponce de Santa Cruz, Antonio. *Tractado de las causas y curacion de las fiebres con secas pestilenciales que han oprimido a Valladolid y otras ciudades de España*. Valladolid: Pedro de Merchan Calderón, 1600.

Pons Ibáñez, Fernando. "Epidemia de peste en Logroño (Año 1599)," *Berceo* 73 (1964), 387–406.

Porcell, Juan Tomás. *Información y curación de la peste de Zaragoza, y preservación contra peste en general*. Zaragoza: Viuda de Bartholomé de Nágera, 1565.

Porras Arboledas, Pedro Andrés. "La práctica mercantil maritima en el Cantábrico Oriental (siglos XV–XIX). Primera parte," *Cuadernos de Historia del Derecho* 7 (2000), 13–127.

Preto, Paolo. *Epidemia, paura e politica nell'Italia moderna*. Rome: Editori Laterza, 1987.

Peste e società a Venezia nel 1576. Vicenza: Neri Pozza Editore, 1978.

Priotti, Jean-Philippe. *Bilbao et ses marchands au XVIe siècle: Genèse d'une croissance*. Villeneuve d'Ascq: Presses Universitaires du Septentrion, 2004.

Los Echávarri: Mercaderes bilbaínos del Siglo de Oro, trans. Fernando Quincoces. Bilbao: Diputación Foral de Bizkaia, 1996.

Pullan, Brian. "Plague and Perceptions of the Poor in Early Modern Italy," in Terence Ranger and Paul Slack, eds. *Epidemics and Ideas: Essays on the Historical Perception of Pestilence*. Past and Present Publications, Cambridge University Press, 1992, 101–23.

Quesada, Santiago. *La idea de ciudad en la cultura hispana de la Edad Moderna*. Barcelona: Universitat de Barcelona, 1992.

Ranger, Terence and Paul Slack, eds. *Epidemics and Ideas: Essays on the Historical Perception of Pestilence*. Past and Present Publications, Cambridge University Press, 1992.

Raoult, Didier, et al. "Plague: history and contemporary analysis," *Journal of Infection* 66 (2013), 18–26.

Redondo, Augustin. "Le pestiféré ou divers aspects du refus de l'Autre au XVIème siecle," in *Les representations de l'Autre dans l'espace ibérique et ibéroamericain*, Augustin Redondo, ed. Paris: Presses de la Sorbonne Nouvelle, 1991, 121–37.

Reher, David S. "Castilla y la crisis del siglo XVII: Contextos demográficos para un ajuste de larga duración," in *Madrid, Felipe II y las ciudades de la Monarquía*, Enrique Martínez Ruiz, ed. vol. 2, 347–74. Madrid: Actas, 2000.

"Relación de la antigüedad y sitio de Medina del Campo y sus ferias y de la contratación de ellas, y del estado que tienen hasta hoy 18 de octubre de 1606," in *Colección de documentos inéditos para la historia de España*, vol. 17. Madrid: Imprenta la Viuda de Calero, 1850, 541–74.

Reyes Leoz, José Luis de los. "Madrid, laboratorio de pobres: Asistencia y control social en la Corte de los Austrias," PhD diss., Universidad Autónoma de Madrid, 2003.

Ribadeneira, Pedro. *Tratado de la religión y virtudes que debe tener el príncipe christiano para gobernar y conservar sus estados. Contra lo que Nicolas Machiavello y los políticos deste tiempo enseñan* ... Madrid: P. Madrigal, 1595.

Ringrose, David. *Madrid and the Spanish Economy, 1560–1850*. Berkeley, CA: University of California Press, 1983.

Risse, Guenter B. *Plague, Fear, and Politics in San Francisco's Chinatown*. Baltimore, MD: Johns Hopkins University Press, 2012.

Rodríguez-San Pedro Bezares, Luis Enrique. *Los siglos XVI–XVII: cultura y vida cotidiana*. Madrid: Síntesis, 2000.

Rojo Vega, Anastasio. "La caridad, factor de mortalidad en la epidemia de peste de 1599 en Valladolid," *Medicina y Historia* 30 (1989), 1–16.

Enfermos y sanadores en la Castilla del siglo XVI. Universidad de Valladolid, 1993.

Medicina barroca vallesoletana: Antonio Ponce de Santa Cruz y Alfonso de Santa Cruz. Universidad de Valladolid, 1984.

Rosenberg, Charles E. "Framing disease: illness, society, and history," in *Explaining Epidemics and Other Studies in the History of Medicine*, Charles E. Rosenberg, ed. Cambridge University Press, 1992, 305–18.

Rothschild, Emma. *Economic Sentiments: Adam Smith, Condorcet, and the Enlightenment.* Cambridge, MA: Harvard University Press, 2001.

Rowe, Erin Kathleen. *Saint and Nation: Santiago, Teresa of Ávila, and Plural Identities in Early Modern Spain.* University Park, PA: Pennsylvania State University Press, 2011.

Rueda Fernández, José Carlos. "Aportación al estudio de la extensión geográfica de la epidemia de peste de los años 1596–1602: Un documento inédito del archivo municipal de Zamora," *Studia historica. Historia moderna* 2 (1984), 95–113.

Ruiz Astiz, Javier. "El castigo de destierro en la Navarra moderna: el caso de los implicados en disórdenes públicos." *UNED: Espacio, Tiempo y Forma, series IV, Historia moderna* 23 (2010), 129–51.

Ruiz Martín, Felipe. "Credit procedures for the collection of taxes in the cities of castile during the sixteenth and seventeenth centuries: the case of Valladolid," in *The Castilian Crisis of the Seventeenth Century: New Perspectives on the Economic and Social History of Seventeenth-Century Spain,* I. A. A. Thompson and Bartolomé Yun Casalilla, eds. Past and Present Publications, Cambridge University Press, 1994, 169–81.

Sánchez González, Ramón. "Hambres, pestes y guerras. Elementos de desequilibrio demográfico en la comarca de La Sagra durante la época moderna," *Hispania* 51:2 (1991), 517–58.

Sánchez Sánchez, Andrés. *La beneficiencia en Ávila: Actividad hospitalaria del cabildo catedralicio (Siglos XVI–XIX).* Ávila: Diputación Provincial, Institución Gran Duque de Ávila, 2000.

Schwartz, Stuart B. *Sea of Storms: A History of Hurricanes in the Greater Caribbean from Columbus to Katrina.* Princeton, NJ: Princeton University Press, 2015.

Sepúlveda, Juan Ginés de. "Teófilo," in *Obras completas* vol. 15, José María Núñez González and S. Rus Rufino, eds. Pozoblanco: Ayuntamiento de Pozoblanco, 2010, clxv–cxcii, 193–245.

Serrano de Vargas y Ureña, Juan. *Anacardina espiritual para conservar la memoria de avisos que la Divina Justicia (amonestando enmienda de ofensas) ha enviado a esta ciudad de Málaga.* Málaga: el autor, 1650.

Sewell, William H., Jr. *Logics of History: Social Theory and Social Transformation.* Chicago, IL: University of Chicago Press, 2005.

Siraisi, Nancy G. *History, Medicine, and the Traditions of Renaissance Learning.* Ann Arbor, MI: University of Michigan Press, 2007.

Skaarup, Bjorn Okholm. *Anatomy and Anatomists in Early Modern Spain.* Farnham: Ashgate, 2015.

Slack, Paul. *The Impact of Plague in Tudor and Stuart England.* London: Routledge and Kegan Paul, 1985.

    "Introduction," in *Epidemics and Ideas: Essays on the Historical Perception of Pestilence,* Terence Ranger and Paul Slack, eds. Past and Present Publications, Cambridge University Press, 1992, 1–20.

Soares de Figueroa, Cristóbal. *Plaza universal de todas ciencias y artes...* Madrid: Luis Sánchez, 1615.

Solnit, Rebecca. *A Paradise Built in Hell: The Extraordinary Communities that Arise in Disaster.* New York: Penguin Books, 2009.

Sommerville, Johann P. "The 'New Art of Lying': equivocation, mental reservation, and casuistry," in *Conscience and Casuistry in Early Modern Europe*, Edmund Leites, ed. Cambridge University Press, 1988, 159–84.

Sontag, Susan. "Disease as political metaphor," *New York Review of Books* February 23, 1978.

Soto, Fr. Domingo de and Fr. Juan de Robles. *Deliberación en la causa de los pobres (y réplica de Robles) (1545)*. Madrid: Instituto de Estudios Políticos, 1965.

Stearns, Justin K. *Infectious Ideas: Contagion in Premodern Islamic and Christian Thought in the Western Mediterranean*. Baltimore, MD: Johns Hopkins University Press, 2011.

  "Public health, the state, and religious scholarship: sovereignty in Idris al-Bidlisi's arguments for fleeing the plague," in *The Scaffolding of Sovereignty: Global and Aesthetic Perspectives on the History of a Concept*, Zvi Ben-Dor Benite, Stefanos Geroulanos and Nicole Jerr, eds. New York: Columbia University Press, 2017, 163–85.

Suárez de Figueroa, Cristóbal. *Plaza Universal de Todas Ciencias y Artes...* Madrid: Luis Sánchez, 1615.

Takeda, Junko Thérèse, *Between Crown and Commerce: Marseille and the Early Modern Mediterranean*. Baltimore, MD: Johns Hopkins University Press, 2011.

Tapia, Serafín de, "Los factores de la evolución demográfica de Ávila en el Siglo XVI," *Cuadernos Abulenses* 5, (January–June 1986), 113–200.

Tapia, Serafín de, "Las fuentes demográficas y el potencial humano de Ávila en el siglo XVI," *Cuadernos Abulenses* 2 (July–December 1984), 31–88.

Téllez Alarcia, Diego. "La peste Atlántica en Santo Domingo de la Calzada (1599)," *Berceo* 162 (2012), 85–119.

Testón Núñez, Isabel, et al., "Los problemas del abastecimiento del pan en Extremadura: La ciudad de Trujillo (1550–1610)," *Studia Historica. Historia Moderna* 5 (1987), 159–75.

Thomas, Keith. *Religion and the Decline of Magic*. New York: Charles Scribner's Sons, 1971.

Thompson, I. A. A. "Absolutism, legalism and the law in Castile, 1500–1700," in *Der Absolutismus – ein Mythos? Strukturwandel monarchischer herrschaft*, Ronald G. Asch and Heinz Duchhardt, eds. Cologne: Böhlau Verlag, 1996, 185–228.

  "Oposición política y juicio del gobierno en las Cortes de 1592–98," *Studia Historica. Historia Moderna* 17 (1997), 37–62.

  "Las Alteraciones Granadinas de 1648–1652 a la luz de un nuevo testimonio presencial," in *Homenaje a Don Antonio Domínguez Ortiz*, Juan Luis Castellano Castellano, et al., eds., 3 vols., vol. 2, Granada: Universidad de Granada, 2008, 779–812.

  "El concejo abierto de Alfaro en 1602: La lucha por la democracia municipal en la Castilla seiscientista," *Berceo* (1981), 307–31.

  "Conflictos políticos en las ciudades castellanas en el siglo XVII," in *Ciudades en conflicto (Siglos XVI–XVIII)*, José Ignacio Fortea Pérez and Juan E. Gelabert, eds. Valladolid: Junta de Castilla y León, 2008, 37–55.

Crown and Cortes: Government, Institutions and Representation in Early Modern Castile. London: Variorum, 1993.

"From Reinos to Monarquía: political association in late 16th-century Spain," *TEMPUS: Revista en Historia General* [Medellín] (2016), 91–110.

"The impact of war," in *The European Crisis of the 1590s*, Peter Clark, ed. London: George Allen and Unwin, 1985, 261–84.

"Santiago *v* Santa Teresa – signifying what?," in *Historia en fragmentos: Estudios en homenaje a Pablo Fernández Albaladejo*, Julio A. Pardos, et al., eds. Madrid: Universidad Autónoma de Madrid, 2017, 413–22.

Thompson, I. A. A. and Bartolomé Yun Casalilla, eds. *The Castilian Crisis of the Seventeenth Century: New Perspectives on the Economic and Social History of Seventeenth-Century Spain.* Past and Present Publications, Cambridge University Press, 1994.

Thucydides, *History of the Peloponnesian War*, trans. Rex Warner. London: Penguin Books, 1972.

Tomás y Valiente, Francisco. "La Diputación de las Cortes de Castilla (1525–1601)," in his *Gobierno e instituciones en la España del Antiguo Régimen.* Madrid: Alianza Editorial, 1982, 37–150.

Torrente Pérez, Diego, ed. *Documentos para la historia de San Clemente (Cuenca)*, 2 vols. Madrid: Ayuntamiento de San Clemente, 1975.

Totaro, Rebecca. *Suffering in Paradise: The Bubonic Plague in English Literature from More to Milton.* Pittsburgh, PA: Duquesne University Press, 2005.

Totaro, Rebecca and Ernest B. Gilman, eds. *Representing the Plague in Early Modern England.* New York: Routledge, 2011.

Tracy, James D., ed. *City Walls: The Urban Enceinte in Global Perspective.* Cambridge University Press, 2000.

Trexler, Richard C. *Public Life in Renaissance Florence.* Ithaca, NY: Cornell University Press, 1991.

Trivellato, Francesca. "Is there a future for Italian microhistory in the age of global history?" *California Italian Studies* 2 (1) [2011], http://escholarship .org/uc/item/0z94n9hq (accessed January 2019).

Truchuelo García, Susana. "La incidencia de las relaciones entre Guipúzcoa y el poder real en la conformación de los fueros durante los siglos XVI y XVII," *Manuscrits* 24 (2006), 73–93.

Truman, Ronald W. *Spanish Treatises on Government, Society and Religion in the Time of Philip II: The "de regimine principum" and Associated Traditions.* Leiden: Brill, 1999.

Ulloa, Modesto. *La hacienda real de Castilla en el reinado de Felipe II*, 3rd ed. Madrid: Fundación Universitaria Española, 1986 [1st. ed. 1977].

Valdeon Baruque, Julio. "Reflexiones sobre las murallas urbanas de la Castilla medieval," in *Estudios de historia medieval en homenaje a Luis Suarez Fernández*. Valladolid: Universidad de Valladolid 1991, 509–22.

Valdivielso, Jaime Luis. "Los arrieros burgaleses," *Revista de Folklore* 237 (2000), 105–108.

Varlik, Nükhet, "Plague, conflict, and negotiation: the Jewish broadcloth weavers of Salonica and the Ottoman central administration in the late sixteenth century," *Jewish History* 28 (2014): 261–88.

Plague and Empire in the Early Modern Mediterranean World: The Ottoman Experience, 1347–1600. Cambridge: Cambridge University Press, 2015.

Vaslef, Irene. "The role of St. Roch as a plague saint: a late medieval hagiographic tradition." PhD diss., The Catholic University of America, Washington, DC, 1984.

Vassberg, David. "Life-cycle service as a form of age-specific migration in the 16th and 17th centuries: rural Castile as a case study," in *Les migrations internes et a moyenne distance en Europe, 1500–1900*, Antonio Eiras Roel and Ofelia Rey Castelao, eds., vol. 1, Santiago de Compostela: Xunta de Galicia, 1994, 385–402.

The Village and the Outside World in Golden Age Castile: Mobility and Migration in Everyday Rural Life. Cambridge: Cambridge University Press, 1996.

Vilar Berrogain, Jean. *Literatura y economía: La figura satírica del arbitrista en el Siglo de Oro*, trans. Francisco Bustelo and Gerónima del Real. Madrid: Revista de Occidente, 1973.

Villalba, Joaquin de. *Epidemiologia española, o historia cronológica de las pestes, contagios, epidemias y epizootias que han acaecido en España desde la venida de los Cartagineses hasta el año 1801*, Antonio Carreras Panchón, ed. Universidad de Málaga, 1984. [Madrid 1803].

Villalpando Martinez, Manuela "Tres noticias de la Segovia antigua: Un brote de peste en la Segovia de 1653," *Estudios Segovianos* 95 (1997), 17–26.

Villuga, Pero Juan. *Reportorio de todos los caminos de España hasta ahora nunca visto en el que allará qualquier viaje que quiera andar muy aprovechoso para todos los caminantes*. Facs. ed., Hispanic Society of America, New York: De Vinne Press, 1902 [Medina del Campo, 1546].

Vincent, Bernard. "La peste atlantica de 1596–1602," *Asclepio* 28 (1976), 5–25.

"Les épidémies dans l'Espagne des années 1555–1570," in *Le corps dans la société espagnole des XVI et XVIIeme siècles*, Agustin Redondo, ed. Paris: Publications de la Sorbonne, 1990, 141–52.

Viñas, Carmelo and Ramón Paz, eds. *Relaciones histórico-geográfico-estadísticas de los pueblos de España hechas por iniciativa de Felipe II. Ciudad Real*. Madrid: Instituto de Sociología Balmes [CSIC], 1971.

Viñas y Mey, Carmelo and Ramón Paz, eds. *Relaciones de los pueblos de España ordenadas por Felipe II*. [Provincia de Madrid y Reino de Toledo], 4 vols. in 3. Madrid: Instituto Balmes de Sociologia [CSIC], 1949.

Viñes Ibarrola, José. *Una epidemia de peste bubonica en el siglo XVI*. Pamplona: Editorial Aramburu, 1947.

Virgil. *The Aeneid*, trans. Robert Fagles. New York: Viking, 2006.

Walker, Mack. *German Home Towns: Community, State, and General Estate, 1648–1871*. Ithaca, NY: Cornell University Press, 1971.

Wallis, Patrick. "A dreadful heritage: interpreting epidemic disease at Eyam, 1666–2000," *History Workshop Journal* 61 (Spring 2006), 31–56.

"Plagues, morality and the place of medicine in early modern England," *The English Historical Review* 121:490 (February 2006), 1–24.

Weber, Alison. *Teresa of Avila and the Rhetoric of Femininity*. Princeton, NJ: Princeton University Press, 1996.

Weisser, Michael R. *The Peasants of the Montes: The Roots of Rural Rebellion in Spain*. Chicago, IL: University of Chicago Press, 1976.

Whittles, Lilith K. and Xavier Didelot, "Epidemiological Analysis of the Eyam Plague Outbreak of 1665–1666," *Proceedings of the Royal Society* http://rspb .royalsocietypublishing.org/content/283/1830/20160618 (accessed January 2019).

Williams, Patrick. *The Great Favourite: The Duke of Lerma and the Court and Government of Philip III of Spain, 1598–1621*. Manchester: Manchester University Press, 2006.

"Philip III and the restoration of Spanish Government, 1598–1603," *The English Historical Review* 88:349 (October 1973), 751–69.

Wilson, F. P. *The Plague in Shakespeare's London*. Oxford: Clarendon Press, 1927.

Wing, John T. *Roots of Empire: Forests and State Power in Early Modern Spain, c. 1500–1750*. Leiden: Brill, 2015.

Woodward, Kenneth L. *Making Saints: How the Catholic Church Determines Who Becomes a Saint, Who Doesn't, and Why*. New York: Simon and Schuster, 1990.

Woolf, Virginia. *A Writer's Diary*, Leonard Woolf, ed. New York: Harcourt Brace Jovanovich, 1954.

Wright, Elizabeth. *Pilgrimage to Patronage: Lope de Vega and the Court of Philip III, 1598–1621*. Lewisburg, PA: Bucknell University Press, 2001.

Ximénez Savariego, Juan. *Tratado de peste, donde se contienen las causas, preservación, y cura...* Antequera: Claudio Bolan, 1602.

Zabala Aguirre, Pilar. *Las alcabalas y la hacienda real en Castilla*. Santander: Universidad de Cantabria, 2000.

Zamudio de Alfaro, Andrés. *Orden para la cura y preservación de las secas y carbuncos...* Madrid: Luis Sánchez, 1599.

Regimiento curativo y preservativo de pestilencia. Madrid, 1599.

Zarco-Bacas y Cuevas, Eusebio Julián, ed. *Relaciones de pueblos del obispado de Cuenca hechas por orden de Felipe II*, 2 vols. Cuenca: Biblioteca Diocesana Conquense, 1927.

Index